Discovery of Marine Natural Products in China: Selected Papers from the 16th National Annual Conference and 2023 International Symposium on Marine Drugs (16-NASMD) Conference

Discovery of Marine Natural Products in China: Selected Papers from the 16th National Annual Conference and 2023 International Symposium on Marine Drugs (16-NASMD) Conference

Editors

Hong Wang
Huawei Zhang
Bin Wei

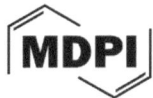

Basel • Beijing • Wuhan • Barcelona • Belgrade • Novi Sad • Cluj • Manchester

Editors

Hong Wang
College of Pharmaceutical Science and Jianxing Honors College
Zhejiang University of Technology
Hangzhou
China

Huawei Zhang
College of Pharmaceutical Science
Zhejiang University of Technology
Hangzhou
China

Bin Wei
College of Pharmaceutical Science
Zhejiang University of Technology
Hangzhou
China

Editorial Office
MDPI AG
Grosspeteranlage 5
4052 Basel, Switzerland

This is a reprint of articles from the Special Issue published online in the open access journal *Marine Drugs* (ISSN 1660-3397) (available at: https://www.mdpi.com/journal/marinedrugs/special_issues/OH944SNPQZ).

For citation purposes, cite each article independently as indicated on the article page online and as indicated below:

Lastname, A.A.; Lastname, B.B. Article Title. *Journal Name* **Year**, *Volume Number*, Page Range.

ISBN 978-3-7258-2207-2 (Hbk)
ISBN 978-3-7258-2208-9 (PDF)
doi.org/10.3390/books978-3-7258-2208-9

© 2024 by the authors. Articles in this book are Open Access and distributed under the Creative Commons Attribution (CC BY) license. The book as a whole is distributed by MDPI under the terms and conditions of the Creative Commons Attribution-NonCommercial-NoDerivs (CC BY-NC-ND) license.

Contents

About the Editors vii

Zijun Liu, Wenyan Sun, Zhe Hu, Wei Wang and Huawei Zhang
Marine *Streptomyces*-Derived Novel Alkaloids Discovered in the Past Decade
Reprinted from: *Mar. Drugs* 2024, 22, 51, doi:10.3390/md22010051 1

Gang-Ao Hu, Yue Song, Shi-Yi Liu, Wen-Chao Yu, Yan-Lei Yu, Jian-Wei Chen, et al.
Exploring the Diversity and Specificity of Secondary Biosynthetic Potential in *Rhodococcus*
Reprinted from: *Mar. Drugs* 2024, 22, 409, doi:10.3390/md22090409 27

Cancan Wang, Ye Fan, Chenjie Wang, Jing Tang, Yixian Qiu, Keren Xu, et al.
Discovery of Prenyltransferase-Guided Hydroxyphenylacetic Acid Derivatives from Marine Fungus *Penicillium* sp. W21C371
Reprinted from: *Mar. Drugs* 2024, 22, 296, doi:10.3390/md22070296 42

Jie Wang, Yue-Lu Yan, Xin-Yi Yu, Jia-Yan Pan, Xin-Lian Liu, Li-Li Hong and Bin Wang
Meroterpenoids from Marine Sponge *Hyrtios* sp. and Their Anticancer Activity against Human Colorectal Cancer Cells
Reprinted from: *Mar. Drugs* 2024, 22, 183, doi:10.3390/md22040183 54

Shaoshuai Xin, Mengqi Zhang, Peihai Li, Lizhen Wang, Xuanming Zhang, Shanshan Zhang, et al.
Marine-Fungus-Derived Natural Compound 4-Hydroxyphenylacetic Acid Induces Autophagy to Exert Antithrombotic Effects in Zebrafish
Reprinted from: *Mar. Drugs* 2024, 22, 148, doi:10.3390/md22040148 65

Zimin Xiao, Jian Cai, Ting Chen, Yilin Wang, Yixin Chen, Yongyan Zhu, et al.
Two New Sesquiterpenoids and a New Shikimic Acid Metabolite from Mangrove Sediment-Derived Fungus *Roussoella* sp. SCSIO 41427
Reprinted from: *Mar. Drugs* 2024, 22, 103, doi:10.3390/md22030103 82

Yongna Cao, Fenghua Xu, Qing Xia, Kechun Liu, Houwen Lin, Shanshan Zhang and Yun Zhang
The Peptide LLTRAGL Derived from *Rapana venosa* Exerts Protective Effect against Inflammatory Bowel Disease in Zebrafish Model by Regulating Multi-Pathways
Reprinted from: *Mar. Drugs* 2024, 22, 100, doi:10.3390/md22030100 92

Mingxia Zhao, Zhiqiang Yang, Xinyue Li, Yaqi Liu, Yingying Zhang, Mengqian Zhang, et al.
Development of Integrated Vectors with Strong Constitutive Promoters for High-Yield Antibiotic Production in Mangrove-Derived *Streptomyces*
Reprinted from: *Mar. Drugs* 2024, 22, 94, doi:10.3390/md22020094 109

Tingting Jiang, Bing Zhang, Haixing Zhang, Mingjun Wei, Yue Su, Tuo Song, et al.
Purification and Properties of a Plasmin-like Marine Protease from Clamworm (*Perinereis aibuhitensis*)
Reprinted from: *Mar. Drugs* 2024, 22, 68, doi:10.3390/md22020068 120

Chun-Ju Lu, Li-Fen Liang, Geng-Si Zhang, Hai-Yan Li, Chun-Qing Fu, Qin Yu, et al.
Carneusones A-F, Benzophenone Derivatives from Sponge-Derived Fungus *Aspergillus carneus* GXIMD00543
Reprinted from: *Mar. Drugs* 2024, 22, 63, doi:10.3390/md22020063 136

Zhou Wang, Jianglin Yin, Meng Bai, Jie Yang, Cuiping Jiang, Xiangxi Yi, et al.
New Polyene Macrolide Compounds from Mangrove-Derived Strain *Streptomyces hiroshimensis* GXIMD 06359: Isolation, Antifungal Activity, and Mechanism against *Talaromyces marneffei*
Reprinted from: *Mar. Drugs* **2024**, *22*, 38, doi:10.3390/md22010038 . . . . **147**

Zheng-Biao Zou, Tai-Zong Wu, Long-He Yang, Xi-Wen He, Wen-Ya Liu, Kai Zhang, et al.
Hepialiamides A–C: Aminated Fusaric Acid Derivatives and Related Metabolites with Anti-Inflammatory Activity from the Deep-Sea-Derived Fungus *Samsoniella hepiali* W7
Reprinted from: *Mar. Drugs* **2023**, *21*, 596, doi:10.3390/md21110596 . . . . **165**

Yan Peng, Xianwen Yang, Riming Huang, Bin Ren, Bin Chen, Yonghong Liu and Hongjie Zhang
Diversified Chemical Structures and Bioactivities of the Chemical Constituents Found in the Brown Algae Family Sargassaceae
Reprinted from: *Mar. Drugs* **2024**, *22*, 59, doi:10.3390/md22020059 . . . . **177**

About the Editors

Hong Wang

Hong Wang received her PhD degree in Organic Chemistry from Lanzhou University in 2002. Afterward, she conducted postdoctoral research at the Institute of Organic and Pharmaceutical Chemistry, Zhejiang University. In 2004, she joined the College of Pharmaceutical Science at the Zhejiang University of Technology, where she remains to date. During this period, she has established her own marine drugs laboratory and published over 150 scientific papers, book chapters, and patents. Her research focuses on antibiotic/antitumor resistance and the development of novel antimicrobial agents and antitumor agents.

Huawei Zhang

Huawei Zhang received his BS in Food Sciences in 2000 and his MS in Food Chemistry in 2003 from Northwest A&F University (China) and his PhD in Natural Products Chemistry in 2006 from Nanjing University (China) under the supervision of professor Renxiang Tan. After acting as a Postdoctoral Fellow at Nanjing University for two years, he was appointed as a faculty member of the Zhejiang University of Technology (China) in April 2008. He spent one year as a visiting scientist with Phillip Crews (the University of California Santa Cruz, USA) for one year. He has published over 120 articles and holds 20 patents. He is member of the Professional Committee of China Medicinal Fungus Society and of the Marine Pharmacology Committee of China Pharmacology Society. His research interest mainly focuses on bioactive secondary metabolites from microbes and their biosynthetic analyses.

Bin Wei

Bin Wei received his PhD degree in biomedical science from the University of Macau, Macau, China, in 2018. Bin Wei is a member of the Youth Committee of the Professional Committee of Marine Drugs of the Chinese Pharmaceutical Association and is currently working as a lecturer at the Collaborative Innovation Center of Yangtze River Delta Region Green Pharmaceuticals, the Zhejiang University of Technology. His research focuses on novel discovery strategies for microbial natural products. He has published over 80 academic papers in journals such as *Microbiome, Biotechnology Advances,* and *Marine Drugs*.

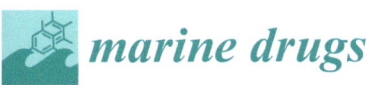

Review

Marine *Streptomyces*-Derived Novel Alkaloids Discovered in the Past Decade

Zijun Liu, Wenyan Sun, Zhe Hu, Wei Wang and Huawei Zhang *

School of Pharmaceutical Sciences, Zhejiang University of Technology, Hangzhou 310014, China; 17857693513@163.com (Z.L.); 202005140518@zjut.edu.cn (W.S.); 18098450998@163.com (Z.H.); 2112107012@zjut.edu.cn (W.W.)
* Correspondence: hwzhang@zjut.edu.cn; Tel.: +86-571-8832-0913

Abstract: Natural alkaloids originating from actinomycetes and synthetic derivatives have always been among the important suppliers of small-molecule drugs. Among their biological sources, *Streptomyces* is the highest and most extensively researched genus. Marine-derived *Streptomyces* strains harbor unconventional metabolic pathways and have been demonstrated to be efficient producers of biologically active alkaloids; more than 60% of these compounds exhibit valuable activity such as antibacterial, antitumor, anti-inflammatory activities. This review comprehensively summarizes novel alkaloids produced by marine *Streptomyces* discovered in the past decade, focusing on their structural features, biological activity, and pharmacological mechanisms. Future perspectives on the discovery and development of novel alkaloids from marine *Streptomyces* are also provided.

Keywords: marine *Streptomyces*; alkaloid; indole; pyrrole; pyridine; amide; anti-microbial effect; anti-inflammation; cytotoxicity

1. Introduction

Extensive marine habitats differ greatly from the land in terms of temperature, pressure and inorganic salt content, thereby providing a wealth of ecological and biogenetic diversity [1]. Benefiting from technological advances in deep-sea resource extraction and microbial culture methods, the number of new microbial species with unique metabolisms has constantly expanded in recent years [2]. Natural products of marine microbial origin are more likely to have novel skeletons and significant pharmacological activity [3]. It is estimated that at least 30,000 compounds with therapeutic potential have been isolated from marine microorganisms; some of these substances have been used as lead compounds or biomaterials in new therapies such as drug-resistant cancer treatment [4,5]. Actinomycetes are one of the largest phyla of bacterial groups and are ubiquitous in both terrestrial and marine ecosystems [6]. Their biosynthetic gene clusters (BGCs) have well-known abilities in the metabolization of complex natural products [7]. *Streptomyces*, as the largest and most advanced genus of actinomycetes, is the source of 60% of natural antibiotics, and classic examples widely are used in clinical practice, including erythromycin, streptomycin and rifamycin [8,9]. In the past thirty years, the number of novel metabolites produced with marine *Streptomyces* as a percentage of the total source has increased from 23.0% to 40.1% per decade (Figure 1), suggesting that these *Streptomyces* strains play an increasingly important role in the production of new natural products.

Alkaloids are the main chemical constituents in the secondary metabolites (SMs) of actinomycetes, and one of the compounds known to have the highest degree of druggability [10]. Most of these nitrogen-containing molecules have complex ring structures with promising pharmacological activity [11]. It has been demonstrated that marine alkaloids have widely clinical application value in the treatment of cancer, microbial infection, cardiovascular disease, inflammation, etc [12]. With the development of microbial genomics

Citation: Liu, Z.; Sun, W.; Hu, Z.; Wang, W.; Zhang, H. Marine *Streptomyces*-Derived Novel Alkaloids Discovered in the Past Decade. *Mar. Drugs* **2024**, *22*, 51. https://doi.org/10.3390/md22010051

Academic Editor: Patrizia Diana

Received: 18 December 2023
Revised: 21 January 2024
Accepted: 21 January 2024
Published: 22 January 2024

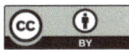

Copyright: © 2024 by the authors. Licensee MDPI, Basel, Switzerland. This article is an open access article distributed under the terms and conditions of the Creative Commons Attribution (CC BY) license (https://creativecommons.org/licenses/by/4.0/).

and metabonomics, the biosynthetic potential of marine *Streptomyces* has been deeply explored in the past decade. This review first provides a comprehensive overview of all new alkaloids produced by marine *Streptomyces* strains reported between January 2013 and June 2023. Three core databases (Web of Science, SciFinder and Dictionary of Natural Products) were used to search the targeted literature pertaining to specific topics related to marine and *Streptomyces* as well as novel or new alkaloids. According to their chemical structures, these metabolites (**1–261**) are grouped into nine types including indole, pyrrole, oxazole and thiazole, pyridine, pyrazine and piperazine, phenazine and phenoxazine, indolizidine and pyrrolizidine, amide and miscellaneous alkaloids. It is notable that indole, pyrrole, pyridine and amide are the major types, accounting for 72.9% of marine *Streptomyces*-derived novel alkaloids (Figure 2a). Detailed information for these substances is summarized in Table S1. In addition, *Streptomyces* strains isolated from marine sediments have a numerical advantage (Figure 2b); the number of new alkaloids produced by marine *Streptomyces* had a short-lived upward trend, but has fallen in the last two years (Figure 2c).

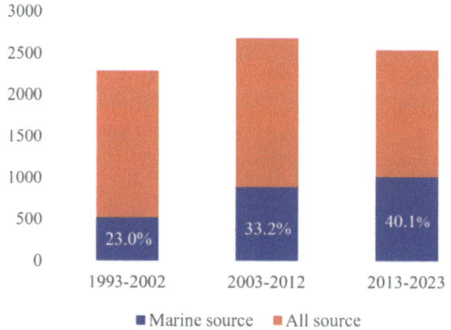

Figure 1. Source and statistics of new compounds from *Streptomyces* over the past three decades.

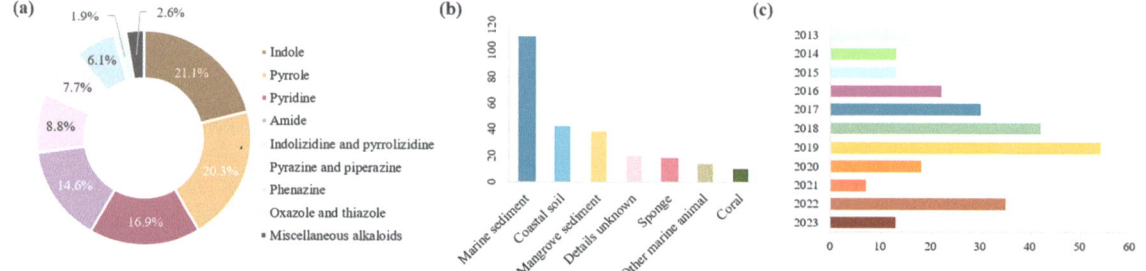

Figure 2. (**a**) Structural classes of marine *Streptomyces*-derived alkaloids reported in January 2013–June 2023; (**b**) sources of marine *Streptomyces* strains; and (**c**) number of new alkaloids discovered between January 2013–June 2023.

2. Indoles

Indoles are bicyclic alkaloids that usually use tryptophan or tryptamine as biosynthetic precursors [13]. They are common and grow rapidly in the SMs of marine-derived microorganisms with a wide range of biological activities [14]. Compounds **1–55** have been described as indole alkaloid derivatives of marine *Streptomyces* origin, including bisindole, indole sesquiterpenoid, and other miscellaneous indoles.

2.1. Bisindoles

Bisindole alkaloids represent a family formed by the oxidation and polymerization of two L-tryptophan molecules, which have more pronounced biological activities compared to the indole monomer structure [15]. These alkaloids have been reported to have cytotoxic, antibacterial, and antiviral activities; bisindole derivatives containing triazine groups have been used as targeted pyruvate dehydrogenase kinase (PDK) inhibitors in the treatment of pancreatic ductal adenocarcinoma [16,17]. This chapter highlights marine *Streptomyces*-derived staurosporine analogues and chlorinated bisindoles.

2.1.1. Staurosporines

The potent protein kinase C (PKC) inhibitor (IC$_{50}$ = 2.7 nM) staurosporine containing the indolo[2,3-*a*]carbazole structure was first discovered in *S. staurosporeus* in 1977 [18]. Lately, several analogues have been isolated and approved for clinical use, such as midostaurin and lestaurtinib [19]. Compounds **1–4** (Figure 3) are marine *Streptomyces'* staurosporine derivatives with significant selective inhibition of Rho-associated protein kinase (ROCK2), PKC and Brution tyrosine kinase (BTK) [20,21]. A biosynthesis study indicated that the C-N bond linking the aglycone and deoxysugar moiety of staurosporine is catalyzed by cytochrome P450 enzymes [22]. Twelve holyrine A derivatives (**5–16**, Figure 3) displayed strongly or moderately cytotoxic and enzyme-inhibitory activity, with IC$_{50}$ values ranging from 0.0057 to 16.6 μM [21,23–25]. When cultured in a liquid medium with 5-hydroxy-L-tryptophan precursors, strain *Streptomyces* sp. OUCMDZ-3118 was shown to produce another analogue 3-hydroxy-K252d (**17**, Figure 3), which demonstrated cytotoxicity against A549 and MCF-7 cell lines with IC$_{50}$ values of 1.2 ± 0.05 μM, 1.6 ± 0.09 μM, respectively [26].

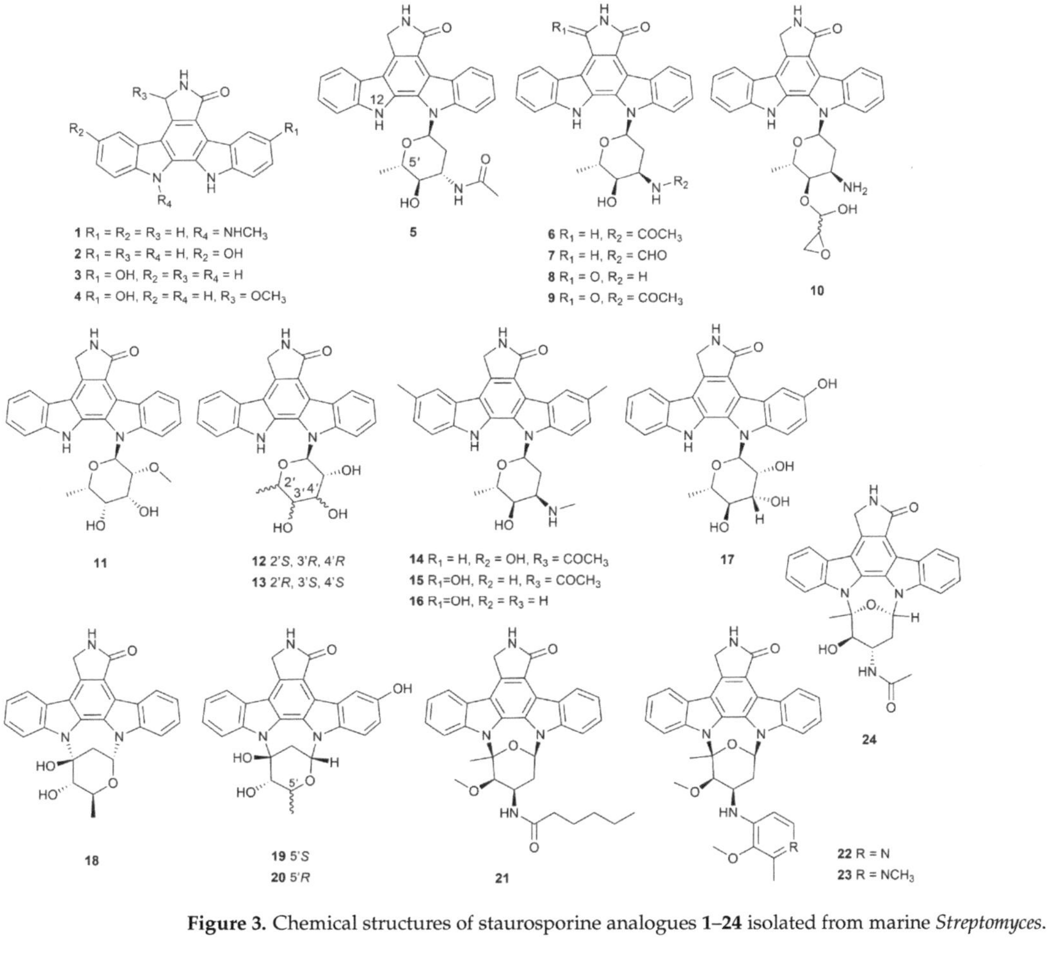

Figure 3. Chemical structures of staurosporine analogues **1–24** isolated from marine *Streptomyces*.

Moreover, streptocarbazoles C–H (**18–23**, Figure 3) were extracted from *Streptomyces* sp. DT-A65, DT-A61 and OUCMDZ-5380 [21,25,27]. Streptocarbazoles D and E rarely contained a hydroxyl group at the C-3 position. Compound **20** inhibited a PC3 cell line with an IC_{50} value of 5.6 μM, while compounds **21–23** inhibited acute myeloid leukemia cell line MV4-11 (IC_{50} = 0.81–1.88 μM). In addition, strain DT-A61 collected another staurosporine analogue (**24**, Figure 3), which exhibited extremely potent cytotoxic activity against PC3 cells with an IC_{50} value of 0.16 μM [21]. The structure–activity relationship (SAR) analysis showed that staurosporine analogs with a glycosyl unit double-linked to the aromatic aglycone by two C-N bonds displayed better biological effects.

2.1.2. Halogenated Bisindoles

To the best of our knowledge, all bisindoles from marine *Streptomyces* are chlorinated (**25–39**, Figure 4). Indimicins A−E (**25–29**) and lynamicins F−G (**30** and **31**) were obtained from a deep-sea-derived *Streptomyces* sp. SCSIO 03032 by solid phase extraction with XAD-16 resin [28]. These compounds had unusual 1′,3′-dimethyl-2′-hydroindole structures. Only dimethyl-substituted indimicin B (**26**) was seen to have antitumor activity against the MCF-7 cell line with an IC_{50} value of 10.0 μM. In order to characterize the function of gene *spmH*, which was predicted to be an L-Trp 5-halogenase, the authors inactivated this gene in strain SCSIO 03032 and obtained four bisindoles without a halogen substituent named spiroindimicins G–H (**32–33**) and indimicins F–G (**34–35**) [29]. It was confirmed that *spmH* functioned as halogenase and acted in early biosynthesis using L-Trp as a substrate. Compounds **32** and **33** showed various degrees of cytotoxicity against four cancer cell lines (SF-268, MCF-7, HepG2 and A549) and the presence or absence of chlorine atoms had no significant effect on the cytotoxic activity.

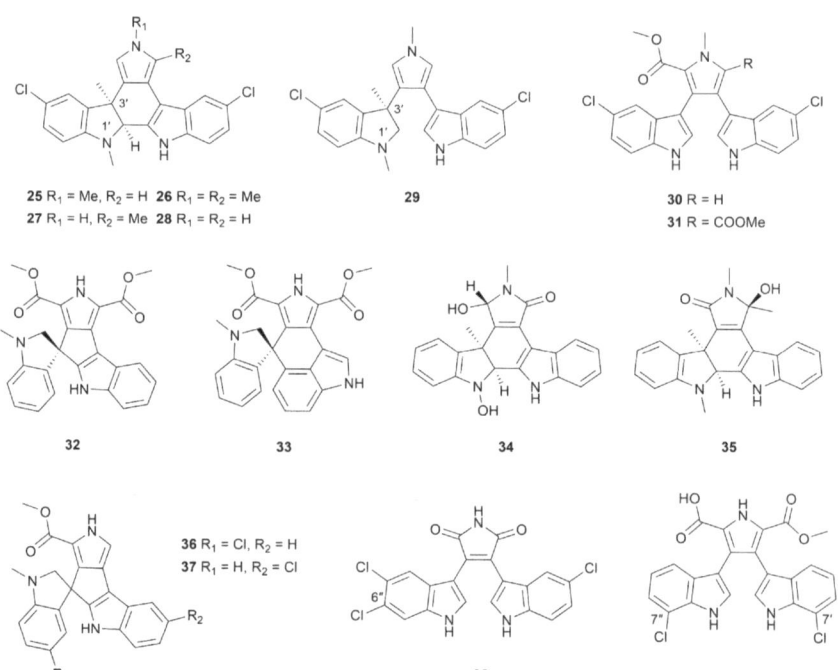

Figure 4. Chemical structures of halogenated bisindoles **25–39** isolated from marine *Streptomyces*.

Two non-typical bisindole spiroindimicins E and F (**36** and **37**) were purified from the metabolites of strain MP131-18 with cluster 36 being predicted to be the gene cluster responsible for bisindole biosynthesis [30]. Only compound **36** showed weak cytotoxic activity against T24 bladder cancer cells, while **36–37** had no antimicrobial activity due to this type of effect was proportional to the amount of halogenation. In addition, *Streptomyces* sp. SCSIO 11791 produced two chlorinated bisindoles (**38** and **39**), which displayed moderate cytotoxicity against four tumor cells with IC_{50} values ranging from 2.9 μM to 19.4 μM [31]. Compound **38** additionally exhibited cytotoxic activity against MDA-MB-231 and NCI-H460 cell lines as well as inhibition of Gram-positive bacteria. The structure–activity relationship suggested that the substitution of the C-6″ position by the chlorine atom was more beneficial to the biological activity.

2.2. Indole Sesquiterpenoids

The first bacterial-derived indole sesquiterpenoid alkaloid, named xiamycin, was isolated from an endophytic *Streptomyces* sp. from *B. gymnorrhiza* in 2010 [32]. In recent years, compounds of this family have been found in marine *Streptomyces*, and have attracted attention because of their antibacterial, anti-human-immunodeficiency-virus (HIV) and anti-tumor activities [33]. Xiamycins C–E (**40–42**, Figure 5) were isolated from *Streptomyces* sp. HK-18 [34]. Compounds **41** and **42** exhibited strong activity against the replication of porcine epidemic diarrhea virus (PEDV) in a dose-dependent manner, with EC_{50} values of 0.93 μM and 2.89 μM, respectively. The mechanism of action inhibited the synthesis of key structural proteins for PEDV to prevent virus replication. The methyl ester group was an important functional group to maintain activity. Overexpression of the *orf2011* gene encoding the LuxR family regulator in the *Streptomyces* sp. HK-18 resulted in the production of two members of the xiamycins family containing an N-O bone linked aliphatic chain structure named lipoxiamycins A and B (**43** and **44**, Figure 5) as well as increased production of xiamycins dimers dixiamycins A and C (**45** and **46**, Figure 5) [35]. An anti-inflammatory assay showed that compounds **43** and **45** could significantly inhibit the production of lipopolysaccharide-induced NO with IC_{50} values of 9.89 ± 0.92 and 4.12 ± 0.22 μM, respectively.

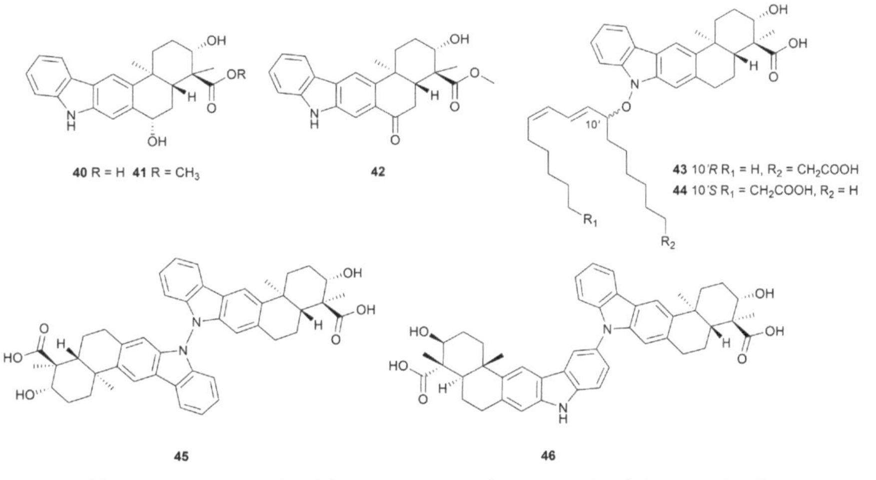

Figure 5. Chemical structures of Indole sesquiterpenoids **40–46** isolated from marine *Streptomyces*.

2.3. Other Indoles

The first naturally derived indolinone-naphthofuran alkaloids, (±)-Pratensilins A–C (**47–49**, Figure 6), were isolated from *Streptomyces pratensis* KCB-132 obtained from a marine sediment from the Bohai Sea, China [36]. Only compound **47** displayed moderate cytotoxicity against eight human cancer cell lines (IC_{50} = 2.4 μM–67.4 μM), with small steric substituents in R_2 and R_3. After adding 50 μM of lanthanum chloride to the liquid medium, an indolinone-naphthofuran analogue (±)-Pratensilin D (**50**, Figure 4) was detected in the metabolites [37]. (-)-Pratensilin D (**50**) exhibited more potent biological activity against

Gram-positive bacteria, yeast and five human cancer cell lines. One anthranilate-containing alkaloid, anthranosides C (**51**, Figure 6), was separated from a sponge-derived *Streptomyces* sp. CMN-62 (Naozhou Island, China) and exhibited a 171 μM IC_{50} against the influenza A H_1N_1 virus [38]. Four indole alkaloids streptoindoles A–D (**52–55**, Figure 6) were obtained from *Streptomyces* sp. ZZ1118 rice solid medium derived from a gut sample of marine shrimp (*Penaeus* sp.) [39]. Compound **54** potently inhibited *E. coli* and *C. albicans* (MIC = 7 μg/mL) and compound **55** was weakly active against methicillin-resistant *Staphylococcus aureus* (MRSA) only (MIC = 25 μg/mL). Compounds **52** and **53** were effective against all three pathogens, with MIC values of 7–25 μg/mL.

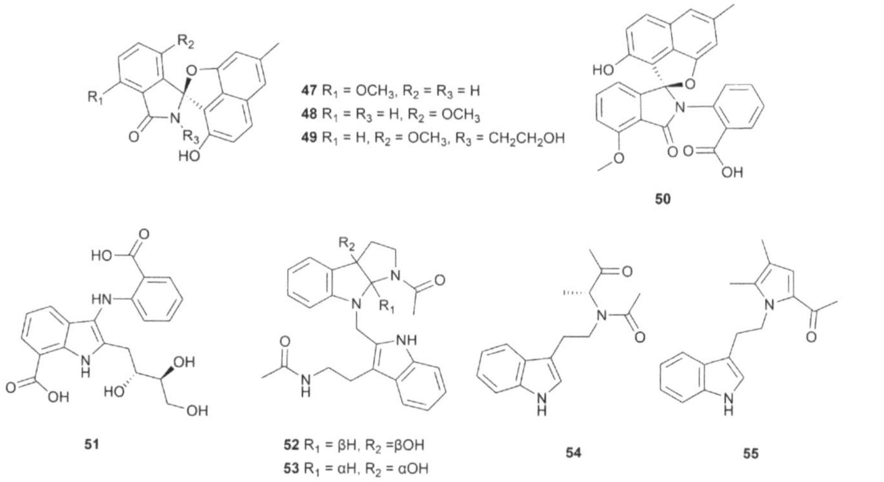

Figure 6. Chemical structures of other indoles **47–55** isolated from marine *Streptomyces*.

3. Pyrroles

Pyrrole alkaloids have more potential to be designed as lead compounds due to their property of easily forming hydrogen bonds [40]. Marine pyrrole derivatives usually have more unique structures and significant pharmacological activities such as antimicrobial, antiproliferative, anti-inflammatory and antiviral activities [41].

3.1. Pyrrolones and Pyrrolidones

This part describes cases in which pyrrole or pyrrolidine pentacyclic rings are replaced by carbonyl groups. The formed pyrrolone and pyrrolidone structures are crucial heterocyclic pharmacophores in medicinal chemistry, with significant biological activities [42]. The tirandamycins are a class of bacterial RNA polymerase (RNAP) inhibitors containing dienoyl tetramic acid and 2,4-pyrrolidinedione structures [43]. Two tirandamycin analogues tirandamycin K and isotirandamycin B (**56** and **57**, Figure 7), together with two known derivatives (**58** and **59**, Figure 7), were produced from marine *Streptomyces* strains [44,45]. Compound **56** was the first linear tirandamycin derivative that avoided bicyclic ketal ring formation due to the inability of the C-9S hydroxyl group to be nucleophilically attacked by C-13. In a pathogenic bacterial inhibitory activity assay, compounds **57–59** showed obvious antibacterial activity against *S. agalactiae* with MIC values of 2.5–5.0 μg/mL. However, compound **56** was inactive, therefore the authors deduced that the bicyclic ketal ring moiety was a necessary RNA polymerase target.

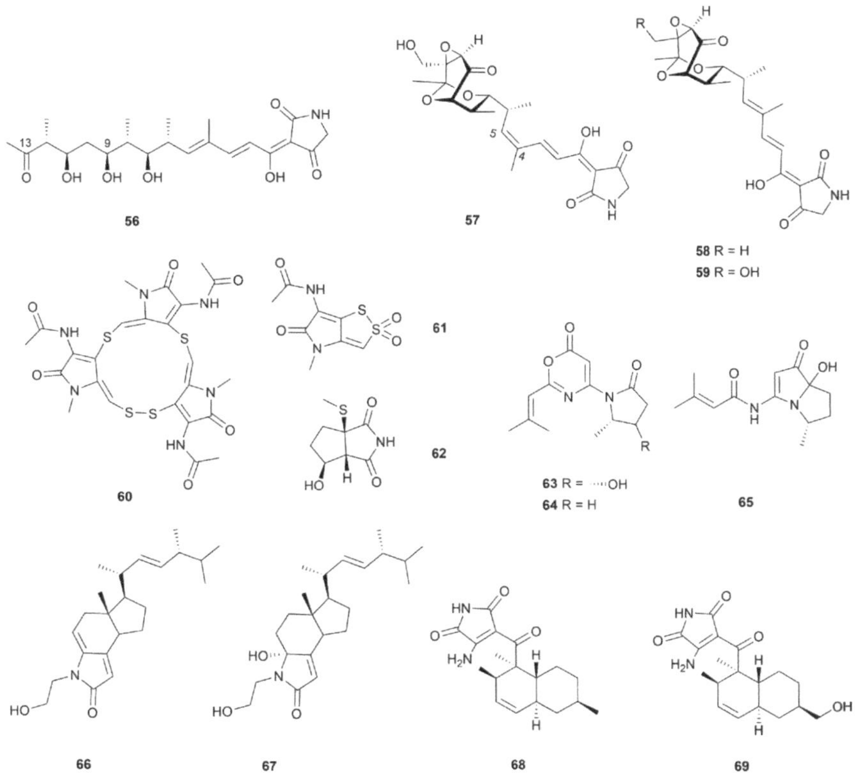

Figure 7. Chemical structures of pyrrolone and pyrrolidone alkaloids **56–69** isolated from marine *Streptomyces*.

Three thio-containing pyrrolone-based alkaloids (**60–62,** Figure 7) were discovered from two marine *Streptomyces* [46,47]. Thiolopyrrolone A (**60**) had an unusual macrocyclic skeleton and also inhibited Bacille Calmette–Guérin (BCG), *M. tuberculosis*, and *S. aureus*, with MIC values of 10, 10 and 100 μg/mL, respectively. Bacillimide (**62**) had a rare cyclopenta[c]pyrrole-1,3-dione structure bearing a methylsulfide group. This pyrrolidone alkaloid was an isocitrate lyase (ICL) enzyme moderate inhibitor under C_2-carbon-utilizing conditions, demonstrating an IC_{50} value of 44.24 μM against *C. albicans*. In addition, *Streptomyces* sp. KMF-004 yielded two unusual pyrrolidinyl-oxazinone alkaloids, Salinazinones A and B (**63** and **64**, Figure 7) [48]. Compound **64** showed an inhibitory effect on lipopolysaccharide (LPS)-induced NO production by BV-2 microglia cells (an IC_{50} value of 17.7 μM). The authors speculated that the oxazinone structure was synthesized by amide cyclization and gave a possible biosynthetic intermediate named bohemamine D (**65**). Anandins A and B (**66** and **67**, Figure 7), as two unique pyrrolidone-containing steroidal alkaloids, were isolated from *Streptomyces anandii* H41-59 derived from mangrove sediments [49]. The compound **66** showed moderate inhibitory effects against cancer cell lines MCF-7, SF-268 and NCI-H460 (IC_{50} = 7.5–7.9 μg/mL, respectively). Two pyrrolidone derivatives, ligiamycins A and B (**68** and **69**, Figure 7), were obtained by co-culture of two marine-derived strains *Streptomyces* sp. GET02.ST and *Achromobacter* sp. GET02.AC [50]. A biological evaluation showed that compound **68** exhibited moderate effects against *S. aureus* and *S. enterica* (both MIC values of 16 μg/mL), while compound **69** was cytotoxic against HCT116 cancer cells (IC_{50} = 20.1 μM). The presence of the hydroxyl group in compound **69** had an opposite effect on antitumor activity and antibacterial activity.

3.2. Pyrrolobenzodiazepines

Pyrrolo[1,4]benzodiazepines (PBDs, Figure 8) are tricyclic alkaloids that can be divided into [2,1-c][1,4], [1,2-a][1,4] and [1,2-d][1,4] structural types according to the different positions of the pyrrole ring-binding [51]. Natural PBDs are originally derived from *Streptomyces* as DNA alkylating antitumor drugs, and the classical representatives are anthramycin, sibiromycin and tomaymycin [52]. A pyrrolobenzodiazepine alkaloid, oxoprothracarcin (**70**), was produced by *Streptomyces* sp. M10946 obtained from a mangrove sediment [53]. Compound **70** had antiproliferative effects against MDA-MB-231 cells and A549 cells at 10 μM, with growth inhibition rates of 10.2% and 7.3%. An unusual PBD derivative, 7-methoxy-8-hydroxy cycloanthranilylproline (**71**), along with a known analogue (**72**), was isolated from marine *S. cacaoi* 14CM034 and displayed antimicrobial effects on *E. coli*, MRSA, *E. faecium*, *P. aeruginosa* and *C. albicans*, with MIC values ranging from 8.75 to 32 μg/mL [54]. It seems that methoxy substitution on the benzene ring of PBD diminished the antimicrobial effect.

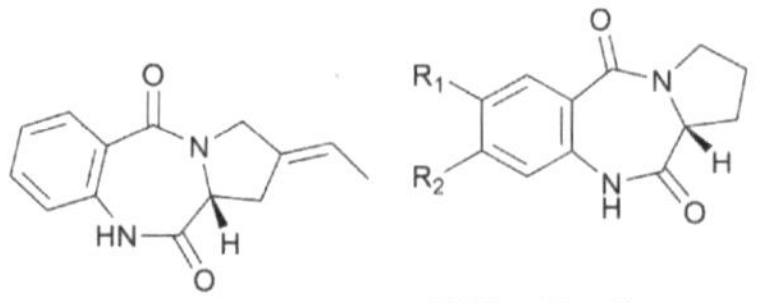

Figure 8. Chemical structures of pyrrolobenzodiazepines **70**–**72** isolated from marine *Streptomyces*.

3.3. Ansamycins

Ansamycins are a class of important macrocyclic lactam alkaloids obtained mainly from actinomycetes, of which the more representative include the anti-tuberculosis drug laofomycin, Hsp90 inhibitor geldamycin, and anticancer drug ansamitocin P-3 [55]. According to the different aromatic cores, ansamycins can be divided into benzene series and naphthalene series [56]. Hygrocins are a subclassification of naphthalenic ansamycins, whose amides are five-membered or seven-membered nitrogen heterocycles [57]. After knocking out the gene *gdmAI* responsible for the synthesis of the high-yield ansamycin analogue geldanamycin in *Streptomyces* sp. LZ35, hygrocins C−F (**73**–**76**, Figure 9) were produced and characterized [58]. In 2015, strain LZ35 was genetically modified by overexpression of *hgc1*, a LAL-type activator, and was found to produce three hygrocin derivatives, hygrocins H−J (**77**–**79**, Figure 9) [59]. Compounds **73**, **74**, **76** and **77** were shown to be cytotoxic to MDA-MB-231, PC3 and HeLa cell lines, with IC_{50} values of 0.5–5.0 μM. *Streptomyces* sp. ZZ1956 afforded nine derivatives named hygrocins K–S (**80**–**88**, Figure 9) [60]. Compounds **83**, **86** and **87** showed antiproliferative activity against human glioma U87MG and U251 cells with IC_{50} values of 7.04-10.46 μM. In addition, compounds **83**, **84**, and **87** displayed antibacterial activity against MRSA and *E. coli* (MIC = 8–24 μg/mL). The *E* configuration of C-3 and C-4 double bond and the existence of the *ansa* ring in these molecules are the keys to their strong biological activity.

Three ansamycin derivatives with unprecedented skeletons, ansalactams B–D (**89**–**91**, Figure 9), were isolated from marine sediment-derived *Streptomycetes* sp. CNH189 [61]. Antibacterial activity tests showed that compounds **89**–**91** had weak inhibitory activity against MRSA, with MIC values of 31.2, 31.2, and 62.5 μg/mL, respectively. A chemical study of the strain *Streptomyces* sp. KFD18 produced four ansamycin analogues named divergolides T–W (**92**–**95**, Figure 9) [62]. All these substances showed various degrees of cytotoxic activity against cancer cell lines SGC-7901, K562, Hela and A549; compounds with hydroxylation of C-7 and *R* configuration of C-2 exhibited weak cytotoxic effect.

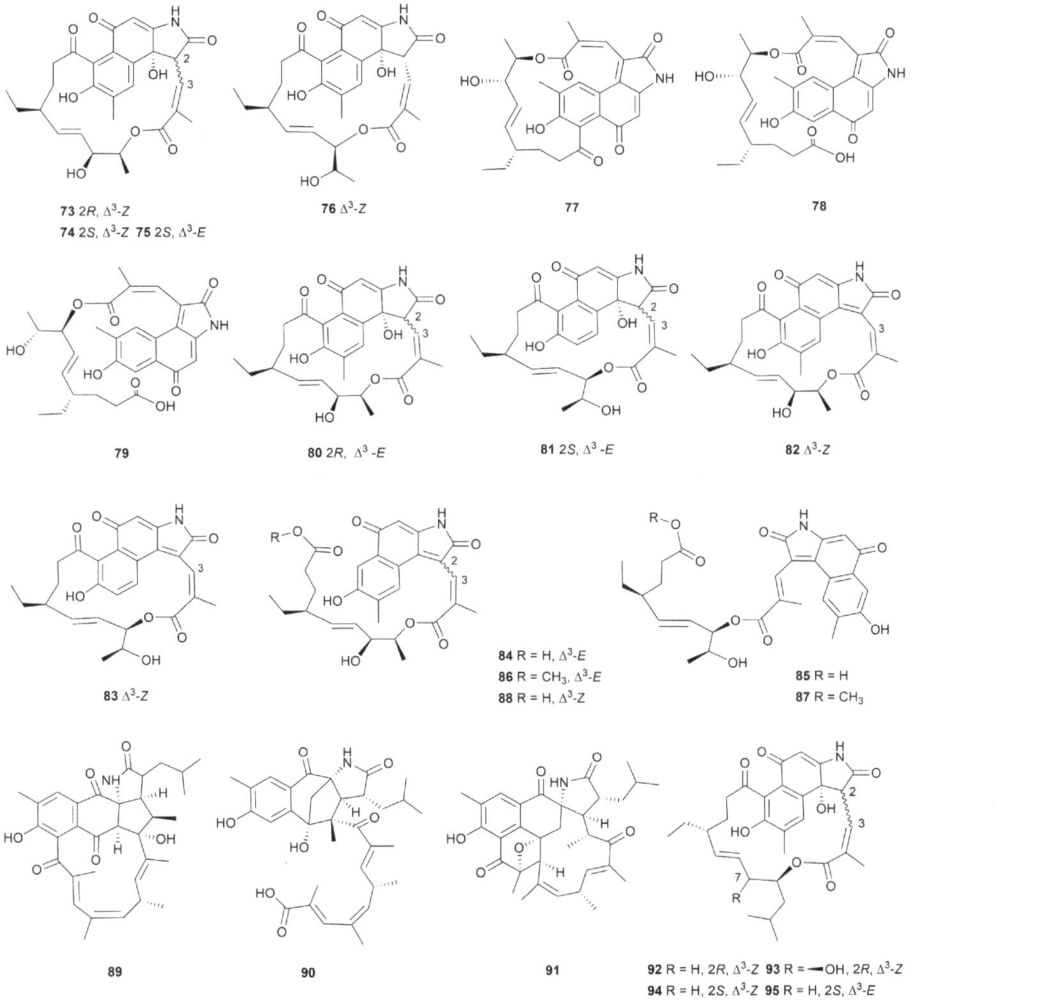

Figure 9. Chemical structures of ansamycin analogues **73–95** isolated from marine *Streptomyces*.

3.4. Other Pyrroles

Chlorizidine A (**96**, Figure 10), biosynthesized based on the non-ribosomal peptide synthetases/polyketide synthases (NRPS/PKS) pathway, was an unprecedented alkaloid containing chlorinated 5H-pyrrolo[2,1-*a*]isoindol-5-one fragment [63]. It exhibited an IC$_{50}$ value of 3.2–4.9 μM against the HCT-116 adenocarcinoma cell line with the pyrrole isoindolone ring moiety as a key pharmacophore. Isolated from marine sediment samples, the *S. zhaozhouensis* 208DD-064 produced two halogenated pyrroles, streptopyrroles B and C (**97** and **98**, Figure 10) [64]. Compounds **97** and **98** showed promising activity with three Gram-positive bacteria (MIC = 0.7–2.9 μM), with inverse correlation to the number of halogen substituents. Moreover, streptopyrrole B (**97**) exhibited moderate activity against six cancer cell lines. Three pyrrole ether compounds of the indanomycin family (**99–102**, Figure 10) were isolated from *S. antibioticus* PTZ0016 extracts based on antimicrobial activity [65]. A biological evaluation showed that compounds **99–102** inhibited the growth of *S. aureus* with MIC values of 4.0–8.0 μg/mL. Nitricquinomycins A–C (**103–105**, Figure 10) arethe first example of naphthopyrroledione derivatives containing an angolosamine moiety and **105** had a significantly inhibitory effect on A2780 cell lines (IC$_{50}$ = 4.77 μM) and moderate activity against *E. coli*, *S. aureus* and *C. albicans* (MIC values of 20–40 µM) [66]. In 2021, a nitricquinomycin analogue, bhimamycin J (**106**), was purified from *Streptomyces* sp. MS180069 and demonstrated 79.7% inhibition of angiotensin converting enzyme 2 (ACE2) at 25 µg/mL [67]. Isolated from a deep-sea floor, the *Streptomyces* sp. GGS53 produced two pyrrolosesquiterpenes glaciapyrroles, D and E (**107** and **108**, Figure 7) [68]. Influenza A viruses were used to infect Mardin–Darby canine kidney cells; **108** exhibited significant antiviral activity, resulting in the reduction of the viral titer by 70%.

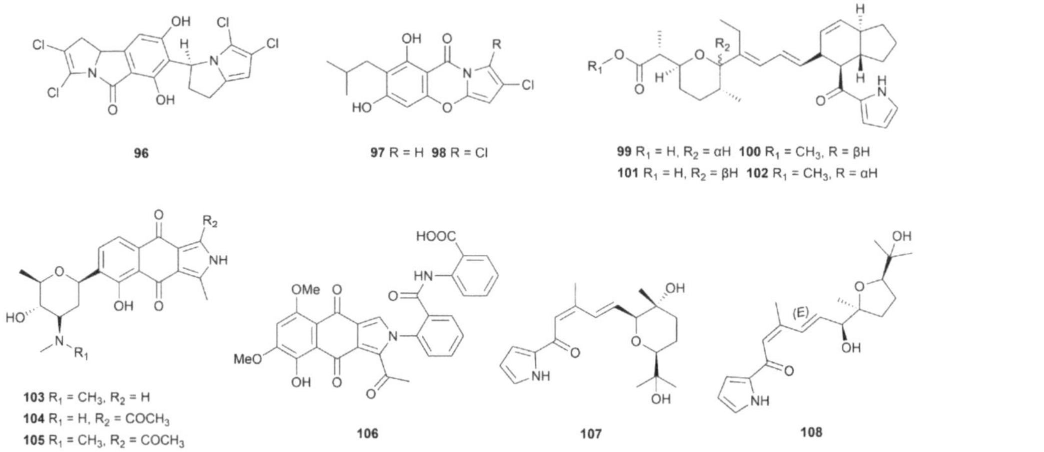

Figure 10. Chemical structures of other pyrroles **96–108** isolated from marine *Streptomyces*.

4. Oxazoles and Thiazoles

Oxazole and thiazole rings exhibit a wide range of pharmacological activities, such as antiproliferative, anti-inflammatory and antimicrobial activity, by binding non-covalently to many enzyme and receptor targets [69,70]. Most of these alkaloids have been mentioned in other chapters, and this chapter summarizes the remaining five compounds **109–113** (Figure 11). Under LC-MS/MS molecular networking guidance, five siderophores containing oxazole or thiazole rings were isolated from *S. diastaticus* NBU2966 collected from marine sponge *Axinellida* sp. [71]. However, none of these metabolites demonstrated activity against *S. aureus*, MRSA, *B. subtilis*, and *P. aeruginosa*.

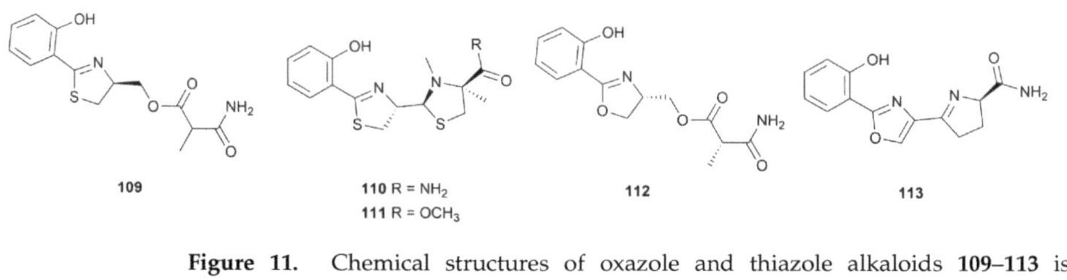

Figure 11. Chemical structures of oxazole and thiazole alkaloids **109–113** isolated from marine *Streptomyces*.

5. Pyridines

Pyridine alkaloids are a class of important skeletons for maintaining the pharmacological activity of drugs [72]. This chapter summarizes pyridine and its derivatives of marine *Streptomyces* sp., including pyridone, benzopyridine (quinoline), and the saturated variant, piperidine.

5.1. Piericidins

Piericidins are a class of 4-pyridinol alkaloids decorated with methylated polyene side chains, mostly isolated from actinomycetes of soil, marine or bio-symbiotic origin [73]. Due to structural similarities with coenzyme Q, some piericidins exhibit NADH−ubiquinone oxidoreductase inhibitory activity [74]. Moreover, insecticidal, cytotoxic, and bactericidal effects of piericidins have been reported. When a mangrove soil-derived *Streptomyces* sp. CHQ-64 was knocked out of the gene *rdmF*, a positive regulatory gene for reedsmycins (polyol polyene macrolides), one mutant strain was shown to produce a piericidin analogue (**114**, Figure 12), which displayed prominent cytotoxicity against the HeLa, NB4, A549 and H1975 cell lines (IC_{50} values of 0.003–0.56 μM). Seventeen piericidin derivatives (**115–131**, Figure 12) purified from *S. psammoticus* SCSIO NS126 from mangrove sediment samples showed strong or moderate activity against renal cell (RCC) carcinoma cell line ACHN with IC_{50} values of 0.31–60 μM [75]. A mechanism-of-action (MOA) study revealed that compounds **115–131** could increase the expression of peroxiredoxin 1 (PRDX1), decreasing the level of reactive oxygen species in cells. The piericidin glycosides (**119–131**) were more effective in binding to PRDX1 than the aglycones (**115–118**), although ultimately there was no significant difference in antitumor activity. Piericidin A5 (**132**) together with G1 (**133**) produced by strain SCSIO 40063 exhibited antitumor activity against SF-268, MCF-7, HepG2 and A549 tumor cell lines, with IC_{50} values ranging from 10.0 to 12.7 μM [76].

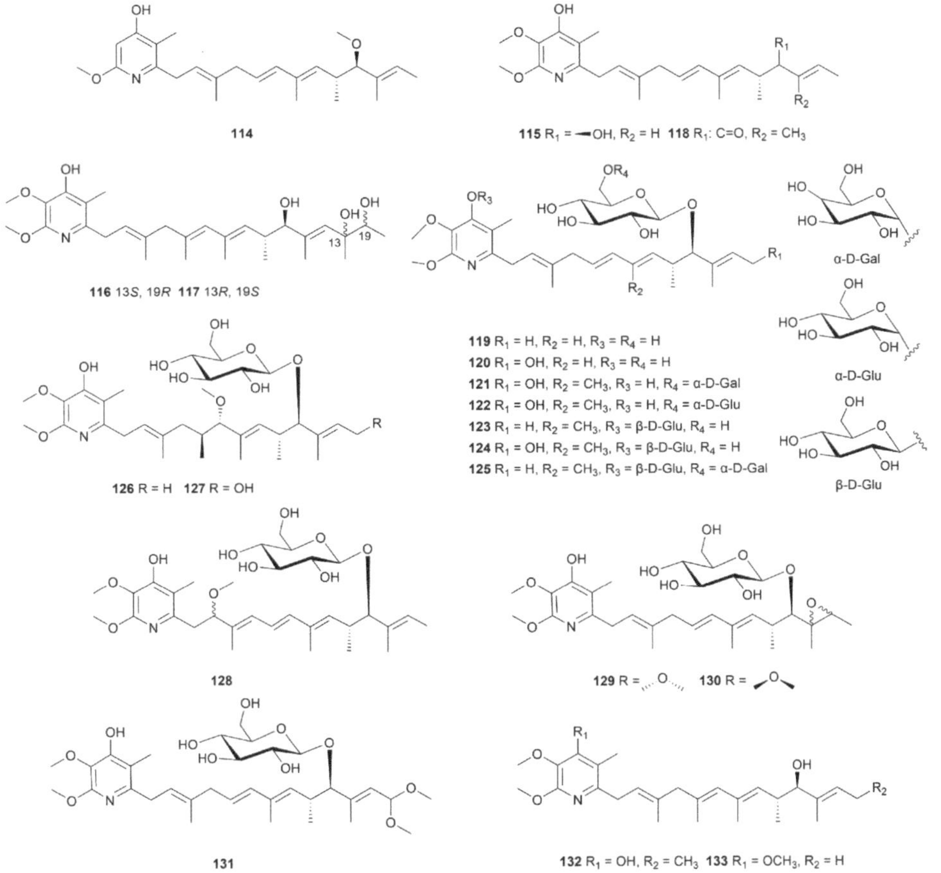

Figure 12. Chemical structures of piericidin analogues **114–133** isolated from marine *Streptomyces*.

5.2. Quinolines

Quinolines have been designed as important skeletons in drug structures for more than two centuries [77]. Classic examples are quinine, the first effective antimalarial drug in history, and the broad-spectrum antibiotic fluoroquinolone [78]. This subsection provides an overview of quinoline alkaloids of marine *Streptomyces* sp. origin and their derivatives isoquinolines and quinolones. Compounds **134–141** (Figure 13) were identified as simple quinoline alkaloids purified from marine *Streptomyces*. Strain CNP975 produced two rare quinoline derivatives containing 3-hydroxyquinaldic acid (3HQA) fragments, named actinoquinolines A and B (**134** and **135**), with stronger inhibitory activity against cyclooxygenases-2 (COX-2, IC_{50} of 2.13 and 1.42 µM, respectively) compared to cyclooxygenases-1 (COX-1, IC_{50} of 7.6 and 4.9 µM, respectively) [79]. The cyclization of the hydroxyl group increases the activity of the compounds against COX-1/2. Three amino-acid-substituted quinoline derivatives (**136–138**) were isolated by *S. cyaneofuscatus* M-157 collected from coral samples containing serine, glutamine, and cysteine residues unit, respectively [80]. Only compound **137** displayed weak cytotoxicity against human tumor cell line HepG2, with IC_{50} value of 51.5 µM. Diazaquinomycins E–G (**139–141**) were unusual diazaanthracene alkaloids, and compound **139**, with double substitution, had cytotoxic activity against the ovarian cancer cell line OVCAR5 by upregulating the cell cycle inhibitor p21 and impairing DNA (IC_{50} value of 9.0 µM) [81]. Antichlamydial activity-guided purification of a chlorinated quinolone ageloline A (**142**, Figure 13) was isolated from *Streptomyces* sp. SBT345 collected from the Mediterranean sponge *Agelas oroides* [82]. Compound **142** dose-dependently exhibited inhibition of *Chlamydia trachomatis* growth (IC_{50} value of 9.54 ± 0.36 µM) by inhibiting reactive oxygen species (ROS) production during the early stages of infection. The high-yield extract medium of strain B1848 afforded three isoquinolinequinone alkaloids, mansouramycins E–G (**143–145**, Figure 13) [83]. In a cytotoxicity assay against 36 tumor cells, compound **144** exhibited selective moderate cytotoxic activity (mean IC_{50} value of 7.92 µM), while compound **143** exhibited weak effect.

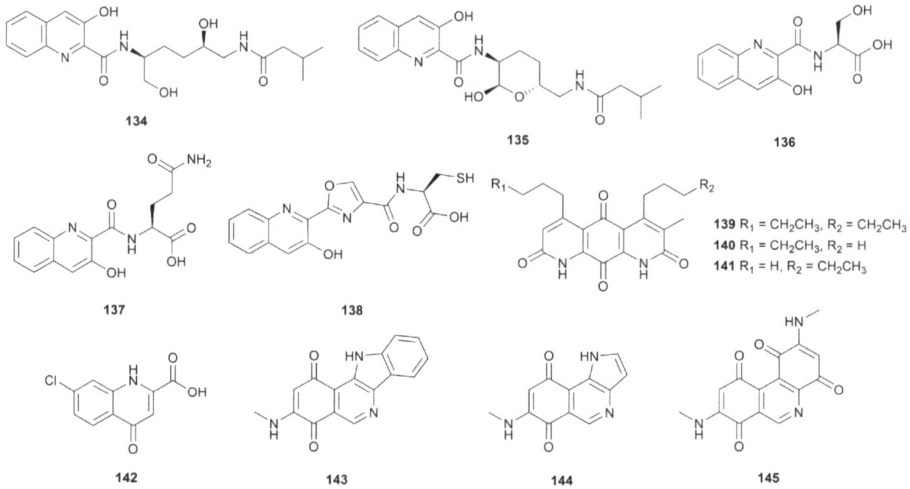

Figure 13. Chemical structures of quinolines **134–145** isolated from marine *Streptomyces*.

5.3. Other Pyridines

Two pyridine derivatives, strepchazolins A and B (**146** and **147**, Figure 14), were purified from *S. chartreusis* NA02069 [84]. Compound **146** inhibited a 64.0 µM MIC value against *B. subtilis* and a 50.6 µM IC_{50} value against acetylcholinesterase. Compound **147** was inactive, indicating that steric configuration affected biological activity. Isolated from a marine mud sample, *Streptomyces* sp. ZZ741 afforded ten glutarimide analogues named streptoglutarimides A–J (**148–157**, Figure 14) [85]. All analogues were effective against MRSA

(MIC = 9–11 µg/mL), *E. coli* (MIC = 8–12 µg/mL) and *C. albicans* (MIC = 8–20 µg/mL). The five-membered and six-membered rings in C-4 substituents had no significant effect on pharmacological activity. Moreover, **155** displayed promising antiproliferative activity against glioma cells U87MG and U251 with IC_{50} values of 3.8 ± 0.6 µM and 1.5 ± 0.1 µM, respectively.

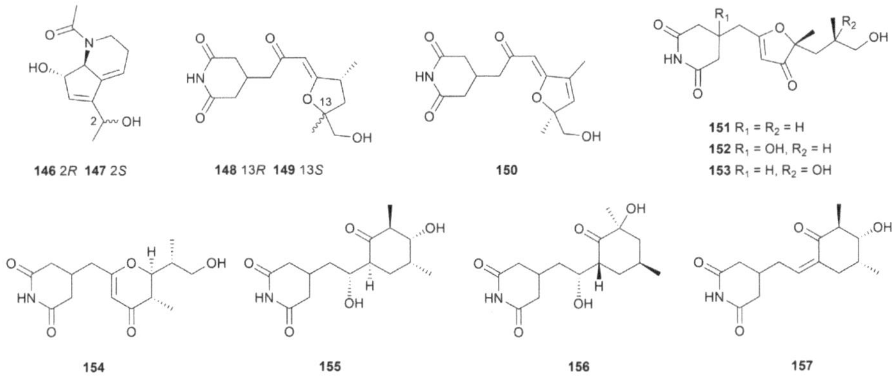

Figure 14. Chemical structures of other pyridines **146–157** isolated from marine *Streptomyces*.

6. Pyrazines and Piperazines

6.1. Pyrazines

Owing to nitrogen atoms acting as hydrogen bonding acceptors and the structure being conducive to nucleophilic reaction, pyrazine is commonly used as a classical pharmacophore [86]. Pyrazine derivatives have been reported for applications as antitumor drugs, diuretics, anti-inflammatory and anti-infective drugs [87]. Griseusrazin A (**158**, Figure 15) was isolated from a strain *S. griseus* subsp. *griseus* 09-0144 and activated the expression of heme oxygenase 1 which inhibits the upstream NF-κB pathway [88]. Therefore, it could downregulate the expression of related enzymes inducible nitric oxide synthase (iNOS) and COX-2 at the transcriptional level as well as the production of inflammatory mediators NO and PGE_2. Compounds **159–161** (Figure 15) were purified by *Streptomyces* sp. Did-27 isolated from the marine tunicate *Didemnum* sp., from which **159** and **161** showed weak cytotoxicity against HCT-116 and MCF-7 cancer cell lines with IC_{50} of 25–35 µg/mL [89]. Collected from a sample of coastal soil from Zhoushan Islands, China, the *Streptomyces* sp. ZZ446 afforded four pyrazinones of streptopyrazinones A–D (**162–165**, Figure 15) [90]. These compounds exhibit 35.0-60.0 µg/mL MIC values against *C. albicans* and 58.0-65.0 µg/mL MIC values against MRSA. In 2022, two pyrazines named actinopolymorphs E and F (**166** and **167**, Figure 15) were obtained from marine sediment-derived strain CNP-944 and only compound **167** exhibited weak activity against *K. rhizophila*, *B. subtilis* and *S. aureus* with MIC values of 16–64 µg/mL [91]. Compound **166** was inactive, which indicated that the carbonyl was the key active moiety.

6.2. Diketopiperazines

Piperazine alkaloids of biological origin are most commonly of the 2,5-diketopiperazines (2,5-DKPs) type, with a cyclodipeptide structure formed by condensation of two amino acids [92]. These simple dipeptides reported for multiple biological activities have a flexible skeleton with multiple chiral centers and four hydrogen bonding sites [93].

A variety of 2,5-DKPs alkaloids (**168–177**, Figure 16) had been isolated and characterized from several marine *Streptomyces* spp. Compounds **168–170** were condensed with leucine and phenylalanine residues and purified by a *Streptomyces* sp. MNU FJ-36 obtained from the intestinal fabric of *Katsuwonus* sp. [94]. All compounds were weakly inhibitory to A549 and HCT-116 cell lines. Streptodiketopiperazines A (**171**) and B (**172**) containing phenylalanine residues were isolated from the Mariana Trench source *Streptomyces* sp.

SY1965 [95]. Biological evaluation showed that **171** and **172** showed weak antifungal activity against *C. albicans* (MIC = both 42 μg/mL). A 2,5-DKPs dimer naseseazine C (**173**) had moderate inhibitory activity against chloroquine-sensitive *Plasmodium falciparum* (average IC_{50} value = 3.52 ± 1.2 μM) [96]. This dimer was connected by an unconventional C-6′/C-3 linkage and thus promoted antimalarial activity. Actinozine A (**174**) and cyclo(2-OH-D-Pro-L-Leu) (**175**) as two 2,5-DKP alkaloids were produced by *Streptomyces* sp. Call-36 from the Red Sea sponge *Callyspongia* sp. [97]. Compound **174** had a special hydroperoxy moiety on the proline residue. Antimicrobial assays against *S. aureus* and *C. albicans* revealed that **174** and **175** showed inhibition zones of 16–23 mm. Furthermore, a glycosylated 2,5-DKP (**176**) and its aglycone (**177**) showed inhibitory activity against MRSA, *E. coli* and *C. albicans* (MIC = 26.0–37.0 μg/mL) [98].

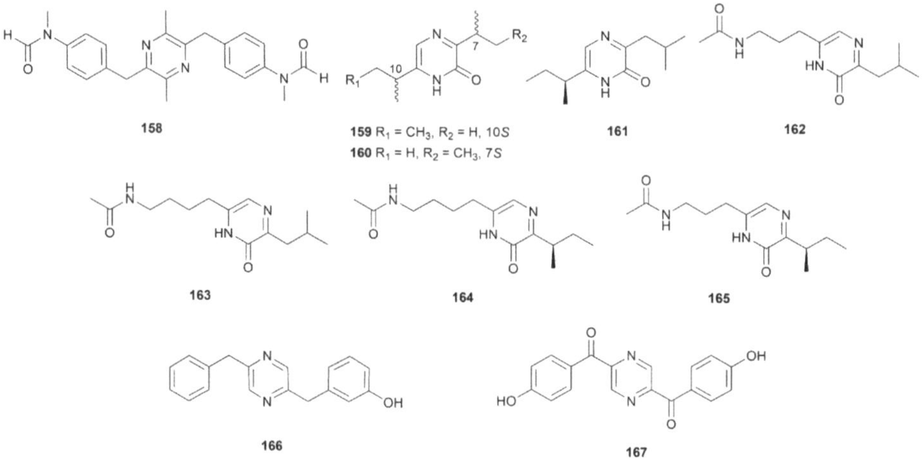

Figure 15. Chemical structures of pyrazines **158–167** isolated from marine *Streptomyces*.

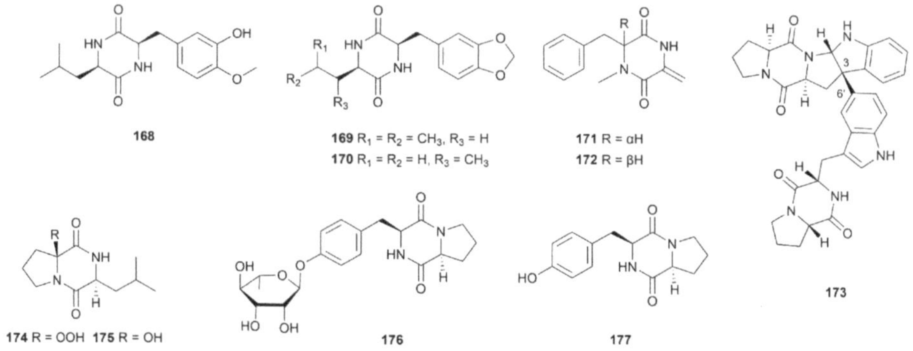

Figure 16. Chemical structures of diketopiperazines **168–177** isolated from marine *Streptomyces*.

7. Phenazines and Phenoxazines

To the best of our knowledge, phenazines and phenoxazines are mainly derived from SMs of *Streptomyces* and *Pseudomonas* isolated from soil or marine habitats [99]. Most of these alkaloids are characterized by promising biological activities such as antibacterial, antiviral, antitumor and antiparasitic effects [100]. Six antitumor phenoxazines venezuelines A–E (**178–182**, Figure 17) and maroxazinone (**183**, Figure 17) were isolated from two sediments-derived *Streptomyces* [101,102]. Compound **179** showed moderate antitumor activity against five cancer cell lines with IC_{50} values of 5.74–9.67 μM and weak activity against human hepatoma cell Bel 7042 (IC_{50} >10 μM). Notably, the cytotoxicity of this compound may be explained by significant upregulation of the orphan nuclear receptor Nur77 (apoptosis-associated) expression. **183** showed moderate antiproliferative activity against MCF7, HEPG2 and HCT116 cell lines with IC$_{50}$ values of 4.32, 2.90 and 8.51 μg/mL, respectively. Cytotoxic activity of phenoxazinones was stronger than phenoxazines and the increase of substituents weakened the activity. Sponges can host microorganisms colonization due to their porous structure, therefore the metabolites of sponge symbiotic microorganisms are important sources of marine natural products [103]. *Streptomyces* sp. HB202 was isolated from the sponge *Halichondria panicea* and yielded three phenazine alkaloids streptophenazines I–K (**184–186**, Figure 17) [104]. These compounds inhibited the activity of inflammatory response associated enzyme phosphodiesterase (PDE 4B) with IC$_{50}$ values ranging from 11.6 to 12.2 μM. In addition, compound **186** had antibacterial activity against *B. subtilis* and *S. epidermidis* (IC$_{50}$ = 21.6 ± 6.8 μM and 14.5 ± 2.0 μM, respectively).

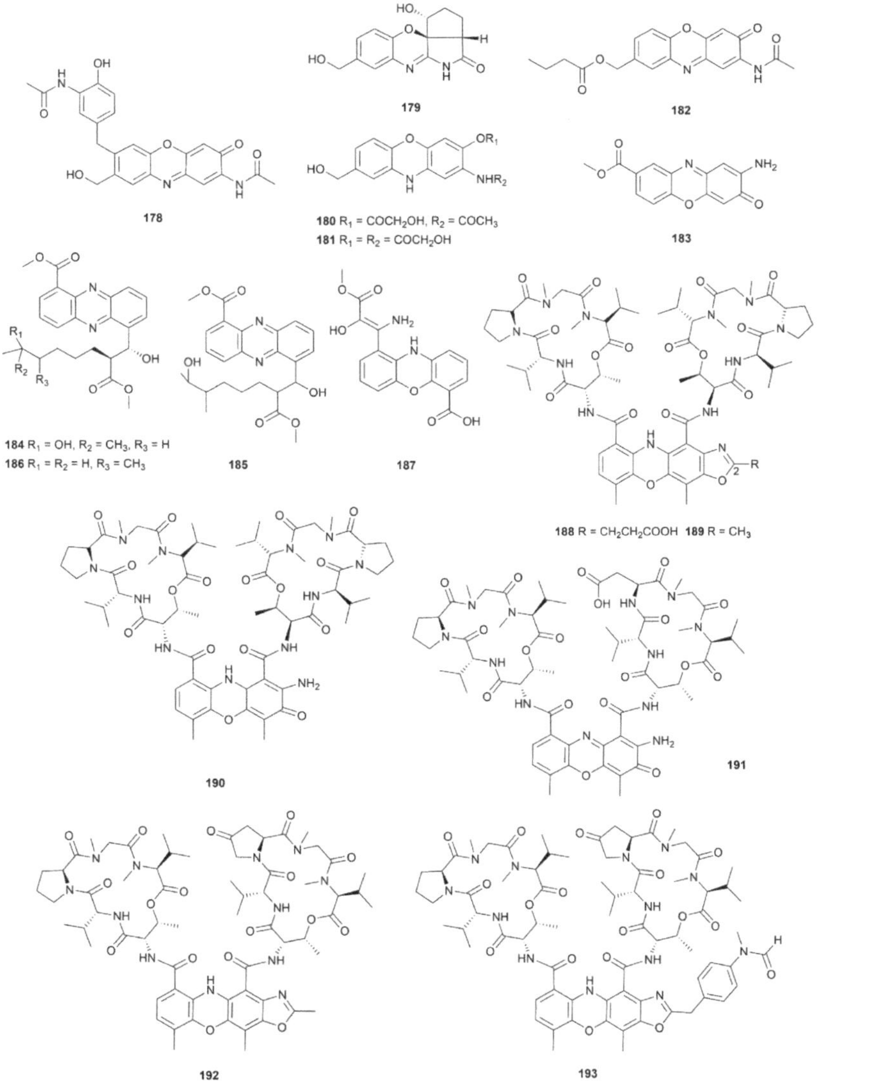

Figure 17. Chemical structures of phenazine and phenoxazine alkaloids **178–193** isolated from marine *Streptomyces*.

One phenoxazine derivative strepoxazine A (**187**, Figure 17) was produced by a strain SBT345 obtained from the mediterranean sponge *Agelas oroides* [105]. The IC_{50} value for **187** against promyelocytic leukemia cells HL-60 was 16 µg/mL. Actinomycin analogues (**188–193**, Figure 17) are a class of tetracyclic 5H-oxazolo[4,5-b]phenoxazine alkaloids [106,107]. Neo-actinomycin A (**188**) exhibited promising cytotoxic activity against HCT116 and A549 cancer cell lines (IC_{50} = 38.7 nM and 65.8 nM, respectively), as well as the biosynthetic pathways of **188** and **189** were the condensation of actinomycin D (**190**) with α-ketoglutarate or pyruvate. Actimomycin S (**191**) and neo-actinomycins C–D (**192–193**) were bacteriostatic against five common pathogenic bacteria (MIC = 2.5–80.0 µg/mL) and exhibited potent cytotoxic activity against HepG2 liver carcinoma cell line by blocking the G0/G1 phase cell cycle. The different substituents at C-2 position of oxazole ring showed great difference in biological activity.

8. Indolizidines and Pyrrolizidines

8.1. Indolizidines

Indolizidine were reported to have broad biological activity, such as antitumor activity, anti-infective system disease activity, and anti-inflammatory activity [108]. Most indolizidines are obtained from plants and animals, rarely from microbial sources [109].

Eight indolizidine alkaloids cyclizidines B–I (**194–201**, Figure 18) were detected in the EtOAc extracts of the strain *Streptomyces* sp. HNA39 [110]. Cyclizidine C (**195**) showed the most promising activity against PC-3 and HCT-116 cancer cell lines, with IC_{50} values of 0.52 ± 0.03 µM and 8.3 ± 0.1 µM, respectively. Moreover, compounds **195**, **198**, **200** and **201** exhibited moderate inhibitory activities against protein kinase ROCK2. In another report, a low-yielding indolizidine named cyclizidine J (**202**, Figure 18) was detected in strain HNA39 [111]. This compound had an uncommon chlorine atom substitution at the C-8 position. However, **202** lacked inhibitory activity against cancer cell line PC-3 and protein kinase. A stress culture of marine hydrothermal vent actinomycetes with heavy metal ions can activate silent biosynthetic pathways [112]. After the addition of 100 µmol/L Ni^{2+} to the medium of metal-resistant *Streptomyces* sp. WU20, a cyclizidine analogue (**203**, Figure 18) that was absent before addition was purified [113]. The authors hypothesized that the ring opening of the five-membered ring in the structure of alkaloid **203** was due to the inhibition of normal biosynthesis by heavy metal stress. Compound **203** was bacteriostatic against *B. subtilis* with MIC of around 32 µg/mL. Chemical analysis of symbiotic strain *Streptomyces* sp. HZP-2216E from fresh sea lettuce *Ulva pertusa* led to the discovery of an indolizinium alkaloid, streptopertusacin A (**204**, Figure 18), which had a 40 mg/mL MIC value against MRSA [114]. The antitumor activity of alkaloids was enhanced when C-8 was replaced by a hydroxyl group, but the cytotoxicity was lost after the aromatization of the indolizidine core.

8.2. Pyrrolizidines

Pyrrolizidines are mainly derived from plants as toxic components of chemical defense [115]. Bacterial-derived pyrrolizidines have been reported less frequently, with a total of 12 species and about 60 compounds of this class identified as of 2021 [116]. These Pyrrolizidines are commonly biosynthesized by multidomain NRPS gene clusters and are post-modified as well by flavine adenosine dinucleotide (FAD)-dependent monooxygenases [117].

Bohemamine is a rare pyrrolizidine subtype derived only from actinomycetes [118]. The fermentation broth of strain *S. spinoverrucosus* SNB-048 purified two bohemamine-type pyrrolizidines named spithioneines A and B (**205** and **206**, Figure 18) with rare ergothioneine moiety [119]. In the same year, six derivatives of bohemamines D−I (**207–212**, Figure 18) were again isolated from strain SNB-048 [120]. Unfortunately, none of the compounds showed significant activity. Tracing the cytotoxic activity of *S. spinoverrucosus* SNB-032 metabolites led to the isolation of an analogue, 5-Br-bohemamine C (**213**, Figure 18), as well as three dimeric bohemamines dibohemamines A–C (**214–216**, Figure 18) [121]. The authors confirmed that the dimer formation was a non-enzymatic Baylis–Hillman addition reaction of monomeric compounds using formaldehyde in the medium. Compounds **215** and **216** exhibited potent cytotoxicity against an NSCLC cell line A549 with IC$_{50}$ values of 0.140 and 0.145 µM, respectively. In addition, compound **216** showed moderate activity against an HCC1171 cell line (IC$_{50}$ = 1.2 µM). Bohemamine-type pyrrolizidines exhibited significant cytotoxic activity due to the polymerization of dimer.

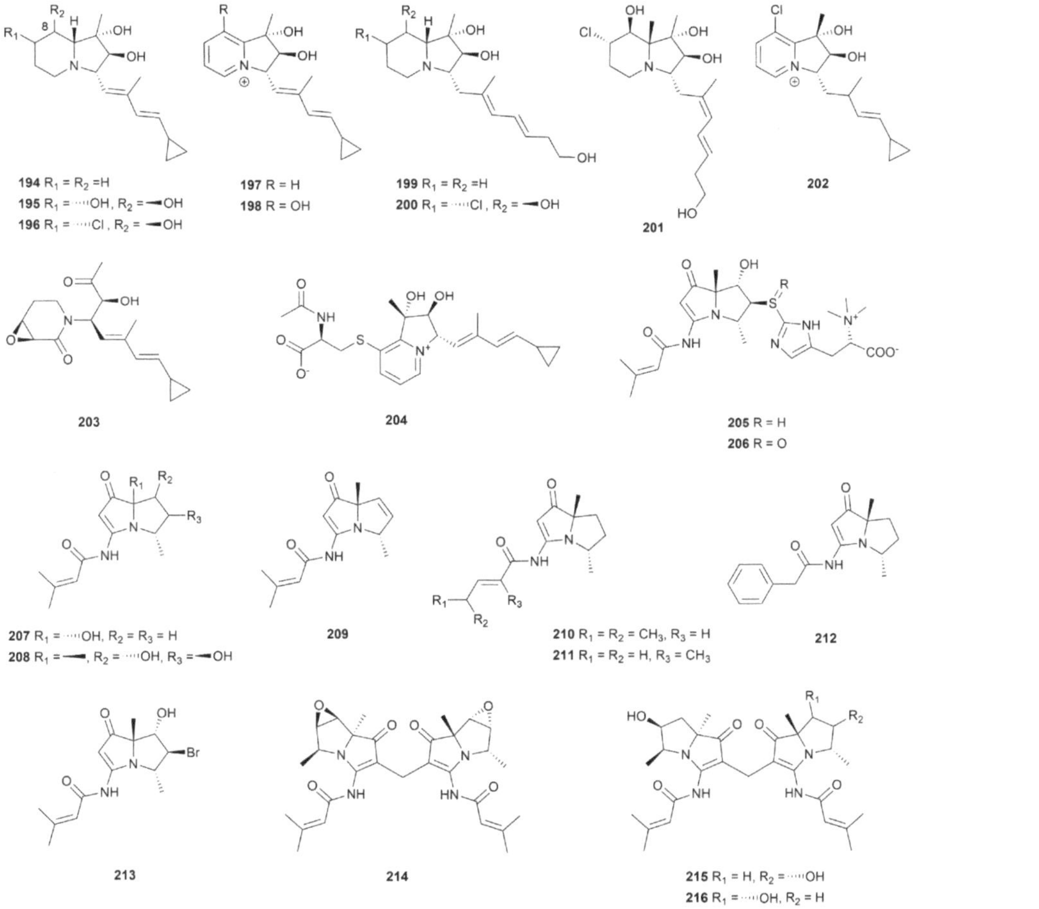

Figure 18. Chemical structures of indolizidine and pyrrolizidine alkaloids **194–216** isolated from marine *Streptomyces*.

9. Amides

9.1. Linear Amides

Marine sediment-derived *Streptomyces* sp. SNE-011 afforded three acylated arylamine alkaloids named carpatamides A–C (**217–219**, Figure 19) [122]. Compounds **217** and **219** displayed positive activity against HCC366, A549 and HCC44 cell lines (IC$_{50}$ = 2.2–8.4 µM). For compound **218**, the authors hypothesized that the reason for its inactivity was the inability of the structure to pass through the cell membrane. Antimycin is an antibiotic with antibacterial, insecticidal and anticancer activity, consisting of a rare nine-membered dilactone core [123]. Antimycins E–H (**220–223**, Figure 19) were isolated from *Streptomyces* sp. THS-55, and showed extremely significant cytotoxic activity against the HeLa cell line (IC$_{50}$ < 0.1 µM) by downregulating the levels of E6/E7 oncoproteins [124]. The potency was dependent on the long-chain substituent of R_2 and the acyl group of R_3. In addition, neoantimycins A and B (**224** and **225**, Figure 19) were isolated from *S. antibioticus* and exhibited weak cytotoxic activity against the SF-268 cancer cell line [125]. Bagremycin is a phenol ester formed from *p*-hydroxystyrene and *p*-hydroxybenzoic acid with antimicrobial activity [126]. Bagremycins C and D (**226** and **227**, Figure 19) were isolated in 2017 from *Streptomyces* sp. Q22 [127]. The following year, bagremycins F and G (**228** and **229**, Figure 19) were purified from coastal mud-sourced *Streptomyces* sp. ZZ745 [128]. Compound **226** inhibited the G_0/G_1 cell cycle in four glioma cells (U87MG, U251, SHG44 and C6) with IC_{50} values of 2.2 to 6.4 µM. Furthermore, compounds **228** and **229** showed 41.8 and 67.1 µM MIC values against *E. coli*. One N-acetyl macrolide analogue N-acetylborrelidin B (**230**, Figure 19) was detected by a strain *S. mutabilis* MII with stronger activity against *Staphylococcus warneri* (18 mm zone of inhibition) [129].

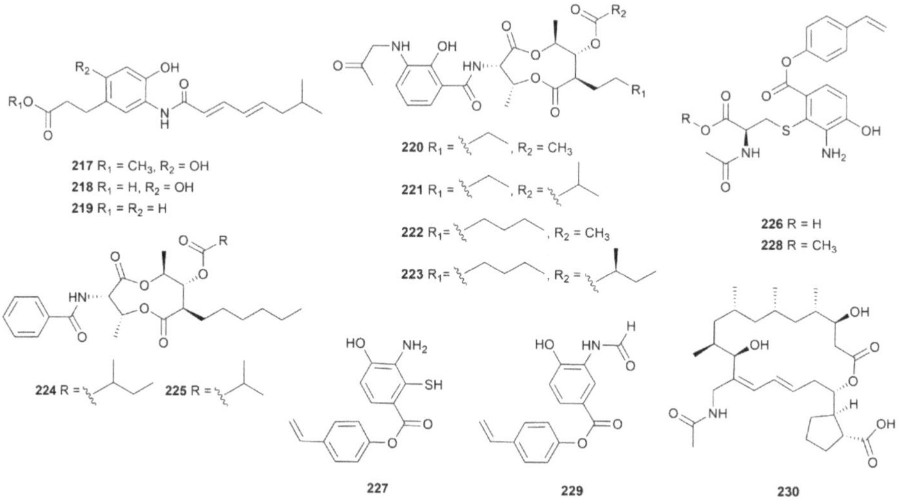

Figure 19. Chemical structures of linear amides **217–230** isolated from marine *Streptomyces*.

9.2. Macrolactams

Macrolactams are a class of macrocyclic compounds in which amide units are integrated into a polyketide skeleton above twelve carbons [130]. These compounds often contain an azacyclic core skeleton or azacyclic substituent modifications that result in alkalinity [131].

Polycyclic tetramate macrolactams (PTMs) are polycyclic macrolactam examples encoded by the PKS/NRPS heterozygous gene cluster [132]. Three PTMs (**231–233**, Figure 20) were purified from *S. zhaozhouensis* CA-185989 [133]. Compounds **231** and **232** had the most promising activity against MRSA, *C. albicans* and *A. fumigatus* (MIC = 1–8 µg/mL). The addition of the strong promoter *ermE**p to the PTM gene cluster of the deep-sea-derived *S. pactum* SCSIO 02999 activated the generation of six antitumor active PTMs, pactamides A–F (**234–239**, Figure 20) [134]. Compound **234** exhibited 0.24–0.51 µM IC_{50} values against four cancer cell lines. In addition, some atypical structural PTMs (Figure 20) with moderate cytotoxic activity, such as chlorinated derivatives chlokamycin (**240**) and H-10/H-11 *trans*-oriented PTM (**241–246**), have been reported in recent years from marine *Streptomyces* metabolites [135,136]. The substituent class of the side-chain tricyclic ring significantly affected the biological activity of the compounds. Moreover, a simple macrolactam JBIR-150 (**247**, Figure 20) exhibited cytotoxic activity against human malignant mesothelioma MESO-1 (IC_{50} = 2.3 µM) and human T-lymphoma Jurkat cells (IC_{50} = 0.9 µM) [137]. Another similar substance, muanlactam (**248**, Figure 20) was targeted for purification from *Streptomyces* sp. MA159 through combined genomic library and spectral characterization; and its IC_{50}

value against the HCT116 cell line was 1.58 µM [138]. *Streptomyces* sp. OUCMDZ-4348 is an extreme habitat microbe collected from Antarctica and was shown to produce two bicyclic macrolactams (**249** and **250**, Figure 20) [139]. Only **249** exhibited a moderate IC$_{50}$ value (9.8 µM) against the gastric carcinoma cell line N87. In another polar actinomyces, *S. somaliensis* 1107, four macrocyclic lactam containing furan rings (**251–254**, Figure 20) were isolated, one of which, compound **251** had anti-inflammatory activity [140].

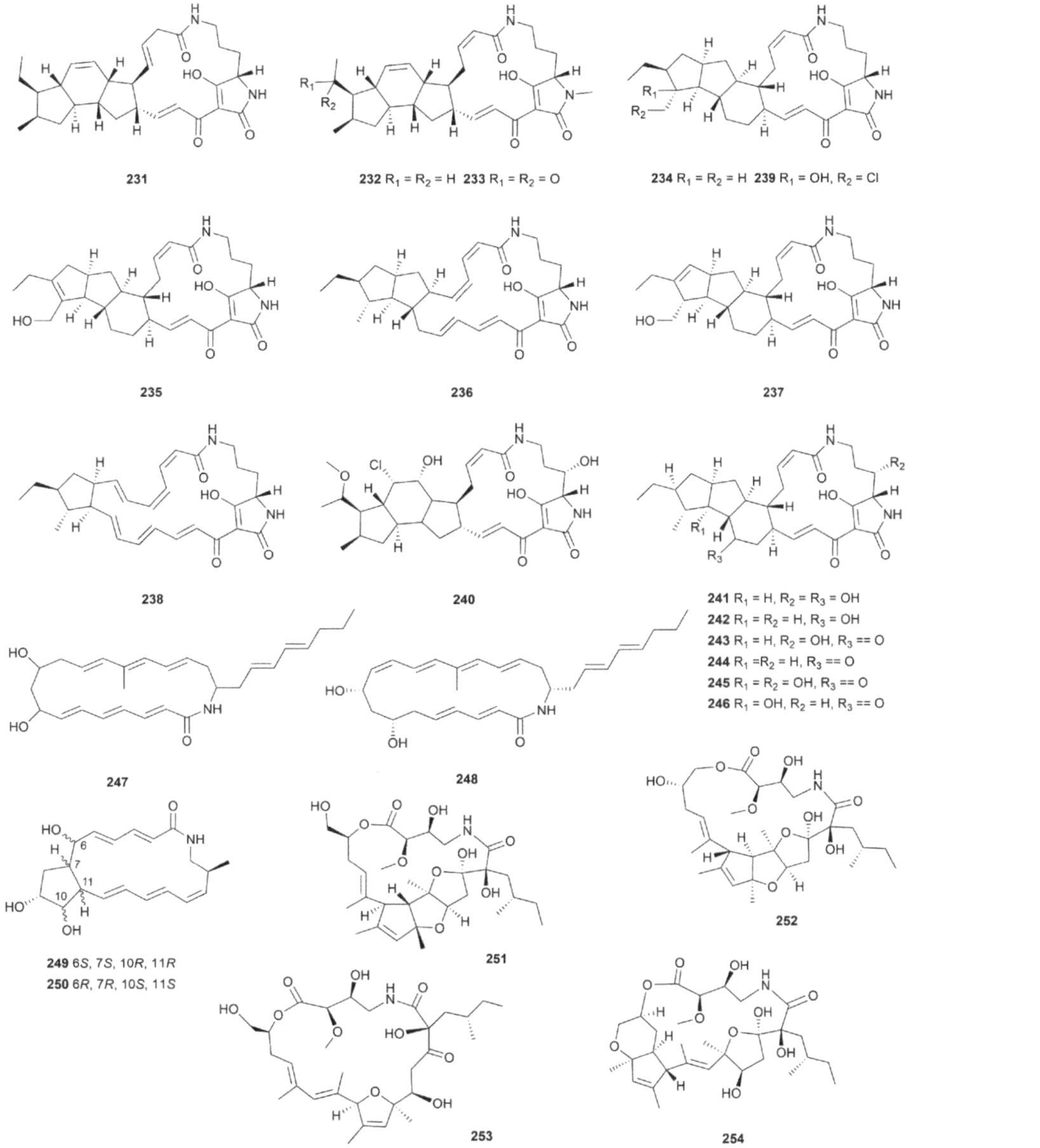

Figure 20. Chemical structures of macrolactams **231–254** isolated from marine *Streptomyces*.

10. Miscellaneous Alkaloids

Niphimycin (NM) is a class of guanidylpolyol macrolide antibiotics with extensive antibacterial activity against fungi and Gram-positive bacteria [141]. Four niphimycins derivatives (**255–258**, Figure 21) were obtained from *Streptomyces* sp. IMB7-145 and **255**,

257 and **258** displayed antibacterial effects on MRSA and vancomycin-resistant enterococci (VRE) with MIC values of 8–64 µg/mL [142]. Moreover, compound **255** exhibited significant anti-*M. tuberculosis* activity (MIC = 32 µg/mL) and significantly inhibited the growth of the phytopathogenic fungus *Fusarium oxysporum* f. sp.*cubense* (EC$_{50}$ = 1.20 µg/mL) as well as demonstrating cytotoxic activity against nasopharyngeal carcinoma cell lines TW03 and 5-8F (IC$_{50}$ = 12.24 µg/mL and 9.44 µg/mL, respectively) [143,144]. The increase in malonyl substituents had a negative effect on its biological activity. Antartin (**259**, Figure 21) was a zizaane-type sesquiterpene produced by strain *Streptomyces* sp. SCO736 and showed promising cytotoxic activity against twelve human cancer cells, with 50% growth inhibition (GI$_{50}$) of 4–8 µg/mL and inhibited the production of solid lung tumor cells [145]. Penzonemycins A and B (**260–261**, Figure 21) were two phenylhydrazones, in which their hydrazone moiety was synthesized by a non-enzymatic Japp−Klingemann coupling reaction [146]. Compound **260** inhibited cancer cell lines SF-268, MCF-7, A549 and HepG-2, with IC$_{50}$ values ranging from 30.44 to 61.92 µM.

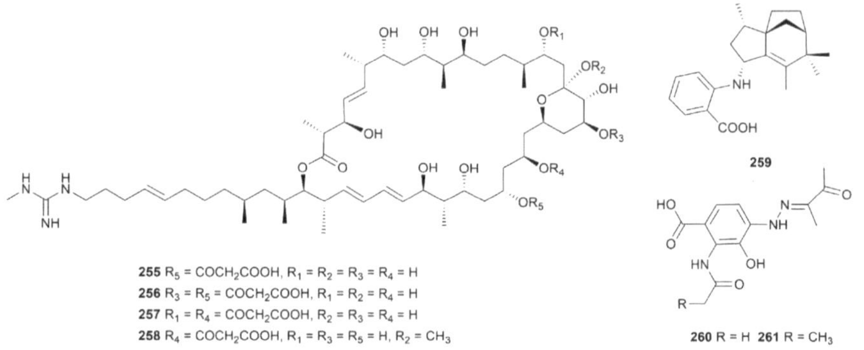

255 R$_5$ = COCH$_2$COOH, R$_1$ = R$_2$ = R$_3$ = R$_4$ = H
256 R$_3$ = R$_5$ = COCH$_2$COOH, R$_1$ = R$_2$ = R$_4$ = H
257 R$_1$ = R$_4$ = COCH$_2$COOH, R$_2$ = R$_3$ = R$_4$ = H
258 R$_4$ = COCH$_2$COOH, R$_1$ = R$_3$ = R$_5$ = H, R$_2$ = CH$_3$

260 R = H 261 R = CH$_3$

Figure 21. Chemical structures of miscellaneous alkaloids **255–261** isolated from marine *Streptomyces*.

11. Conclusions and Future Perspectives

Microorganisms in special habitats have cryptic and extraordinary potential for biosynthesizing unique SMs with diverse biological properties. Marine *Streptomyces* as an excellent producer of therapeutic agents has become a global hotspot in natural product research and continue to play a paramount role in the production of new alkaloids for drug discovery. This review comprehensively summarizes as many as 261 new alkaloids discovered in marine *Streptomyces* in the past decade (January 2013–June 2023). Among these metabolites, 199 compounds have promising therapeutic effects. For instance, compounds **38**, **41**, **42**, **97**, **98**, **142** and **193** exhibited excellent antimicrobial activity, and **114**, **188** and **220–239** displayed remarkable cytotoxic effects. In addition, compounds **5–16** showed significant selective inhibition on protein kinases PKC, ROCK2 and BTK. This work will pave the way for further development of marine *Streptomyces*-derived alkaloids.

Although strategies for the isolation of marine microbial metabolites have been revolutionized over the past decades, there are still difficulties to overcome. Traditional means of separating natural products are subject to randomization. The efficient isolation of novel natural products and removal of inactive known compounds have been thorny issues hindering the development of natural medicinal chemistry. The annotation of BGCs, as well as LC-MS/MS-based metabolite structure prediction methods, will remain hot research topics in this field in the future. BGCs of marine microorganisms often have low or no expression under routine laboratory culture conditions. BGC activation techniques, such as OSMAC strategy, strain co-culture, ribosome engineering, heterologous expression of gene clusters and overexpression/knockout of regulatory genes and ribosome engineering, provide methodological references to break this bottleneck. In addition to the discovery of these therapeutic agents, it is crucial to solve the problem of compound supply. Currently, in addition to the total synthesis route design of natural products, the modification of industrial production strains using genetic engineering approaches and optimization of microbial fermentation and extraction, as well as purification processes at various levels, should be employed in the preparation of these substances.

Supplementary Materials: The following supporting information can be downloaded at: https://www.mdpi.com/article/10.3390/md22010051/s1, Table S1: detailed information for new alkaloids from marine *Streptomyces* discovered in 2013–June 2023.

Author Contributions: Conceptualization, H.Z.; investigation, Z.L., W.S. and Z.H.; visualization, Z.L. and W.W.; writing—original draft, Z.L.; writing—review and editing, H.Z. All authors have read and agreed to the published version of the manuscript.

Funding: This work was financially supported by the National Key Research and Development Program of China (2022YFC2804203).

Institutional Review Board Statement: Not applicable.

Data Availability Statement: The data presented in this study are available in the Supplementary Material.

Conflicts of Interest: The authors declare no conflicts of interest.

References

1. Konig, G.M.; Kehraus, S.; Seibert, S.F.; Abdel-Lateff, A.; Muller, D. Natural products from marine organisms and their associated microbes. *Chembiochem* **2006**, *7*, 229–238. [CrossRef] [PubMed]
2. Yang, Z.; He, J.; Wei, X.; Ju, J.; Ma, J. Exploration and genome mining of natural products from marine *Streptomyces*. *Appl. Microbiol. Biotechnol.* **2020**, *104*, 67–76. [CrossRef] [PubMed]
3. Hu, Y.; Chen, S.; Yang, F.; Dong, S. Marine indole alkaloids—Isolation, structure and bioactivities. *Mar. Drugs* **2021**, *19*, 658. [CrossRef] [PubMed]
4. Bérdy, J. Thoughts and facts about antibiotics: Where we are now and where we are heading. *J. Antibiot.* **2012**, *65*, 385–395. [CrossRef] [PubMed]
5. Fernandes, A.S.; Oliveira, C.; Reis, R.L.; Martins, A.; Silva, T.H. Marine-inspired drugs and biomaterials in the perspective of pancreatic cancer therapies. *Mar. Drugs* **2022**, *20*, 689. [CrossRef]
6. Barka, E.A.; Vatsa, P.; Sanchez, L.; Gaveau-Vaillant, N.; Jacquard, C.; Meier-Kolthoff, J.P.; Klenk, H.P.; Clement, C.; Ouhdouch, Y.; van Wezel, G.P. Taxonomy, physiology, and natural products of *Actinobacteria*. *Microbiol. Mol. Biol. Rev.* **2016**, *80*, 1–43. [CrossRef]
7. Ngamcharungchit, C.; Chaimusik, N.; Panbangred, W.; Euanorasetr, J.; Intra, B. Bioactive metabolites from terrestrial and marine actinomycetes. *Molecules* **2023**, *28*, 5915. [CrossRef]
8. Donald, L.; Pipite, A.; Subramani, R.; Owen, J.; Keyzers, R.A.; Taufa, T. *Streptomyces*: Still the biggest producer of new natural secondary metabolites, a current perspective. *Microbiol. Res.* **2022**, *13*, 418–465. [CrossRef]
9. Zhang, S.; Chen, Y.; Zhu, J.; Lu, Q.; Cryle, M.J.; Zhang, Y.; Yan, F. Structural diversity, biosynthesis, and biological functions of lipopeptides from *Streptomyces*. *Nat. Prod. Rep.* **2023**, *40*, 557–594. [CrossRef]
10. Huang, T.; Zhou, Z.; Liu, Q.; Wang, X.; Guo, W.; Lin, S. Biosynthetic mechanisms of alkaloids from actinomycetes. *Prog. Chem.* **2018**, *30*, 692–702.
11. Netz, N.; Opatz, T. Marine indole alkaloids. *Mar. Drugs* **2015**, *13*, 4814–4914. [CrossRef] [PubMed]
12. Munekata, P.E.S.; Pateiro, M.; Conte-Junior, C.A.; Domínguez, R.; Nawaz, A.; Walayat, N.; Movilla Fierro, E.; Lorenzo, J.M. Marine alkaloids: Compounds with in vivo activity and chemical synthesis. *Mar. Drugs* **2021**, *19*, 374. [CrossRef] [PubMed]
13. Rosales, P.F.; Bordin, G.S.; Gower, A.E.; Moura, S. Indole alkaloids: 2012 until now, highlighting the new chemical structures and biological activities. *Fitoterapia* **2020**, *143*, 104558. [CrossRef]
14. Holland, D.C.; Carroll, A.R. Marine indole alkaloid diversity and bioactivity. What do we know and what are we missing? *Nat. Prod. Rep.* **2023**, *40*, 1595–1607. [CrossRef] [PubMed]
15. Xu, M.; Peng, R.; Min, Q.; Hui, S.; Chen, X.; Yang, G.; Qin, S. Bisindole natural products: A vital source for the development of new anticancer drugs. *Eur. J. Med. Chem.* **2022**, *243*, 114748. [CrossRef] [PubMed]
16. Carbone, D.; De Franco, M.; Pecoraro, C.; Bassani, D.; Pavan, M.; Cascioferro, S.; Parrino, B.; Cirrincione, G.; Dall'Acqua, S.; Moro, S.; et al. Discovery of the 3-amino-1,2,4-triazine-based library as selective PDK1 inhibitors with therapeutic potential in highly aggressive pancreatic ductal adenocarcinoma. *Int. J. Mol. Sci.* **2023**, *24*, 3679. [CrossRef] [PubMed]
17. Carbone, D.; De Franco, M.; Pecoraro, C.; Bassani, D.; Pavan, M.; Cascioferro, S.; Parrino, B.; Cirrincione, G.; Dall'Acqua, S.; Sut, S.; et al. Structural manipulations of marine natural products inspire a new library of 3-amino-1,2,4-triazine PDK inhibitors endowed with antitumor activity in pancreatic ductal adenocarcinoma. *Mar. Drugs* **2023**, *21*, 288. [CrossRef]
18. Gani, O.A.; Engh, R.A. Protein kinase inhibition of clinically important staurosporine analogues. *Nat. Prod. Rep.* **2010**, *27*, 489–498. [CrossRef]
19. Kapoor, R.; Saini, A.; Sharma, D. Indispensable role of microbes in anticancer drugs and discovery trends. *Appl. Microbiol. Biotechnol.* **2022**, *106*, 4885–4906. [CrossRef]

20. Cheng, X.; Zhou, B.; Liu, H.; Huo, C.; Ding, W. One new indolocarbazole alkaloid from the *Streptomyces* sp. A22. *Nat. Prod. Res.* **2018**, *32*, 2583–2588. [CrossRef]
21. Wang, J.N.; Zhang, H.J.; Li, J.Q.; Ding, W.J.; Ma, Z.J. Bioactive indolocarbazoles from the marine-derived *Streptomyces* sp. DT-A61. *J. Nat. Prod.* **2018**, *81*, 949–956. [CrossRef] [PubMed]
22. Onaka, H.; Asamizu, S.; Igarashi, Y.; Yoshida, R.; Furumai, T. Cytochrome P450 homolog is responsible for C-N bond formation between aglycone and deoxysugar in the staurosporine biosynthesis of *Streptomyces* sp. TP-A0274. *Biosci. Biotechnol. Biochem.* **2005**, *69*, 1753–1759. [CrossRef] [PubMed]
23. Qin, L.; Zhou, B.; Ding, W.; Ma, Z. Bioactive metabolites from marine-derived *Streptomyces* sp. A68 and its Rifampicin resistant mutant strain R-M1. *Phytochem. Lett.* **2018**, *23*, 46–51. [CrossRef]
24. Zhou, B.; Hu, Z.J.; Zhang, H.J.; Li, J.Q.; Ding, W.J.; Ma, Z.J. Bioactive staurosporine derivatives from the *Streptomyces* sp. NB-A13. *Bioorg. Chem.* **2019**, *82*, 33–40. [CrossRef]
25. Zhou, B.; Qin, L.; Ding, W.; Ma, Z. Cytotoxic indolocarbazoles alkaloids from the *Streptomyces* sp. A65. *Tetrahedron* **2018**, *74*, 726–730. [CrossRef]
26. Wang, C.; Monger, A.; Wang, L.; Fu, P.; Piyachaturawat, P.; Chairoungdua, A.; Zhu, W. Precursor-directed generation of indolocarbazoles with topoisomerase IIα inhibitory activity. *Mar. Drugs* **2018**, *16*, 168. [CrossRef]
27. Cui, T.; Lin, S.; Wang, Z.; Fu, P.; Wang, C.; Zhu, W. Cytotoxic indolocarbazoles from a marine-derived *Streptomyces* sp. OUCMDZ-5380. *Front. Microbiol.* **2022**, *13*, 957473. [CrossRef]
28. Zhang, W.; Ma, L.; Li, S.; Liu, Z.; Chen, Y.; Zhang, H.; Zhang, G.; Zhang, Q.; Tian, X.; Yuan, C.; et al. Indimicins A–E, bisindole alkaloids from the deep-sea-derived *Streptomyces* sp. SCSIO 03032. *J. Nat. Prod.* **2014**, *77*, 1887–1892. [CrossRef]
29. Liu, Z.; Ma, L.; Zhang, L.; Zhang, W.; Zhu, Y.; Chen, Y.; Zhang, W.; Zhang, C. Functional characterization of the halogenase SpmH and discovery of new deschloro-tryptophan dimers. *Org. Biomol. Chem.* **2019**, *17*, 1053–1057. [CrossRef]
30. Paulus, C.; Rebets, Y.; Tokovenko, B.; Nadmid, S.; Terekhova, L.P.; Myronovskyi, M.; Zotchev, S.B.; Ruckert, C.; Braig, S.; Zahler, S.; et al. New natural products identified by combined genomics-metabolomics profiling of marine *Streptomyces* sp. MP131-18. *Sci. Rep.* **2017**, *7*, 42382. [CrossRef]
31. Song, Y.; Yang, J.; Yu, J.; Li, J.; Yuan, J.; Wong, N.K.; Ju, J. Chlorinated *bis*-indole alkaloids from deep-sea derived *Streptomyces* sp. SCSIO 11791 with antibacterial and cytotoxic activities. *J. Antibiot.* **2020**, *73*, 542–547. [CrossRef] [PubMed]
32. Ding, L.; Munch, J.; Goerls, H.; Maier, A.; Fiebig, H.H.; Lin, W.H.; Hertweck, C. Xiamycin, a pentacyclic indolosesquiterpene with selective anti-HIV activity from a bacterial mangrove endophyte. *Bioorg. Med. Chem. Lett.* **2010**, *20*, 6685–6687. [CrossRef] [PubMed]
33. Munda, M.; Nandi, R.; Gavit, V.R.; Kundu, S.; Niyogi, S.; Bisai, A. Total syntheses of naturally occurring antiviral indolosesquiterpene alkaloids, xiamycins C-F via Csp(3)-H functionalization. *Chem. Sci.* **2022**, *13*, 11666–11671. [CrossRef]
34. Kim, S.H.; Ha, T.K.; Oh, W.K.; Shin, J.; Oh, D.C. Antiviral indolosesquiterpenoid xiamycins C-E from a halophilic actinomycete. *J. Nat. Prod.* **2016**, *79*, 51–58. [CrossRef]
35. Park, J.; Cho, H.S.; Moon, D.H.; Lee, D.; Kal, Y.; Cha, S.; Lee, S.K.; Yoon, Y.J.; Oh, D.-C. Discovery of new indolosesquiterpenoids bearing a N-O linkage by overexpression of LuxR regulator in a marine bacterium *Streptomyces* sp. *Front. Mar. Sci.* **2023**, *10*, 1140516. [CrossRef]
36. Zhang, S.; Yang, Q.; Guo, L.; Zhang, Y.; Feng, L.; Zhou, L.; Yang, S.; Yao, Q.; Pescitelli, G.; Xie, Z. Isolation, structure elucidation and racemization of (+)- and (−)-pratensilins A-C: Unprecedented spiro indolinone-naphthofuran alkaloids from a marine *Streptomyces* sp. *Chem. Commun.* **2017**, *53*, 10066–10069. [CrossRef] [PubMed]
37. Guo, L.; Zhang, L.; Yang, Q.; Xu, B.; Fu, X.; Liu, M.; Li, Z.; Zhang, S.; Xie, Z. Antibacterial and cytotoxic bridged and ring cleavage angucyclinones from a marine *Streptomyces* sp. *Front. Chem.* **2020**, *8*, 586. [CrossRef]
38. Che, Q.; Qiao, L.; Han, X.; Liu, Y.; Wang, W.; Gu, Q.; Zhu, T.; Li, D. Anthranosides A-C, anthranilate derivatives from a sponge-derived *Streptomyces* sp. CMN-62. *Org. Lett.* **2018**, *20*, 5466–5469. [CrossRef]
39. Newaz, A.W.; Yong, K.; Lian, X.; Zhang, Z. Streptoindoles A–D, novel antimicrobial indole alkaloids from the marine-associated actinomycete *Streptomyces* sp. ZZ1118. *Tetrahedron* **2022**, *104*, 132598. [CrossRef]
40. Zhang, Y.; Hou, S.; Zhang, M.; Wu, Y. Research progress in biosynthesis of five-membered heterocyclic rings in natural products. *J. Microbiol.* **2019**, *39*, 1–12.
41. Seipp, K.; Geske, L.; Opatz, T. Marine pyrrole alkaloids. *Mar. Drugs* **2021**, *19*, 514. [CrossRef] [PubMed]
42. Asif, M.; Alghamdi, S. An overview on biological importance of pyrrolone and pyrrolidinone derivatives as promising Sscaffolds. *Russ. J. Org. Chem.* **2021**, *57*, 1700–1718. [CrossRef]
43. Mo, X.; Wang, Z.; Wang, B.; Ma, J.; Huang, H.; Tian, X.; Zhang, S.; Zhang, C.; Ju, J. Cloning and characterization of the biosynthetic gene cluster of the bacterial RNA polymerase inhibitor tirandamycin from marine-derived *Streptomyces* sp. SCSIO1666. *Biochem. Biophys. Res. Commun.* **2011**, *406*, 341–347. [CrossRef] [PubMed]
44. Zhang, X.; Li, Z.; Du, L.; Chlipala, G.E.; Lopez, P.C.; Zhang, W.; Sherman, D.H.; Li, S. Identification of an unexpected shunt pathway product provides new insights into tirandamycin biosynthesis. *Tetrahedron Lett.* **2016**, *57*, 5919–5923. [CrossRef] [PubMed]
45. Cong, Z.; Huang, X.; Liu, Y.; Liu, Y.; Wang, P.; Liao, S.; Yang, B.; Zhou, X.; Huang, D.; Wang, J. Cytotoxic anthracycline and antibacterial tirandamycin analogues from a marine-derived *Streptomyces* sp. SCSIO 41399. *J. Antibiot.* **2019**, *72*, 45–49. [CrossRef]

46. Song, F.; Hu, J.; Zhang, X.; Xu, W.; Yang, J.; Li, S.; Xu, X. Unique cyclized thiolopyrrolones from the marine-derived *Streptomyces* sp. BTBU20218885. *Mar. Drugs* **2022**, *20*, 214. [CrossRef]
47. Chung, B.; Hwang, J.Y.; Park, S.C.; Kwon, O.S.; Cho, E.; Lee, J.; Lee, H.S.; Oh, D.C.; Shin, J.; Oh, K.B. Inhibitory effects of nitrogenous metabolites from a marine-derived *Streptomyces bacillaris* on isocitrate lyase of *Candida albicans*. *Mar. Drugs* **2022**, *20*, 138. [CrossRef]
48. Kim, M.C.; Lee, J.H.; Shin, B.; Subedi, L.; Cha, J.W.; Park, J.S.; Oh, D.C.; Kim, S.Y.; Kwon, H.C. Salinazinones A and B: Pyrrolidinyl-oxazinones from solar saltern-derived *Streptomyces* sp. KMF-004. *Org. Lett.* **2015**, *17*, 5024–5027. [CrossRef]
49. Zhang, Y.M.; Liu, B.L.; Zheng, X.H.; Huang, X.J.; Li, H.Y.; Zhang, Y.; Zhang, T.T.; Sun, D.Y.; Lin, B.R.; Zhou, G.X. Anandins A and B, two rare steroidal alkaloids from a marine *Streptomyces anandii* H41-59. *Mar. Drugs* **2017**, *15*, 355. [CrossRef]
50. Lim, H.J.; An, J.S.; Bae, E.S.; Cho, E.; Hwang, S.; Nam, S.J.; Oh, K.B.; Lee, S.K.; Oh, D.C. Ligiamycins A and B, decalin-aminomaleimides from the co-culture of *Streptomyces* sp. and *Achromobacter* sp. Isolated from the marine wharf roach, *Ligia exotica*. *Mar. Drugs* **2022**, *20*, 83. [CrossRef]
51. Varvounis, G. An update on the synthesis of pyrrolo[1,4]benzodiazepines. *Molecules* **2016**, *21*, 154. [CrossRef]
52. Pavlikova, M.; Kamenik, Z.; Janata, J.; Kadlcik, S.; Kuzma, M.; Najmanova, L. Novel pathway of 3-hydroxyanthranilic acid formation in limazepine biosynthesis reveals evolutionary relation between phenazines and pyrrolobenzodiazepines. *Sci. Rep.* **2018**, *8*, 7810. [CrossRef] [PubMed]
53. Han, Y.; Li, Y.Y.; Shen, Y.; Li, J.; Li, W.J.; Shen, Y.M. Oxoprothracarcin, a novel pyrrolo[1,4]benzodiazepine antibiotic from marine *Streptomyces* sp. M10946. *Drug Discov. Ther.* **2013**, *7*, 243–247. [CrossRef] [PubMed]
54. Çetinel Aksoy, S.; Küçüksolak, M.; Uze, A.; Bedir, E. Benzodiazepine derivatives from marine-derived *Streptomyces cacaoi* 14CM034. *Rec. Nat. Prod.* **2021**, *15*, 602–607. [CrossRef]
55. Kang, Q.; Shen, Y.; Bai, L. Biosynthesis of 3,5-AHBA-derived natural products. *Nat. Prod. Rep.* **2012**, *29*, 243–263. [CrossRef] [PubMed]
56. Li, S.; Wang, H.; Li, Y.; Deng, J.; Lu, C.; Shen, Y.; Shen, Y. Biosynthesis of hygrocins, antitumor naphthoquinone ansamycins produced by *Streptomyces* sp. LZ35. *Chembiochem* **2014**, *15*, 94–102. [CrossRef]
57. Cai, P.; Kong, F.; Ruppen, M.E.; Glasier, G. Hygrocins A and B, naphthoquinone macrolides from *Streptomyces hygroscopicus*. *J. Nat. Prod.* **2005**, *68*, 1736–1742. [CrossRef]
58. Lu, C.; Li, Y.; Deng, J.; Li, S.; Shen, Y.; Wang, H.; Shen, Y. Hygrocins C-G, cytotoxic naphthoquinone ansamycins from gdmAI-disrupted *Streptomyces* sp. LZ35. *J. Nat. Prod.* **2013**, *76*, 2175–2179. [CrossRef]
59. Li, S.; Lu, C.; Ou, J.; Deng, J.; Shen, Y. Overexpression of hgc1 increases the production and diversity of hygrocins in *Streptomyces* sp. LZ35. *RSC Adv.* **2015**, *5*, 83843–83846. [CrossRef]
60. Yi, W.; Newaz, A.W.; Yong, K.; Ma, M.; Lian, X.Y.; Zhang, Z. New Hygrocins K-U and streptophenylpropanamide A and bioactive compounds from the marine-associated *Streptomyces* sp. ZZ1956. *Antibiotics* **2022**, *11*, 1455. [CrossRef]
61. Le, T.C.; Yang, I.; Yoon, Y.J.; Nam, S.J.; Fenical, W. Ansalactams B-D illustrate further biosynthetic plasticity within the ansamycin pathway. *Org. Lett.* **2016**, *18*, 2256–2259. [CrossRef] [PubMed]
62. Zhou, L.M.; Kong, F.D.; Xie, Q.Y.; Ma, Q.Y.; Hu, Z.; Zhao, Y.X.; Luo, D.Q. Divergolides T-W with apoptosis-inducing activity from the mangrove-derived actinomycete *Streptomyces* sp. KFD18. *Mar. Drugs* **2019**, *17*, 219. [CrossRef] [PubMed]
63. Alvarez-Mico, X.; Jensen, P.R.; Fenical, W.; Hughes, C.C. Chlorizidine, a cytotoxic 5H-pyrrolo[2,1-a]isoindol-5-one-containing alkaloid from a marine *Streptomyces* sp. *Org. Lett.* **2013**, *15*, 988–991. [CrossRef] [PubMed]
64. Heo, C.S.; Kang, J.S.; Kwon, J.H.; Anh, C.V.; Shin, H.J. Pyrrole-containing alkaloids from a marine-derived actinobacterium *Streptomyces zhaozhouensis* and their antimicrobial and cytotoxic activities. *Mar. Drugs* **2023**, *21*, 167. [CrossRef] [PubMed]
65. Lian, X.Y.; Zhang, Z. Indanomycin-related antibiotics from marine *Streptomyces antibioticus* PTZ0016. *Nat. Prod. Res.* **2013**, *27*, 2161–2167. [CrossRef] [PubMed]
66. Zhou, B.; Huang, Y.; Zhang, H.; Li, J.; Ding, W. Nitricquinomycins A-C, uncommon naphthopyrroledones from the *Streptomyces* sp. ZS-A45. *Tetrahedron* **2019**, *75*, 3958–3961. [CrossRef]
67. Song, F.; Yang, N.; Khalil, Z.G.; Salim, A.A.; Han, J.; Bernhardt, P.V.; Lin, R.; Xu, X.; Capon, R.J. Bhimamycin J, a rare benzo[*f*]isoindole-dione alkaloid from the marine-derived actinomycete *Streptomyces* sp. MS180069. *Chem. Biodivers.* **2021**, *18*, e2100674. [CrossRef] [PubMed]
68. Ko, K.; Kim, S.H.; Park, S.; Han, H.S.; Lee, J.K.; Cha, J.W.; Hwang, S.; Choi, K.Y.; Song, Y.J.; Nam, S.J.; et al. Discovery and photoisomerization of new pyrrolosesquiterpenoids glaciapyrroles D and E, from deep-sea sediment *Streptomyces* sp. *Mar. Drugs* **2022**, *20*, 281. [CrossRef]
69. Guerrero-Pepinosa, N.Y.; Cardona-Trujillo, M.C.; Garzon-Castano, S.C.; Veloza, L.A.; Sepulveda-Arias, J.C. Antiproliferative activity of thiazole and oxazole derivatives: A systematic review of in vitro and in vivo studies. *Biomed. Pharmacother.* **2021**, *138*, 111495. [CrossRef]
70. Davyt, D.; Serra, G. Thiazole and oxazole alkaloids: Isolation and synthesis. *Mar. Drugs* **2010**, *8*, 2755–2780. [CrossRef]
71. Liu, Y.; Ding, L.; Deng, Y.; Wang, X.; Cui, W.; He, S. Feature-based molecular networking-guided discovery of siderophores from a marine mesophotic zone *Axinellida* sponge-associated actinomycete *Streptomyces diastaticus* NBU2966. *Phytochemistry* **2022**, *196*, 113078. [CrossRef] [PubMed]

72. Zhang, X.; Tao, F.; Cui, T.; Luo, C.; Zhou, Z.; Huang, Y.; Tan, L.; Peng, W.; Wu, C. Sources, transformations, syntheses, and bioactivities of monoterpene pyridine alkaloids and cyclopenta[c]pyridine derivatives. *Molecules* **2022**, *27*, 7187. [CrossRef] [PubMed]
73. Zhou, X.; Fenical, W. The unique chemistry and biology of the piericidins. *J. Antibiot.* **2016**, *69*, 582–593. [CrossRef] [PubMed]
74. Azad, S.M.; Jin, Y.; Ser, H.-L.; Goh, B.-H.; Thawai, L.-H.I.C.; He, Y.-W. Biological insights into the piericidin family of microbial metabolites. *J. Appl. Microbiol.* **2022**, *132*, 772–784. [CrossRef]
75. Zhou, X.; Liang, Z.; Li, K.; Fang, W.; Tian, Y.; Luo, X.; Chen, Y.; Zhan, Z.; Zhang, T.; Liao, S.; et al. Exploring the natural piericidins as anti-renal cell carcinoma agents targeting peroxiredoxin 1. *J. Med. Chem.* **2019**, *62*, 7058–7069. [CrossRef]
76. Peng, J.; Zhang, Q.; Jiang, X.; Ma, L.; Long, T.; Cheng, Z.; Zhang, C.; Zhu, Y. New piericidin derivatives from the marine-derived *Streptomyces* sp. SCSIO 40063 with cytotoxic activity. *Nat. Prod. Res.* **2022**, *36*, 2458–2464. [CrossRef]
77. Heeb, S.; Fletcher, M.P.; Chhabra, S.R.; Diggle, S.P.; Williams, P.; Camara, M. Quinolones: From antibiotics to autoinducers. *FEMS Microbiol. Rev.* **2011**, *35*, 247–274. [CrossRef]
78. Senerovic, L.; Opsenica, D.; Moric, I.; Aleksic, I.; Spasic, M.; Vasiljevic, B. Quinolines and quinolones as antibacterial, antifungal, anti-virulence, antiviral and anti-parasitic agents. *Adv. Exp. Med. Biol.* **2020**, *1282*, 37–69. [CrossRef]
79. Hassan, H.M.; Boonlarppradab, C.; Fenical, W. Actinoquinolines A and B, anti-inflammatory quinoline alkaloids from a marine-derived *Streptomyces* sp., strain CNP975. *J. Antibiot.* **2016**, *69*, 511–514. [CrossRef]
80. Ortiz-Lopez, F.J.; Alcalde, E.; Sarmiento-Vizcaino, A.; Diaz, C.; Cautain, B.; Garcia, L.A.; Blanco, G.; Reyes, F. New 3-hydroxyquinaldic acid derivatives from cultures of the marine derived actinomycete *Streptomyces cyaneofuscatus* M-157. *Mar. Drugs* **2018**, *16*, 371. [CrossRef]
81. Mullowney, M.W.; Ó hAinmhire, E.; Shaikh, A.; Wei, X.; Tanouye, U.; Santarsiero, B.D.; Burdette, J.E.; Murphy, B.T. Diaza-quinomycins E-G, novel diaza-anthracene analogs from a marine-derived *Streptomyces* sp. *Mar. Drugs* **2014**, *12*, 3574–3586. [CrossRef]
82. Cheng, C.; Othman, E.M.; Reimer, A.; Grüne, M.; Kozjak-Pavlovic, V.; Stopper, H.; Hentschel, U.; Abdelmohsen, U.R. Ageloline A, new antioxidant and antichlamydial quinolone from the marine sponge-derived bacterium *Streptomyces* sp. SBT345. *Tetrahedron Lett.* **2016**, *57*, 2786–2789. [CrossRef]
83. Shaaban, M.; Shaaban, K.A.; Kelter, G.; Fiebig, H.H.; Laatsch, H. Mansouramycins E–G, cytotoxic isoquinolinequinones from marine *Streptomycetes*. *Mar. Drugs* **2021**, *19*, 715. [CrossRef] [PubMed]
84. Yang, C.L.; Wang, Y.S.; Liu, C.L.; Zeng, Y.J.; Cheng, P.; Jiao, R.H.; Bao, S.X.; Huang, H.Q.; Tan, R.X.; Ge, H.M. Strepchazolins A and B: Two new alkaloids from a marine *Streptomyces chartreusis* NA02069. *Mar. Drugs* **2017**, *15*, 244. [CrossRef] [PubMed]
85. Zhang, D.; Yi, W.; Ge, H.; Zhang, Z.; Wu, B. Bioactive streptoglutarimides A-J from the marine-derived *Streptomyces* sp. ZZ741. *J. Nat. Prod.* **2019**, *82*, 2800–2808. [CrossRef]
86. Hou, W.; Dai, W.; Huang, H.; Liu, S.-L.; Liu, J.; Huang, L.-J.; Huang, X.-H.; Zeng, J.-L.; Gan, Z.-W.; Zhang, Z.-Y.; et al. Pharmacological activity and mechanism of pyrazines. *Eur. J. Med. Chem.* **2023**, *258*, 115544. [CrossRef]
87. Dolezal, M.; Zitko, J. Pyrazine derivatives: A patent review (June 2012-present). *Expert Opin. Ther. Pat.* **2015**, *25*, 33–47. [CrossRef]
88. Lee, D.S.; Yoon, C.S.; Jung, Y.T.; Yoon, J.H.; Kim, Y.C.; Oh, H. Marine-derived secondary metabolite, griseusrazin A, suppresses inflammation through heme oxygenase-1 induction in activated RAW264.7 macrophages. *J. Nat. Prod.* **2016**, *79*, 1105–1111. [CrossRef]
89. Shaala, L.A.; Youssef, D.T.; Badr, J.M.; Harakeh, S.M. Bioactive 2(1*H*)-pyrazinones and diketopiperazine alkaloids from a tunicate-derived actinomycete *Streptomyces* sp. *Molecules* **2016**, *21*, 1116. [CrossRef]
90. Chen, M.; Chai, W.; Zhu, R.; Song, T.; Zhang, Z.; Lian, X. Streptopyrazinones A-D, rare metabolites from marine-derived *Streptomyces* sp. ZZ446. *Tetrahedron* **2018**, *74*, 2100–2106. [CrossRef]
91. Kim, S.; Hillman, P.F.; Lee, J.Y.; Lee, J.; Lee, J.; Cha, S.-S.; Oh, D.-C.; Nam, S.-J.; Fenical, W. Actinopolymorphols E and F, pyrazine alkaloids from a marine sediment-derived bacterium *Streptomyces* sp. *J. Antibiot.* **2022**, *75*, 619–625. [CrossRef] [PubMed]
92. Sano, S.; Nakao, M. Chemistry of 2,5-diketopiperazine and its bis-lactim ether: A brief review. *Heterocycles* **2015**, *91*, 1349. [CrossRef]
93. Borthwick, A.D. 2,5-Diketopiperazines: Synthesis, reactions, medicinal chemistry, and bioactive natural products. *Chem. Rev.* **2012**, *112*, 3641–3716. [CrossRef] [PubMed]
94. Ou, Y.X.; Huang, J.F.; Li, X.M.; Kang, Q.J.; Pan, Y.T. Three new 2,5-diketopiperazines from the fish intestinal *Streptomyces* sp. MNU FJ-36. *Nat. Prod. Res.* **2016**, *30*, 1771–1775. [CrossRef] [PubMed]
95. Yi, W.; Qin, L.; Lian, X.Y.; Zhang, Z. New antifungal metabolites from the Mariana Trench sediment-associated actinomycete *Streptomyces* sp. SY1965. *Mar. Drugs* **2020**, *18*, 385. [CrossRef]
96. Buedenbender, L.; Grkovic, T.; Duffy, S.; Kurtböke, D.I.; Avery, V.M.; Carroll, A.R. Naseseazine C, a new anti-plasmodial dimeric diketopiperazine from a marine sediment derived *Streptomyces* sp. *Tetrahedron Lett.* **2016**, *57*, 5893–5895. [CrossRef]
97. Shaala, L.A.; Youssef, D.T.A.; Badr, J.M.; Harakeh, S.M.; Genta-Jouve, G. Bioactive diketopiperazines and nucleoside derivatives from a sponge-derived *Streptomyces* species. *Mar. Drugs* **2019**, *17*, 584. [CrossRef]
98. Chen, S.; Zhang, D.; Chen, M.; Zhang, Z.; Lian, X.Y. A rare diketopiperazine glycoside from marine-sourced *Streptomyces* sp. ZZ446. *Nat. Prod. Res.* **2020**, *34*, 1046–1050. [CrossRef]
99. Olyaei, A.; Sadeghpour, M. A review on lawsone-based benzo[a]phenazin-5-ol: Synthetic approaches and reactions. *RSC Adv.* **2022**, *12*, 13837–13895. [CrossRef]

100. Remali, J.; Mohamad Zin, N.; Ng, C.L.; Wan, M.; Aizat, W.M.A.; Tiong, J.J.L. Fenazin sebagai potensi antibiotik baru daripada *Streptomyces kebangsaanensis*. *Sains Malays.* **2019**, *48*, 543–553. [CrossRef]
101. Ren, J.; Liu, D.; Tian, L.; Wei, Y.; Proksch, P.; Zeng, J.; Lin, W. Venezuelines A-G, new phenoxazine-based alkaloids and aminophenols from *Streptomyces venezuelae* and the regulation of gene target Nur77. *Bioorg. Med. Chem. Lett.* **2013**, *23*, 301–304. [CrossRef] [PubMed]
102. Abdelfattah, M.S. A new bioactive aminophenoxazinone alkaloid from a marine-derived actinomycete. *Nat. Prod. Res.* **2013**, *27*, 2126–2131. [CrossRef] [PubMed]
103. Dharmaraj, S.; Sumantha, A. Bioactive potential of *Streptomyces* associated with marine sponges. *World J. Microbiol. Biotechnol.* **2009**, *25*, 1971–1979. [CrossRef]
104. Kunz, A.L.; Labes, A.; Wiese, J.; Bruhn, T.; Bringmann, G.; Imhoff, J.F. Nature's lab for derivatization: New and revised structures of a variety of streptophenazines produced by a sponge-derived *Streptomyces* strain. *Mar. Drugs* **2014**, *12*, 1699–1714. [CrossRef]
105. Cheng, C.; Othman, E.M.; Fekete, A.; Krischke, M. Strepoxazine A, a new cytotoxic phenoxazin from the marine sponge-derived bacterium *Streptomyces* sp. SBT345. *Tetrahedron Lett.* **2016**, *57*, 4196–4199. [CrossRef]
106. Wang, Q.; Zhang, Y.; Wang, M.; Tan, Y.; Hu, X.; He, H.; Xiao, C.; You, X.; Wang, Y.; Gan, M. Neo-actinomycins A and B, natural actinomycins bearing the 5H-oxazolo[4,5-b]phenoxazine chromophore, from the marine-derived *Streptomyces* sp. IMB094. *Sci. Rep.* **2017**, *7*, 3591. [CrossRef] [PubMed]
107. Zhao, W.; Wang, G.; Guo, L.; Wang, J.; Jing, C.; Liu, B.; Zhao, F.; Zhang, S.; Xie, Z. Asp-containing actinomycin and tetracyclic chromophoric analogues from the *Streptomyces* sp. strain S22. *Org. Biomol. Chem.* **2023**, *21*, 1737–1743. [CrossRef]
108. Zhang, J.; Morris-Natschke, S.L.; Ma, D.; Shang, X.F.; Yang, C.J.; Liu, Y.-Q.; Lee, K.-H. Biologically active indolizidine alkaloids. *Med. Res. Rev.* **2020**, *41*, 928–960. [CrossRef]
109. Michael, J.P. Indolizidine and quinolizidine alkaloids. *Nat. Prod. Rep.* **2002**, *19*, 719–741. [CrossRef]
110. Jiang, Y.-J.; Li, J.-Q.; Zhang, H.-J.; Ding, W.-J.; Ma, Z.-J. Cyclizidine-type alkaloids from *Streptomyces* sp. HNA39. *J. Nat. Prod.* **2018**, *81*, 394–399. [CrossRef]
111. Cheng, X.W.; Li, J.Q.; Jiang, Y.J.; Liu, H.Z.; Huo, C. A new indolizinium alkaloid from marine-derived *Streptomyces* sp. HNA39. *J. Asian Nat. Prod. Res.* **2021**, *23*, 913–918. [CrossRef] [PubMed]
112. Jiang, W.; Zhong, Y.; Shen, L.; Wu, X.; Ye, Y.; Chen, C.-T.A.; Wu, B. Stress-driven discovery of natural products from extreme marine environment- Kueishantao hydrothermal vent, a case study of Metal Switch Valve. *Curr. Org. Chem.* **2014**, *18*, 925–934. [CrossRef]
113. Shi, Y.; Pan, C.; Auckloo, B.N.; Chen, X.; Chen, C.A.; Wang, K.; Wu, X.; Ye, Y.; Wu, B. Stress-driven discovery of a cryptic antibiotic produced by Streptomyces sp. WU20 from Kueishantao hydrothermal vent with an integrated metabolomics strategy. *Appl. Microbiol. Biotechnol.* **2017**, *101*, 1395–1408. [CrossRef] [PubMed]
114. Zhang, X.; Chen, L.; Chai, W.; Lian, X.-Y.; Zhang, Z. A unique indolizinium alkaloid streptopertusacin A and bioactive bafilomycins from marine-derived *Streptomyces* sp. HZP-2216E. *Phytochemistry* **2017**, *144*, 119–126. [CrossRef] [PubMed]
115. Fang, Q.; Wu, L.; Urwald, C.; Mugat, M.; Wang, S.; Kyeremeh, K.; Philips, C.; Law, S.; Zhou, Y.; Deng, H. Genomic scanning enabling discovery of a new antibacterial bicyclic carbamate-containing alkaloid. *Synth. Syst. Biotechnol.* **2021**, *6*, 12–19. [CrossRef]
116. Li, S.; Duan, Y.; Huang, Y. Discovery and biosynthesis of bacterial pyrrolizidine alkaloids. *Microbiol. China* **2021**, *48*, 2437–2453.
117. Huang, S.; Tabudravu, J.; Elsayed, S.S.; Travert, J.; Peace, D.; Tong, M.H.; Kyeremeh, K.; Kelly, S.M.; Trembleau, L.; Ebel, R.; et al. Discovery of a single monooxygenase that catalyzes carbamate formation and ring contraction in the biosynthesis of the legonmycins. *Angew. Chem. Int. Ed. Engl.* **2015**, *54*, 12697–12701. [CrossRef] [PubMed]
118. Bugni, T.S.; Woolery, M.; Kauffman, C.A.; Jensen, P.R.; Fenical, W. Bohemamines from a marine-derived *Streptomyces* sp. *J. Nat. Prod.* **2006**, *69*, 1626–1628. [CrossRef]
119. Fu, P.; MacMillan, J.B. Spithioneines A and B, two new bohemamine derivatives possessing ergothioneine moiety from a marine-derived *Streptomyces spinoverrucosus*. *Org. Lett.* **2015**, *17*, 3046–3049. [CrossRef]
120. Fu, P.; La, S.; MacMillan, J.B. 1,3-oxazin-6-one derivatives and bohemamine-type pyrrolizidine alkaloids from a marine-derived *Streptomyces spinoverrucosus*. *J. Nat. Prod.* **2016**, *79*, 455–462. [CrossRef]
121. Fu, P.; Legako, A.; La, S.; MacMillan, J.B. Discovery, Characterization, and Analogue Synthesis of Bohemamine Dimers Generated by Non-enzymatic Biosynthesis. *Chemistry* **2016**, *22*, 3491–3495. [CrossRef] [PubMed]
122. Fu, P.; Johnson, M.; Chen, H.; Posner, B.A.; MacMillan, J.B. Carpatamides A-C, cytotoxic arylamine derivatives from a marine-derived *Streptomyces* sp. *J. Nat. Prod.* **2014**, *77*, 1245–1248. [CrossRef]
123. Yan, Y.; Zhang, L.; Ito, T.; Qu, X.; Asakawa, Y.; Awakawa, T.; Abe, I.; Liu, W. Biosynthetic pathway for high structural diversity of a common dilactone core in antimycin production. *Org. Lett.* **2012**, *14*, 4142–4145. [CrossRef]
124. Zhang, W.; Che, Q.; Tan, H.; Qi, X.; Li, J.; Li, D.; Gu, Q.; Zhu, T.; Liu, M. Marine *Streptomyces* sp. derived antimycin analogues suppress HeLa cells via depletion HPV E6/E7 mediated by ROS-dependent ubiquitin-proteasome system. *Sci. Rep.* **2017**, *7*, 42180. [CrossRef]
125. Hu, C.; Zhou, S.W.; Chen, F.; Zheng, X.H.; Shen, H.F.; Lin, B.R.; Zhou, G.X. Neoantimycins A and B, two unusual benzamido nine-membered dilactones from marine-derived *Streptomyces antibioticus* H12-15. *Molecules* **2017**, *22*, 557. [CrossRef]
126. Bertasso, M.; Holzenkämpfer, M.; Zeeck, A.; Dall'Antonia, F. Bagremycin A and B, novel antibiotics from *Streptomyces* sp. Tü 4128. *J. Antibiot.* **2001**, *54*, 730–736. [CrossRef]

127. Chen, L.; Chai, W.; Wang, W.; Song, T.; Lian, X.Y.; Zhang, Z. Cytotoxic bagremycins from mangrove-derived *Streptomyces* sp. Q22. *J. Nat. Prod.* **2017**, *80*, 1450–1456. [CrossRef]
128. Zhang, D.; Shu, C.; Lian, X.; Zhang, Z. New antibacterial bagremycins F and G from the marine-derived *Streptomyces* sp. ZZ745. *Mar. Drugs* **2018**, *16*, 330. [CrossRef] [PubMed]
129. Hamed, A.; Abdel-Razek, A.S.; Frese, M.; Wibberg, D.; El-Haddad, A.F.; Ibrahim, T.M.A.; Kalinowski, J.; Sewald, N.; Shaaban, M. N-Acetylborrelidin B: A new bioactive metabolite from *Streptomyces mutabilis* sp. MII. *Z. Naturforsch. C* **2018**, *73*, 49–57. [CrossRef] [PubMed]
130. Miyanaga, A.; Kudo, F.; Eguchi, T. Mechanisms of beta-amino acid incorporation in polyketide macrolactam biosynthesis. *Curr. Opin. Chem. Biol.* **2016**, *35*, 58–64. [CrossRef]
131. Hugel, H.M.; Smith, A.T.; Rizzacasa, M.A. Macrolactam analogues of macrolide natural products. *Org. Biomol. Chem.* **2016**, *14*, 11301–11316. [CrossRef]
132. Antosch, J.; Schaefers, F.; Gulder, T.A. Heterologous reconstitution of ikarugamycin biosynthesis in *E. coli*. *Angew. Chem. Int. Ed. Engl.* **2014**, *53*, 3011–3014. [CrossRef]
133. Lacret, R.; Oves-Costales, D.; Gómez, C.; Díaz, C.; de la Cruz, M.; Pérez-Victoria, I.; Vicente, F.; Genilloud, O.; Reyes, F. New ikarugamycin derivatives with antifungal and antibacterial properties from *Streptomyces zhaozhouensis*. *Mar. Drugs* **2014**, *13*, 128–140. [CrossRef]
134. Saha, S.; Zhang, W.; Zhang, G.; Zhu, Y.; Chen, Y.; Liu, W.; Yuan, C.; Zhang, Q.; Zhang, H.; Zhang, L.; et al. Activation and characterization of a cryptic gene cluster reveals a cyclization cascade for polycyclic tetramate macrolactams. *Chem. Sci.* **2017**, *8*, 1607–1612. [CrossRef]
135. Fukudaa, T.; Takahashia, M.; Kasaib, H.; Nagaia, K.; Tomodaa, H. Chlokamycin, a new chloride from the marine-derived *Streptomyces* sp. MA2-12. *Nat. Prod. Commun.* **2017**, *12*, 1223–1226. [CrossRef]
136. Liu, W.; Zhang, W.; Jin, H.; Zhang, Q.; Chen, Y.; Jiang, X.; Zhang, G.; Zhang, L.; Zhang, W.; She, Z.; et al. Genome mining of marine-derived *Streptomyces* sp. SCSIO 40010 leads to cytotoxic new polycyclic tetramate macrolactams. *Mar. Drugs* **2019**, *17*, 663. [CrossRef]
137. Kawahara, T.; Fujiwara, T.; Kagaya, N.; Shin-Ya, K. JBIR-150, a novel 20-membered polyene macrolactam from marine-derived *Streptomyces* sp. OPMA00071. *J. Antibiot.* **2018**, *71*, 390–392. [CrossRef]
138. Shin, Y.H.; Im, J.H.; Kang, I.; Kim, E.; Jang, S.C.; Cho, E.; Shin, D.; Hwang, S.; Du, Y.E.; Huynh, T.H.; et al. Genomic and spectroscopic signature-based discovery of natural macrolactams. *J. Am. Chem. Soc.* **2023**, *145*, 1886–1896. [CrossRef] [PubMed]
139. Shen, J.; Wang, J.; Chen, H.; Wang, Y.; Zhu, W.; Fu, P. Cyclamenols E and F, two diastereoisomeric bicyclic macrolactams with a cyclopentane moiety from an Antarctic *Streptomyces* species. *Org. Chem. Front.* **2020**, *7*, 310–317. [CrossRef]
140. Yang, F.; Sang, M.; Lu, J.R.; Zhao, H.M.; Zou, Y.; Wu, W.; Yu, Y.; Liu, Y.W.; Ma, W.; Zhang, Y.; et al. Somalactams A-D: Anti-inflammatory macrolide lactams with unique ring systems from an Arctic actinomycete strain. *Angew. Chem. Int. Ed. Engl.* **2023**, *62*, e202218085. [CrossRef] [PubMed]
141. Nakayama, K.; Yamaguchi, T.; Doi, T.; Usuki, Y. Synergistic combination of direct plasma membrane damage and oxidative stress as a cause of antifungal activity of polyol macrolide niphimycin. *J. Biosci. Bioeng.* **2002**, *94*, 207–211. [CrossRef]
142. Hu, Y.; Wang, M.; Wu, C.; Tan, Y.; Li, J.; Hao, X.; Duan, Y.; Guan, Y.; Shang, X.; Wang, Y.; et al. Identification and proposed relative and absolute configurations of niphimycins C-E from the marine-derived *Streptomyces* sp. IMB7-145 by genomic analysis. *J. Nat. Prod.* **2018**, *81*, 178–187. [CrossRef]
143. Chen, Y.; Wei, Y.; Cai, B.; Zhou, D.; Qi, D.; Zhang, M.; Zhao, Y.; Li, K.; Wedge, D.E.; Pan, Z.; et al. Discovery of niphimycin C from *Streptomyces yongxingensis* sp. nov. as a promising agrochemical fungicide for controlling banana fusarium wilt by destroying the mitochondrial structure and function. *J. Agric. Food Chem.* **2022**, *70*, 12784–12795. [CrossRef]
144. Huang, Y.; Hu, W.; Huang, S.; Chu, J.; Liang, Y.; Tao, Z.; Wang, G.; Zhuang, J.; Zhang, Z.; Zhou, X.; et al. Taxonomy and anticancer potential of *Streptomyces niphimycinicus* sp. nov. against nasopharyngeal carcinoma cells. *Appl. Microbiol. Biotechnol.* **2023**, *107*, 6325–6338. [CrossRef]
145. Kim, D.; Lee, E.J.; Lee, J.; Leutou, A.S.; Shin, Y.H.; Choi, B.; Hwang, J.S.; Hahn, D.; Choi, H.; Chin, J.; et al. Antartin, a cytotoxic zizaane-type sesquiterpenoid from a *Streptomyces* sp. isolated from an Antarctic marine sediment. *Mar. Drugs* **2018**, *16*, 130. [CrossRef]
146. Liu, W.; Ma, L.; Zhang, L.; Chen, Y.; Zhang, Q.; Zhang, H.; Zhang, W.; Zhang, C.; Zhang, W. Two new phenylhydrazone derivatives from the Pearl River Estuary sediment-derived *Streptomyces* sp. SCSIO 40020. *Mar. Drugs* **2022**, *20*, 449. [CrossRef]

Disclaimer/Publisher's Note: The statements, opinions and data contained in all publications are solely those of the individual author(s) and contributor(s) and not of MDPI and/or the editor(s). MDPI and/or the editor(s) disclaim responsibility for any injury to people or property resulting from any ideas, methods, instructions or products referred to in the content.

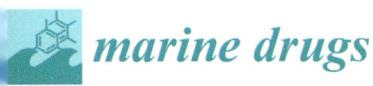

Article

Exploring the Diversity and Specificity of Secondary Biosynthetic Potential in *Rhodococcus*

Gang-Ao Hu [1,†], Yue Song [1,†], Shi-Yi Liu [1], Wen-Chao Yu [1], Yan-Lei Yu [1], Jian-Wei Chen [1], Hong Wang [1,2,*] and Bin Wei [1,2,*]

1. College of Pharmaceutical Science & Collaborative Innovation Center of Yangtze River Delta Region Green Pharmaceuticals, Zhejiang Key Laboratory of Green, Low-Carbon, and Efficient Development of Marine Fishery Resources, Zhejiang University of Technology (ZJUT), Hangzhou 310014, China; 201706030718@zjut.edu.cn (G.-A.H.); 2112107104@zjut.edu.cn (Y.S.); 201906030311@zjut.edu.cn (S.-Y.L.); 2112007282@zjut.edu.cn (W.-C.Y.); yanleiyu@zjut.edu.cn (Y.-L.Y.); cjw983617@zjut.edu.cn (J.-W.C.)
2. Binjiang Institute of Artificial Intelligence, Zhejiang University of Technology (ZJUT), Hangzhou 310051, China
* Correspondence: hongw@zjut.edu.cn (H.W.); binwei@zjut.edu.cn (B.W.)
† These authors contributed equally to this work.

Abstract: The actinomycete genus *Rhodococcus* is known for its diverse biosynthetic enzymes, with potential in pollutant degradation, chemical biocatalysis, and natural product exploration. Comparative genomics have analyzed the distribution patterns of non-ribosomal peptide synthetases (NRPSs) in *Rhodococcus*. The diversity and specificity of its secondary metabolism offer valuable insights for exploring natural products, yet remain understudied. In the present study, we analyzed the distribution patterns of biosynthetic gene clusters (BGCs) in the most comprehensive *Rhodococcus* genome data to date. The results show that 86.5% of the gene cluster families (GCFs) are only distributed in a specific phylogenomic-clade of *Rhodococcus*, with the most predominant types of gene clusters being NRPS and ribosomally synthesized and post-translationally modified peptides (RiPPs). In-depth mining of RiPP gene clusters revealed that *Rhodococcus* encodes many clade-specific novel RiPPs, with thirteen core peptides showing antibacterial potential. High-throughput elicitor screening (HiTES) and non-targeted metabolomics revealed that a marine-derived *Rhodococcus* strain produces a large number of new aurachin-like compounds when exposed to specific elicitors. The present study highlights the diversity and specificity of secondary biosynthetic potential in *Rhodococcus*, and provides valuable information for the targeted exploration of novel natural products from *Rhodococcus*, especially for phylogenomic-clade-specific metabolites.

Keywords: *Rhodococcus*; biosynthetic gene clusters; comparative genomics; high-throughput elicitor screening; non-targeted metabolomics

1. Introduction

Actinobacteria is the major source of natural products in bacteria, with well-known genera such as *Streptomyces*, *Micromonospora*, *Nocardia*, and *Saccharothrix* [1,2]. The genus *Rhodococcus* was first proposed by Zopf in 1891 and contains 55 species with validly published and correct names nowadays [3]. *Rhodococcus* has received widespread attention for its pivotal role in degrading a wide range of natural and xenobiotic compounds, but has received less attention in the discovery of natural products [4]. Currently, only 24 secondary metabolites have been reported to be derived from *Rhodococcus*, including rhodopeptins [5], lariatins [6], aurachins [7], rhodostreptomycin [8], rhodochelin [9], and saframycin [10]; however, these compounds showed excellent and diverse biological activities, such as antibacterial, antifungal, antitrypanosomal, anticancer, and siderophores [4].

McLeod et al. sequenced the complete genome of the first *Rhodococcus* strain (*Rhodococcus jostii* RHA1), and found that the strain encodes up to 24 nonribosomal peptide synthetases (NRPSs) and 7 polyketide synthases (PKSs) [11]. In addition, two recent large-scale genome mining studies have revealed that *Rhodococcus* encodes numerous novel biosynthetic gene clusters (BGCs) for secondary metabolites, highlighting its significant potential in producing novel natural products [12,13]. However, more than 1000 genomes of *Rhodococcus* have been publicly released, and it is crucial to choose the appropriate *Rhodococcus* strain for the exploration of novel secondary metabolites. Our previous research has shown that the distribution patterns of BGCs encoded by multiple genera, such as *Bacillus*, *Allokutzneria*, and *Kibdelosporangium*, exhibit species or genus specificity [14,15]. Furthermore, in-depth exploration of these genomes can help in the targeted discovery of specific types of natural products.

Rhodococcus has been isolated from a wide range of environments, including marine, aquatic, soil, animals, plants, and insects [16]. Based on the study by Agustina Undabarrena et al., phylogenomic analysis of 110 *Rhodococcus* strains indicates that the distribution of *Rhodococcus* species in the evolutionary tree correlates to some extent with their isolation sources. However, eight *Rhodococcus* strains from marine sources are randomly distributed across all four clades of the evolutionary tree [13]. A marine-derived strain, *Rhodococcus* sp. H-CA8f was found to possess a unique BGC distribution within its phylogenomic clade [13]. These findings highlight that *Rhodococcus* strains from marine sources possess greater genetic diversity and more unique secondary metabolite potential.

Therefore, in the present study, we conducted a systematic analysis of the distribution patterns of BGCs and gene cluster families (GCFs) within the most comprehensive *Rhodococcus* genome dataset to date, which were classified into distinct phylogenomic clades. While Undabarrena et al. [13] primarily focused on an in-depth analysis of nonribosomal peptide synthetase (NRPS) GCFs and highlighted the phylogenomic-dependent patterns of NRPS GCFs in *Rhodococcus*, our research expands on this by analyzing the clade-specific distribution of all major BGC types—eight in total. This comprehensive approach provides a broader understanding of the biosynthetic potential within the *Rhodococcus* genus, extending beyond just NRPS clusters. Additionally, we conducted a detailed analysis of the composition of ribosomally synthesized and post-translationally modified peptide (RiPP) GCFs and the metabolite scaffolds they encode. By utilizing deep-learning algorithms, we rapidly identified dozens of novel antimicrobial peptides from the core peptides encoded by RiPP gene clusters. Furthermore, we explored the secondary metabolites of a marine-derived *Rhodococcus* strain through a combined strategy of high-throughput elicitor screening (HiTES) [17] and non-targeted metabolomics. This approach led to intriguing discoveries, including the production of a series of aurachin-like compounds, which have not been previously reported.

2. Results

2.1. The Overall Distribution of BGCs in Rhodococcus

To investigate the diversity and distribution patterns of BGCs in *Rhodococcus*, we retrieved and submitted for bioinformatics analysis all 616 *Rhodococcus* genomes from the NCBI genome database that passed quality filtering. In total, 48% of these genomes have been classified into 37 *Rhodococcus* species levels, while the species information of the other genomes has not been accurately identified. Therefore, the average nucleotide identity (ANI) of pairwise genomes was calculated and used to classify them into different phylogenomic-clades. By optimizing the ANI threshold, we found that at a value of 90, most different *Rhodococcus* species could be classified into distinct phylogenomic clades. At this threshold, the majority of genomes (597 out of 616) were grouped into 29 clades, while the remaining 19 genomes existed as singletons. Subsequently, the hierarchical dendrogram of these genomes was constructed based on the pairwise ANI values, and the genomic features and the number of different classes of BGCs in these genomes were also displayed on the outer ring of the dendrogram. As shown in Figure 1 and Table S1, genomes from different phylogenomic clades are mostly clustered together, and the top ten largest clades contain 494 genomes, accounting for 80.2% of all genomes. Among them, 131 genomes are completely assembled, 257 genomes are assembled at the scaffold level, and 228 genomes are assembled at the contig level. Despite originating from the same genus, these *Rhodococcus* genomes exhibit significant size variation, ranging from approximately 3.7 Mb to 11.7 Mb. For instance, genomes within clade 6 exhibit larger genome sizes, with nearly all surpassing 8 Mb in clade 6, while genomes within clade 4 have smaller genome sizes, generally less than 5 Mb. Additionally, the completeness of the *Rhodococcus* genomes is relatively high, with 85% containing fewer than 100 contigs, indicating a substantial degree of assembly quality.

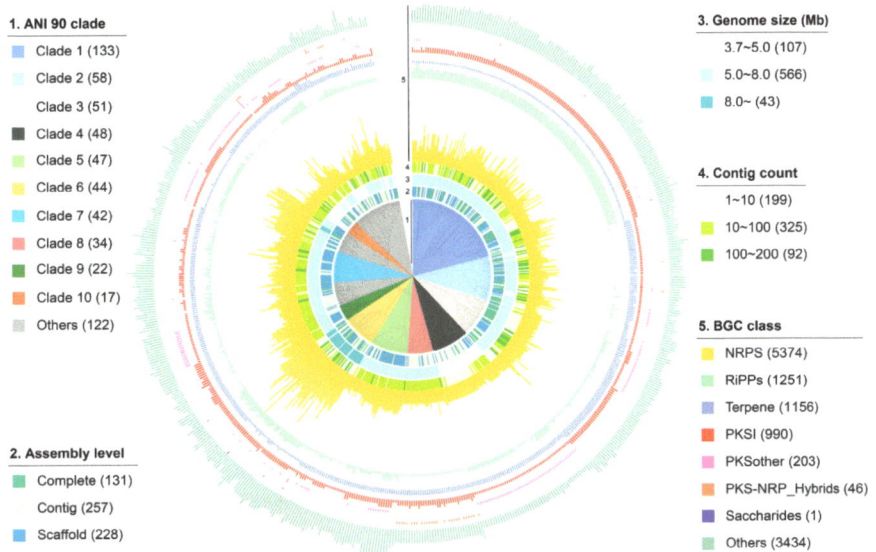

Figure 1. Heatmap and hierarchical clustering based on pairwise ANI values of 616 *Rhodococcus* genomes. Representation of the data (inner to outer layers): phylogenomic clade, assembly level, genome size, contig count, and the numbers of each class of BGCs. The proportions of each subcategory are presented in the figure legends.

All the 616 genomes yield a total of 12,455 BGCs, with lengths ranging from 1.0 to 183.6 kb, resulting in an average of 20 BGCs per *Rhodococcus* genome. The top three dominant classes of BGCs in *Rhodococcus* are NRPS (5374, 43.1%), RiPPs (1251, 10.0%), and Terpene (1156, 9.3%). It is worth noting that the average genome size of clade 6 is significantly larger than that of other clades (9.0 vs. 6.0 Mb), resulting in a notably higher number of BGCs encoded compared to other clades (31.6 vs. 20.2). Interestingly, *Rhodococcus* exhibits significant clade-specificity in gene cluster composition. For instance, the number of terpene gene clusters encoded by strains in clade 1 is significantly lower than those in clade 2 and 3, while the number of RiPP gene clusters is notably higher. Furthermore, genomes in clades 4 contain a higher abundance of PKSother BGCs compared to other clades, whereas genomes in clade 8 stand out for their possession of PKS-NRP_hybrid BGCs.

2.2. The Distribution Pattern of GCFs in Rhodococcus

To accurately assess the specificity of secondary biosynthetic potential in *Rhodococcus*, all the predicted 12,455 BGCs were organized into a gene cluster network comprising 1677 GCFs at the established threshold of 0.3 using BIG-SCAPE. The hierarchical dendrogram of the resulting 1677 GCFs is presented in Figure 2 and Table S2, revealing that 86.5% of GCFs are only distributed in a specific phylogenomic clade of *Rhodococcus*, with the most predominant types of GCFs being NRPS and RiPPs. In total, 762 of these GCFs (45.4%) showed an average cumulative BLAST score of 0 to characterized BGCs from MiBIG and only 491 of GCFs (29.3%) showed an average cumulative BLAST score larger than 1000. In addition, only five GCFs contain BGCs from MiBIG, further implying the novelty of the GCFs encoded by *Rhodococcus*. The network analysis reveals that the GCFs containing BGCs responsible for synthesizing heterobactins, corynecins, rhodochelins, and aurachins include 9, 19, 32, and 4 gene clusters, respectively [13,18–20]. In addition to these, several GCFs exhibit a high degree of similarity to BGCs known to encode compounds such as ectoine and erythrochelin, indicating the potential for the production of similar compounds. Despite including all 616 genomes data from the same genus in this study, only 30 GCFs contained more than 50 BGCs, while 320 GCFs contained between 10 and 50 BGCs. These findings indicate significant diversity and variation in BGCs encoded by *Rhodococcus* species across different strains. The average length of BGCs in about 88% of GCFs was greater than 10 kb, with 25.9% being longer than 50 kb. Additionally, the shorter gene clusters were primarily found in singleton GCFs, indicating that GCFs containing two or more gene clusters had relatively higher completeness and quality. Notably, 40.1% (673 out of 1677) of the representative BGCs were located at the edge of the corresponding contigs and were mainly observed in NRPS GCFs, demonstrating that the fragmentation of genome sequences has significant implications for the mining of NRPS GCFs. Further analysis revealed that the proportion of clade-specific GCFs among the seven categories ranged from 38% to 89%. Specifically, the PKSother category had a higher proportion of clade-specific GCFs at 89%. These findings provide an important reference value for studying the evolutionary patterns of *Rhodococcus* and its secondary metabolic functions.

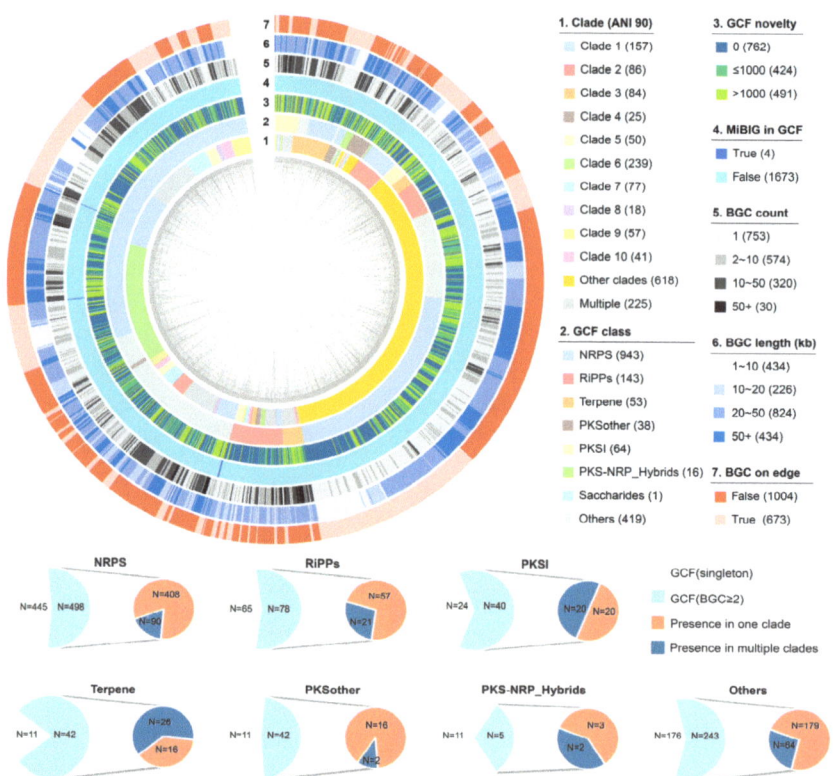

Figure 2. Hierarchical clustering of the 1677 GCFs in *Rhodococcus* genomes. Representation of the data (inner to outer layers): phylogenomic clade, GCF class, the novelty of GCFs, GCF containing BGCs from MiBIG or not, and BGC counts in each GCF. The outer two layers indicate the length and completeness of the representative BGC in each GCF. The proportions of each subcategory of GCFs are presented in the figure legends.

The diversity and specificity of BGCs in *Rhodococcus* were visually demonstrated through the BIG-SCAPE sequence similarity network under mix mode (Figure 3). The NRPS category comprised 53.9% (498) of the total GCFs (≥2 BGCs) in the network, followed by 26.3% (243) others and 8.4% (78) of RiPP GCFs. The distribution of GCF in the top ten phylogenomic clades can be visually distinguished from the network, and the numbers of clade-specific GCFs of different types are also summarized. The results indicate that there is a significant difference in the number of clade-specific GCF encoded by the genomes in these seven categories of GCF. Among them, clades 6 and 1 have the highest number of clade-specific GCFs, mainly distributed in NRPS, others, and RiPP classes of GCFs. In the top ten clades, three lack clade-specific PKSI class GCFs, while six do not encode clade-specific terpene class GCFs, highlighting substantial evolutionary rate disparities among these GCFs.

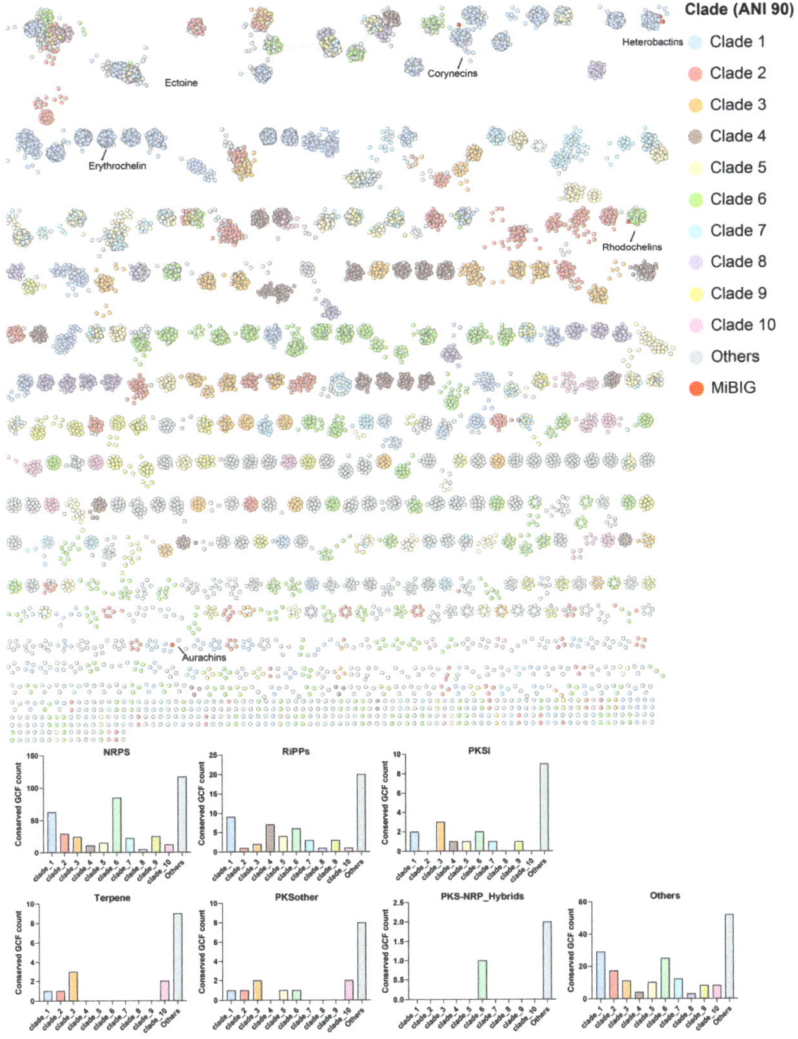

Figure 3. Sequence similarity network of 12,455 BGCs (743 singletons not shown) predicted from 616 *Rhodococcus* genomes. Each node represents one BGC, connected by edges when sharing a raw distance ≤0.3. The network is organized by different categories and the BGCs are colored according to the phylogenomic clade of its source genome.

2.3. Clade Specificity of Rhodococcus in RiPP Biosynthesis

Given that *Rhodococcus* encodes a large number of RiPP gene clusters, which are important sources of antimicrobial peptides, this study further analyzed the diversity and clade-specificity of *Rhodococcus* in RiPP biosynthesis. As shown in Figure 4A, the RiPP category gene clusters defined by BiG-SCAPE exhibit significant diversity and can be classified into subcategories such as RiPP-like (420), Redox cofactor (396), LAP (179), lanthipeptide-class-III (136), lassopeptide (31), and RRE containing (14), with the dominant subcategory being RiPP-like (24.8%). The core peptides of all the 1251 RiPP category gene clusters were predicted by antiSMASH or DeepRiPP, leading to the discovery of 891 core peptides from 459 BGCs, which mainly come from categories such as lanthipeptide-class-III (130), Redox cofactor (117), and RiPP-like (92), lassopeptide (31), LAP (17), RRE containing (11). It is worth noting that all the 460 RiPP gene clusters with predictable core peptides are distributed among 90 GCFs, with 78 being clade-specific, such as GCF_7291 and GCF_7679, which are only observed in *Rhodococcus* genomes of clade 4 (Figure 4B). Among the 78 clade-specific GCFs, 30 of them contain more than two BGCs, with the largest GCF containing 120 lassopeptide gene clusters that are solely distributed in clade 1. All 26 gene clusters in GCF_7291 encoded a single lassopeptide, with the core peptide predicted as APGKSGGKTDGAVFNNIPLGGELTFS. This core peptide exhibited only 42.3% sequence identity to predicted lasso peptides from antiSMASH-DB 3.0, demonstrating the high potential to be a novel lasso peptide. All the 11 gene clusters in GCF_7679 encoded two lassopeptides, with the core peptide predicted as EFIGPNTEAILPFEDHSKE and YGIGGQAEGWNP, respectively. In addition, this gene cluster is probably capable of producing two macrolactams, EFIGPNTE and YGIGGQAE. Both of these two GCFs encode the ABC transporter, asparagine synthetase, and transglutaminase (PF13471), which are essential for lassopeptide biosynthesis. The specific distribution of these gene clusters suggests that *Rhodococcus* strains at similar evolutionary statuses may use different natural weapons for environmental adaptation or defense. To further investigate these core peptides, we utilized two recently reported deep-learning algorithms to predict their activity. These algorithms combine multiple natural language processing neural network models, including LSTM, attention mechanisms, BERT, and XGBoost [21,22]. Consequently, we identified thirteen potential antimicrobial peptides from these core peptides (Table S3), whose antimicrobial activity merits further research and validation.

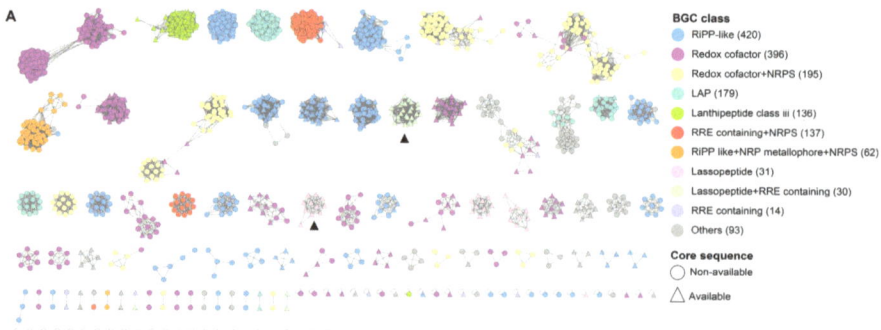

Figure 4. *Cont.*

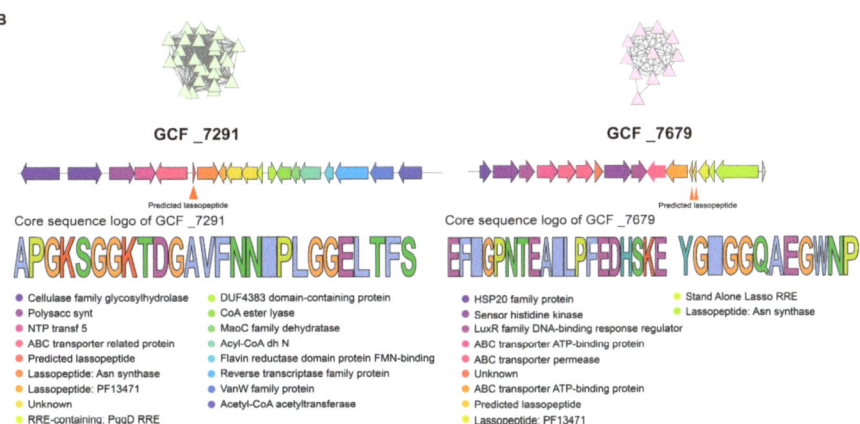

Figure 4. (**A**) A sequence similarity network was constructed for 1251 RiPP gene clusters predicted from 616 *Rhodococcus* genomes. The network also included 442 gene clusters categorized as 'Others' as they exhibit distances below the threshold to RiPP gene clusters. The subclasses of these biosynthetic gene clusters (BGCs) were annotated using the analysis results from antiSMASH, along with the annotation of BGCs predicted with core peptides using DeepRiPP. (**B**) BGC architecture and core peptide sequence logo of two clade-specific gene cluster families (GCF_7291 and GCF_7679).

2.4. Secondary Metabolites of a Marine-Derived Rhodococcus Isolate

Strain 3Y1 was isolated from seawater at a depth of 3000 m in the Massau Trench in the Pacific Ocean at coordinates 148°53.3246′ E, 00°53.8546′ N. The 16S rRNA gene sequence of strain 3Y1 was found to be identical to that of *Rhodococcus qingshengii* JCM 15477^T [23]. According to Lee and Kim [24], this species is a later heterotypic synonym of *Rhodococcus erythropolis*. Therefore, the strain was identified as *Rhodococcus* sp. 3Y1. Secondary metabolites of this strain cultivated under seven different culture media in the presence or absence of six chemical elicitors were comprehensively analyzed using high-resolution liquid chromatography-mass spectrometry. The resulting mass spectra were analyzed using the Global Natural Products Social Molecular Networking (GNPS, https://gnps.ucsd.edu/, accessed on 15 May 2024) workflow, with annotation performed through the Feature-Based Molecular Networking (FBMN) workflow and Dereplicator+. Chemical features detected in the blank samples (culture media) were excluded from the analysis. Using FBMN analysis, a molecular network comprising 1139 features and 451 molecular families was generated. As showed in Figure 5A and Table S4, Dereplicator+ identified a series of aurachin-like compounds. Due to the high structural similarity of these compounds, it was challenging to accurately identify them using solely in silico MS/MS methods. Therefore, unreliable matches were discarded, and manual comparisons were performed to preliminarily identify certain compounds. Additionally, over 90% of the features remained uncharacterized, indicating the presence of potentially novel compounds in *Rhodococcus* that warrant further investigation.

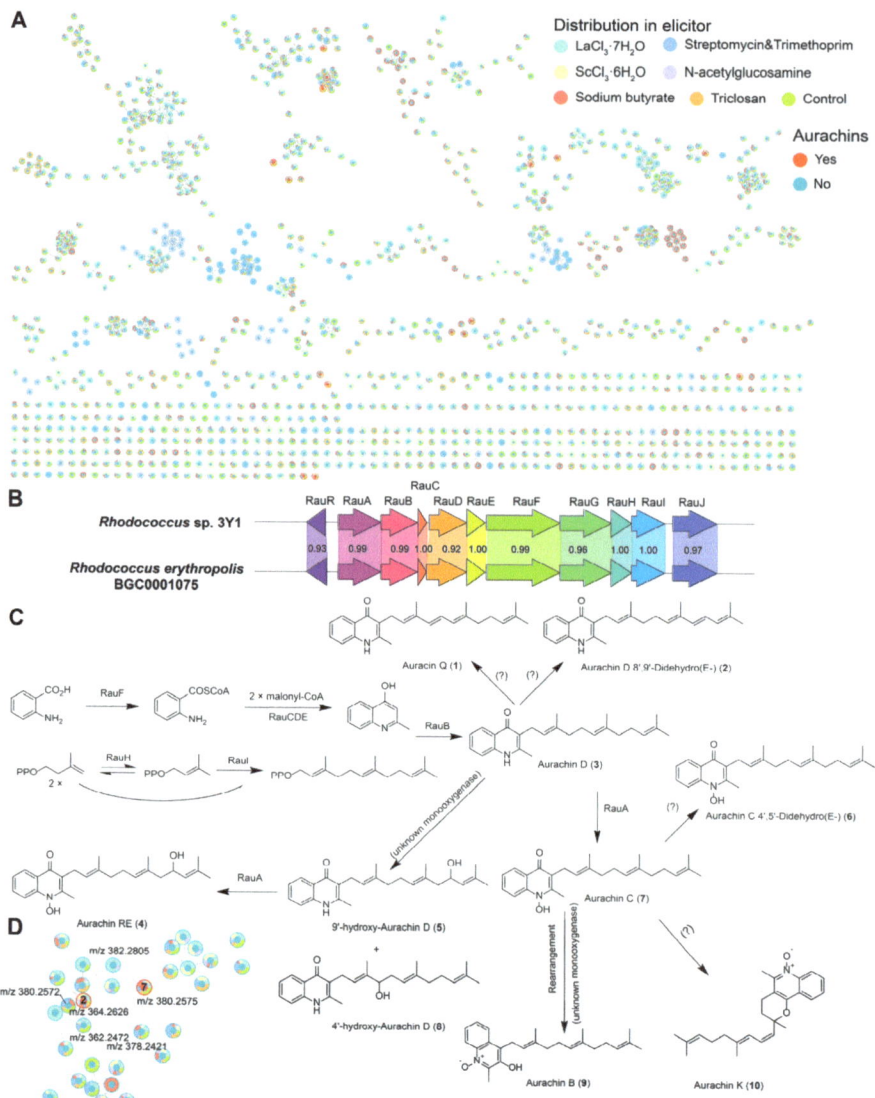

Figure 5. (**A**) Molecular network of crude extracts of *Rhodococcus* sp. 3Y1 cultured under different culture conditions. The pie chart colors on the nodes represent the distribution across different elicitor groups. Node color reflects whether the metabolites could be annotated as Aurachins. (**B**) The putative biosynthetic gene cluster responsible for the biosynthesis of aurachins. (**C**) Chemical structures and biosynthetic pathways of Aurachins, and "?" indicates unknown enzyme. (**D**) A molecular family annotated as Aurachins.

We utilized six different elicitors with various induction mechanisms [25]: lanthanum chloride and scandium chloride as rare metals, N-acetylglucosamine as a oligosaccharides source, sodium butyrate as an HDAC inhibitor, and three antibiotics as competitive agents. Interestingly, under all elicitor conditions, we discovered that the strain *Rhodococcus* sp. 3Y1 produced a series of aurachin-like compounds: Aurachin Q (**1**), Aurachin D 8′,9′-Didehydro (**2**), Aurachin D (**3**), Aurachin RE (**4**), 9′-hydroxy-Aurachin D (**5**), Aurachin C 4′,5′-Didehydro (**6**), Aurachin C (**7**), 4′-hydroxy-Aurachin D (**8**), Aurachin B (**9**) and Aurachin K (**10**). Figure 5D showed a molecular family of aurachin-like compounds, comprising a total of 32 features. Among these, two features have been identified as aurachin-like compounds. One feature was identified as Aurachin C, and another feature was identified as Aurachin D 8′,9′-Didehydro. Several features directly connected to the identified ones may be novel analogs (probably hydrogenation or dehydrogenation) of these identified aurachins. Aurachins and related compounds have been recognized as potent inhibitors of mitochondrial respiration, primarily by blocking NADH oxidation. This inhibitory action is likely attributed to their structural similarity to vitamin K [26]. Aurachin RE, a prenylated quinoline antibiotic first isolated from the genus *Rhodococcus* [27], is biosynthesized by BGC0001075 [19]. Using antiSMASH analysis, we successfully identified the biosynthetic gene cluster responsible for producing aurachins in *Rhodococcus* sp. 3Y1. This BGC shows a high degree of similarity to the previously reported BGC0001075 (Figure 5B). As depicted in Figure 5C, the biosynthetic pathways for compounds **2**, **3**, **4**, **5**, and **6** are relatively well understood and reported [19,28,29]. However, the biosynthetic pathways for compounds **1** and **7** have not yet been clearly identified. Further investigation and exploration into the biosynthetic pathways of these compounds are warranted. Furthermore, under the conditions of sodium butyrate and N-acetylglucosamine, several unique molecular families were detected (Figure 5A). These molecular families have not been annotated, suggesting they may represent novel compounds.

3. Discussion

Rhodococcus is a versatile genus of Gram-stain-positive bacteria known for its remarkable metabolic diversity and ability to thrive in various environments, including soil, water, and even extreme habitats like deep-sea sediments [13]. This genus is of significant interest in the field of natural products due to its extensive secondary metabolite production, which includes antibiotics and other bioactive compounds. With the continuous accumulation of *Rhodococcus* strain resources and microbial natural products, efficiently discovering novel and highly active natural products from *Rhodococcus* has become a significant challenge. This study aims to analyze the diversity and specificity of the secondary biosynthetic potential of *Rhodococcus* from a phylogenomic similarity perspective rather than at the species level, with a particular focus on the potential for synthesizing phylogenomic clade-specific antimicrobial peptides from RiPP gene clusters. Using a deep-sea-derived *Rhodococcus* strain as an example, this study illustrates the discovery of unique and potential novel natural products using LC-MS and HiTES strategies.

Increasing evidence suggests that closely related strains can encode significantly different biosynthetic gene clusters or exhibit substantial differences in the composition of these biosynthetic gene clusters [12–15]. Two recent studies have reported the phylogenomic-dependent patterns of NRPS gene clusters in 30 and 110 *Rhodococcus* genomes, respectively, especially for BGCs predicted to encode the biosynthesis of lipopeptides [12,13]. The present study is the first to systematically and comprehensively analyze the distribution specificity of all eight classes of BGCs in 616 *Rhodococcus* genomes of 48 different phylogenomic-clades. The *Rhodococcus* genome dataset used in this study is about six times larger than those in previous studies. It also provides a detailed revelation of the clade-specific BGCs in the top ten phylogenomic clades of *Rhodococcus*, revealing that *Rhodococcus* may possess various chemical weapons for environmental adaptation or survival maintenance. These findings provide important clues for the targeted discovery of specific types of natural products and offer significant reference value for studying the genetic evolution and metabolic adaptability of *Rhodococcus*.

The quality of genome assembly and the algorithms used for BGC detection significantly impact the accuracy of identifying BGCs. Fragmented genome assemblies can result in the dispersion of genes from the same BGC across different contigs, potentially leading to an overestimation of BGC numbers. Conversely, if a BGC is excessively fragmented, prediction tools may fail to detect it, leading to an underestimation. In recent years, advancements in sequencing and bioinformatics technologies have substantially improved the accuracy and speed of BGC prediction in microorganisms. The most commonly used algorithms for BGC detection involve BLAST and Hidden Markov Model (HMM) comparisons. For instance, the widely utilized tool, antiSMASH [30], employs these methods to efficiently identify BGCs homologous to known clusters through database searches. We reanalyzed the complete genome of the first *Rhodococcus* strain, *Rhodococcus jostii* RHA1 [11], using the latest antiSMASH 7 tool. Our analysis identified 16 NRPS and 2 PKS BGCs, which contrasts with the previously reported 24 NRPS and 7 PKS BGCs. This discrepancy highlights the improvements in tools like antiSMASH, which have greatly enhanced the efficiency and accuracy of BGC prediction, particularly in high-quality genome assemblies. The combination of genome mining techniques and deep-learning algorithms has enabled the targeted discovery of numerous novel and highly active antimicrobial peptides [21,22]. In this study, deep-learning algorithms were used to rapidly predict 13 novel potential antimicrobial peptides from core peptides encoded by RiPP gene clusters of *Rhodococcus*. The activity of these putative antimicrobial peptides awaits experimental validation in future studies. Additionally, the post-translational modification processes of these core peptides may significantly impact the structure and activity of the final metabolites. Therefore, accurate prediction of the products encoded by specific RiPP gene clusters must consider the effects of these modifications.

In this study, we utilized a deep-sea-derived *Rhodococcus* sp. 3Y1 as an example to explore clade-specific natural products through the combination of LC-MS-based untargeted metabolomics with HiTES strategies. We identified a series of aurachin-like compounds and predicted their biosynthetic pathways through genome mining. Aurachins (Aurachin A–L) were first isolated from the myxobacterium *Stigmatella aurantiaca* Sg a15 [28], but their complete biosynthetic pathways remain unclear. Aurachin RE, a prenylated quinoline antibiotic, was first isolated from the genus *Rhodococcus* and exhibits potent antibacterial activity against a variety of Gram-positive bacteria [19]. Further studies isolated two additional aurachin-like compounds (Aurachin Q and Aurachin R) from *Rhodococcus* strains [7]. Aurachin R showed moderate antibacterial activity against *Staphylococcus epidermidis* DSM 20044, *Bacillus subtilis* DSM 347, and *Propionibacterium acnes* DSM 1897, while Aurachin Q did not exhibit antibacterial activity. The present study provides evidence for the targeted discovery of novel aurachin-like compounds, and highlights the structural diversity of aurachins.

4. Materials and Methods

4.1. Genome Collection and Phylogenomic Analysis

Rhodococcus genomes were downloaded from the NCBI web servers, with data up to date as of May 2024. After filtering for genomes with completeness greater than 90%, contamination less than 5%, and fewer than 200 contigs, 616 genomes were retained for further analysis. Assembly information and other relevant details were obtained and organized via FTP from NCBI. The average nucleotide identity between genomes was calculated using the pyANI package [31] to group phylogenomic-close genomes into clades, with an ANI threshold greater than 90%. Based on the ANI similarity matrix of all genomes, a dendrogram of these genomes was constructed using hierarchical clustering in R [32] and visualized with ITOL [33].

4.2. Diversity and Specificity of Biosynthetic Gene Clusters in Rhodococcus

Similar to our previous study [34], all genomes were processed using the command-line version of antiSMASH v7.0.1 with the bacterial setting and default parameters [30]. The number of each class of BGCs and relevant information regarding their architecture were extracted from the HTML files (antiSMASH outputs) using a customized Python toolkit (https://github.com/BioGavin/wlabkit, accessed on 15 May 2024). The diversity and novelty of all eight classes of BGCs were compared with known BGCs in the MiBIG v3.1 database using BIG-SCAPE at the default cut-off of 0.3 [35]. Each node in the network represents a BGC, and BGCs with similar Pfam domain units are connected by edges. Using the parameter -mix, the final analysis produced eight separate networks for each class of BGCs, as well as a mixed network combining all classes. All network was visualized using Cytoscape 3.10.2 [36]. The novelty of GCFs was assessed by calculating the average cumulative BLAST score against known BGCs in the MiBIG database using the antiSMASH function knownclusterblast [30]. For each of the 1677 GCFs, the BGC with the highest total BLAST score and the longest length was selected as the representative BGC. The class of the representative BGC, along with relevant information about them, was used for GCF clustering.

4.3. Diversity and Specificity of Rhodococcus in RiPP Biosynthesis

The putative core peptides of RiPP gene clusters were obtained using the software tools DeepRiPP v1.0.0 [37] and antiSMASH v7.0.1, and used to evaluate the diversity and specificity of *Rhodococcus* in RiPP biosynthesis. The predicted core peptide sequences of RiPP gene clusters in all *Rhodococcus* genomes were extracted from the DeepRiPP output and GBK files (antiSMASH outputs) using a customized Python toolkit (https://github.com/BioGavin/wlabkit, accessed on 15 May 2024). The sequence logo of predicted RiPP core sequence was constructed using TBtools [38]. This antimicrobial activity of the core peptides was predicted using two recently released deep-learning algorithms with the default settings [21,22].

4.4. High-Throughput Elicitor Screening (HiTES)

Rhodococcus sp. 3Y1 was isolated from a depth of 3000 m in the Massau Trench in the Pacific Ocean at coordinates 148°53.3246′ E, 00°53.8546′ N in January 2017. After sampling, 1 L of seawater was stored at 4 °C in a temperature-controlled cold storage. The strain was isolated using B1 isolation medium (0.5 g/L glucose, 0.05 g/L yeast extract, 0.1 g/L K_2HPO_4, 0.005 g/L $MgSO_4 \cdot 7H_2O$, 3% sea salt, 1.5% agar, and 100 mg/L nystatin). The seawater samples were plated and incubated at 28 °C, and single colonies were obtained and stored in 40% glycerol at -80 °C. Genomic DNA was extracted using the Genomic DNA Mini Preparation Kit (Beyotime Institute of Biotechnology, Shanghai, China). The 16S rDNA gene sequence fragment of *Rhodococcus* sp. 3Y1 was amplified using polymerase chain reaction (PCR) with the primer 27F (5′-AGAGTTTGATCCTGGCTCAG-3′). The complete genome was subsequently obtained using a combination of third-generation sequencing with the Oxford Nanopore platform and second-generation sequencing with Illumina. To enhance the reliability of data processing, raw data from both the NovaSeq and GridION X5 platforms were first trimmed using Canu v1.8 [39] to produce high-quality clean reads. The paired-end Illumina reads from second-generation sequencing and the long reads from Nanopore were then assembled using Unicycler v0.4.5 [40], resulting in a high-quality complete genome assembly. The secondary metabolic potential of this strain was comprehensively investigated using a combined strategy of untargeted LC-MS-based metabolomic analysis and high-throughput elicitor screening. The HiTES experiments were conducted under 49 different laboratory culture conditions using seven distinct culture media: M1 (peptone 10 g, yeast extract 5 g, NaCl 10 g for 1 L; pH 7.2), M2 (peptone 5 g, yeast extract 1 g, Fe(III) citrate 0.1 g, NaCl 19.45 g, $MgCl_2$ 5.9 g Na_2SO_4 3.24 g, $CaCl_2$ 1.8 g, KCl 0.55 g, $NaHCO_3$ 0.16 g, KBr 0.08 g, $SrCl_2$ 34 mg, H_3BO_3 22 mg, Na-silicate 2.4 mg, NaF 2.4 mg, $(NH_4)NO_3$ 1.6 mg, Na_2HPO_4 8 mg for 1 L; pH 7.2), M3 (yeast extract 0.5 g, glucose 2 g for 1 L; pH 5–6), M4 (tryptone 5 g, beef extract 3 g, NaCl 5 g for 1 L; pH 7.0), M5 (tryptone 2 g, yeast extract 1 g, glucose 2 g for 1 L; pH 5–6), M6 (peptone 0.5 g, yeast extract 0.5 g, casein peptone 0.5 g, glucose 0.5 g, Soluble amylose 0.5 g, KH_2PO_4 0.3 g, $MgSO_4 \cdot 7H_2O$ 24 mg, sodium pyruvate 0.3 g for 1 L; pH 7.2), M7 (yeast extract 1 g, $MgSO_4 \cdot 7H_2O$ 0.2 g, NaCl 0.4 g, mannitol 10 g for 1 L; pH 7.4). The pre-culture was performed in medium 2216E for 3 days, after which the strain was inoculated into seven different liquid media (M1~M7). Fermentations were carried out in 12 mL cell culture tubes containing 6 mL of medium at 30 °C with shaking at 150 rpm for 3 days. Subsequently, six different elicitors—$LaCl_3 \cdot H_2O$ (2 mM), $ScCl_3 \cdot 6H_2O$ (200 μM), N-acetylglucosamine (100 mM), sodium butyrate (100 mM), streptomycin with trimethoprim (33 µM), and triclosan (5 µM)—were added and the cultures were incubated for an additional 7 days. Blank and control groups were set up for subsequent analysis.

For the extraction of the liquid cultures, 6 mL of culture broth was ultrasonicated and extracted twice with an equal volume of ethyl acetate (EtOAc). The combined EtOAc layers were transferred to a 10 mL sample bottle and dried under vacuum. The resulting crude extracts were re-dissolved in 0.5 mL of methanol (MeOH) and transferred to 1.5 mL centrifuge tubes. These tubes were then concentrated using a termovap sample concentrator. The concentrated extracts were re-dissolved in 50 µL of MeOH and transferred to 1.5 mL vials. The dissolved extracts were centrifuged at 12,000 rpm for 10 min, and the supernatant was filtered through a 0.22 µm nylon syringe filter before injection.

4.5. UPLC-QTOF-MS/MS Analysis

Similar to our recent study [34], the crude extract was analyzed using a SCIEX X500B Q-TOF spectrometer coupled to an ExionLC AC system under the following LC conditions: 1–2 min (10% methanol in H_2O), 2–18 min (10–100% methanol), 18–22 min (100% methanol), and 22.01–25 min (10% methanol) at a flow rate of 0.3 mL/min and a column temperature of 40 °C. The QTOF MS settings during the LC gradient were as follows: positive ion mode mass range 200–1500 m/z, total scan time 0.495 s, maximum candidate ions 5, and ion source temperature 600 °C. MS2 fragmentation was performed with a QTOF mass range of 50–1000 m/z, fixed collision energy of 30 V, fixed collision energy spread of 10 V, and an ion spray voltage of 5.5 kV.

The raw LC-MS data files were converted to mzML format using MSConvert software v3.0.24109 [41] and subsequently processed using MZmine2 software v2.53 [42]. Feature detection, isotope grouping, and alignment were performed following the feature-based molecular networking (FBMN) documentation [43]. The data were filtered by removing all MS/MS peaks from blank media. A CSV file and an MGF file were generated from MZmine2 and uploaded to the FBMN workflow in GNPS (http://gnps.ucsd.edu, accessed on 15 May 2024). Molecular networks were generated with default parameters. Additionally, the MGF file was uploaded to the Dereplicator+ workflow in GNPS (http://gnps.ucsd.edu, accessed on 15 May 2024) with default parameters [44]. The molecular network from FBMN was also visualized using Cytoscape 3.10.2.

5. Conclusions

In conclusion, the current study uncovered that 87.7% of GCFs are uniquely found in a specific phylogenomic clade of *Rhodococcus*, with NRPS and RiPPs being the most prevalent types of gene clusters. Through extensive genome mining and deep-learning analysis, it was revealed that *Rhodococcus* harbors a substantial number of clade-specific novel RiPPs, some of which could exhibit antibacterial properties. The HiTES investigation indicate that certain elicitors can stimulate a marine-derived *Rhodococcus* strain to produce a plethora of potentially new aurachin-like compounds. This study offers valuable insights for targeted exploration of novel natural products from *Rhodococcus*, particularly focusing on clade-specific metabolites.

Supplementary Materials: The following supporting information can be downloaded at: https://www.mdpi.com/article/10.3390/md22090409/s1, Table S1: Genomic features and the antiSMASH results of the 616 *Rhodococcus* genomes; Table S2: Information about the 12,455 BGCs; Table S3: Information about the RiPPs, BGCs and core peptides; Table S4: Metabolite annotation in metabolomic data of *Rhodococcus* sp. 3Y1.

Author Contributions: Formal analysis, G.-A.H.; funding acquisition, H.W. and B.W.; investigation, Y.S.; software, G.-A.H., S.-Y.L. and W.-C.Y.; supervision, H.W. and B.W.; writing—original draft, G.-A.H. and Y.S.; writing—review and editing, Y.-L.Y., J.-W.C. and B.W. All authors have read and agreed to the published version of the manuscript.

Funding: This research was funded by National Key Research and Development Programs (Nos. 2022YFC2804700 and 2022YFC2804104), Fundamental Research Funds for the Provincial Universities of Zhejiang (No. RF-A2022013) and the National Natural Science Foundation of China (No. 42276137).

Institutional Review Board Statement: Not applicable.

Data Availability Statement: The whole genome sequence data reported in this paper have been deposited in the Genome Warehouse of the National Genomics Data Center, China National Center for Bioinformation, under the BioProject accession number PRJCA029818. Additionally, the data are also available in the NCBI under BioProject accession number PRJNA1155922.

Conflicts of Interest: The authors declare no conflicts of interest.

References

1. Vansanten, J.A.; Poynton, E.F.; Dasha, I.; Emily, M.M.; Tylera, A.; Clark, T.N.; Fergusson, C.H.; Fewer, D.P.; Hughes, A.H.; Mccadden, C.A. The Natural Products Atlas 2.0: A Database of Microbially-Derived Natural Products. *Nucleic Acids Res.* **2021**, *50*, D1317–D1323. [CrossRef]
2. Wei, B.; Luo, X.; Zhou, Z.Y.; Hu, G.A.; Li, L.; Lin, H.W.; Wang, H. Discovering the Secondary Metabolic Potential of Saccharothrix. *Biotechnol. Adv.* **2024**, *70*, 108295. [CrossRef]
3. Goodfellow, M.; Alderson, G. The Actinomycete-Genus *Rhodococcus*: A Home for the '*Rhodochrous*' Complex. *Microbiology* **1977**, *100*, 99–122. [CrossRef]
4. Elsayed, Y.; Refaat, J.; Abdelmohsen, U.R.; Fouad, M.A. The Genus *Rhodococcus* as a Source of Novel Bioactive Substances: A Review. *J. Pharmacogn. Phytochem.* **2017**, *6*, 83–92.
5. Chiba, H.; Agematu, H.; Kaneto, R.; Terasawa, T.; Sakai, K.; Dobashi, K.; Yoshioka, T. Rhodopeptins (Mer-N1033), Novel Cyclic Tetrapeptides with Antifungal Activity from *Rhodococcus* sp. I. Taxonomy, Fermentation, Isolation, Physico-Chemical Properties and Biological Activities. *J. Antibiot.* **1999**, *52*, 695–699. [CrossRef]
6. Iwatsuki, M.; Uchida, R.; Takakusagi, Y.; Matsumoto, A.; Jiang, C.L.; Takahashi, Y.; Arai, M.; Kobayashi, S.; Matsumoto, M.; Inokoshi, J.; et al. Lariatins, Novel Anti-Mycobacterial Peptides with a Lasso Structure, Produced by *Rhodococcus Jostii* K01-B017. *J. Antibiot.* **2007**, *60*, 357–363. [CrossRef]
7. Nachtigall, J.; Schneider, K.; Nicholson, G.; Goodfellow, M.; Zinecker, H.; Imhoff, J.F.; Süssmuth, R.D.; Fiedler, H.P. Two new aurachins from *Rhodococcus* sp. Acta 2259. *J. Antibiot. Int. J.* **2010**, *63*, 567–569. [CrossRef]
8. Kurosawa, K.; Ghiviriga, I.; Sambandan, T.G.; Lessard, P.A.; Barbara, J.E.; Rha, C.; Sinskey, A.J. Rhodostreptomycins, Antibiotics Biosynthesized Following Horizontal Gene Transfer from Streptomyces Padanus to *Rhodococcus fascians*. *J. Am. Chem. Soc.* **2008**, *130*, 1126–1127. [CrossRef]
9. Li, L.; Deng, W.; Song, J.; Ding, W.; Zhao, Q.F.; Peng, C.; Song, W.W.; Tang, G.L.; Liu, W. Characterization of the Saframycin A Gene Cluster from Streptomyces Lavendulae NRRL 11002 Revealing a Nonribosomal Peptide Synthetase System for Assembling the Unusual Tetrapeptidyl Skeleton in an Iterative Manner. *J. Bacteriol.* **2007**, *190*, 251–263. [CrossRef] [PubMed]
10. Bosello, M.; Robbel, L.; Linne, U.; Xie, X.; Marahiel, M.A. Biosynthesis of the Siderophore Rhodochelin Requires the Coordinated Expression of Three Independent Gene Clusters in *Rhodococcus jostii* RHA1. *J. Am. Chem. Soc.* **2011**, *133*, 4587–4595. [CrossRef] [PubMed]
11. McLeod, M.P.; Warren, R.L.; Hsiao, W.W.L.; Araki, N.; Myhre, M.; Fernandes, C.; Miyazawa, D.; Wong, W.; Lillquist, A.L.; Wang, D.; et al. The complete genome of *Rhodococcus* sp. RHA1 provides insights into a catabolic powerhouse. *Proc. Natl. Acad. Sci. USA* **2006**, *43*, 15582–15587. [CrossRef]
12. Ana, C.; Lubbert, D.; Mirjan, P.; Medema, M.H. Genome-Based Exploration of the Specialized Metabolic Capacities of the Genus *Rhodococcus*. *BMC Genomics* **2017**, *18*, 593.
13. Undabarrena, A.; Valencia, R.; Cumsille, A.; Zamora-Leiva, L.; Castro-Nallar, E.; Barona-Gómez, F.; Cámara, B. *Rhodococcus* Comparative Genomics Reveals a Phylogenomic-Dependent Non-Ribosomal Peptide Synthetase Distribution: Insights into Biosynthetic Gene Cluster Connection to an Orphan Metabolite. *Microb. Genom.* **2021**, *7*, 000621. [CrossRef] [PubMed]
14. Yin, Q.J.; Ying, T.T.; Zhou, Z.Y.; Hu, G.A.; Yang, C.L.; Hua, Y.; Wang, H.; Wei, B. Species-Specificity of the Secondary Biosynthetic Potential in Bacillus. *Front. Microbiol.* **2023**, *14*, 1271418. [CrossRef]
15. Ma, M.J.; Yu, W.C.; Sun, H.Y.; Dong, B.C.; Hu, G.A.; Zhou, Z.Y.; Hua, Y.; Basnet, B.B.; Yu, Y.L.; Wang, H.; et al. Genus-Specific Secondary Metabolome in *Allokutzneria* and *Kibdelosporangium*. *Synth. Syst. Biotechnol.* **2024**, *9*, 381–390. [CrossRef]
16. Kitagawa, W.; Hata, M. Development of Efficient Genome-Reduction Tool Based on Cre/loxP System in *Rhodococcus erythropolis*. *Microorganisms* **2023**, *11*, 268. [CrossRef] [PubMed]
17. Xu, F.; Wu, Y.; Zhang, C.; Davis, K.M.; Moon, K.; Bushin, L.B.; Seyedsayamdost, M.R. A Genetics-Free Method for High-Throughput Discovery of Cryptic Microbial Metabolites. *Nat. Chem. Biol.* **2019**, *15*, 161–168. [CrossRef]

18. Hofmann, M.; Heine, T.; Malik, L.; Hofmann, S.; Joffroy, K.; Senges, C.H.R.; Bandow, J.E.; Tischler, D. Screening for Microbial Metal-Chelating Siderophores for the Removal of Metal Ions from Solutions. *Microorganisms* **2021**, *9*, 111. [CrossRef]
19. Kitagawa, W.; Ozaki, T.; Nishioka, T.; Yasutake, Y.; Hata, M.; Nishiyama, M. Cloning and Heterologous Expression of the Aurachin RE Biosynthesis Gene Cluster Afford a New Cytochrome P450 for Quinoline N-Hydroxylation. *ChemBioChem* **2013**, *14*, 1085–1093. [CrossRef]
20. Bosello, M.; Zeyadi, M.; Kraas, F.I.; Linne, U.; Marahiel, M.A. Structural Characterization of the Heterobactin Siderophores from *Rhodococcus Erythropolis* PR4 and Elucidation of Their Biosynthetic Machinery. *J. Nat. Prod.* **2013**, *76*, 2282–2290. [CrossRef]
21. Huang, J.; Xu, Y.; Xue, Y.; Huang, Y.; Li, X.; Chen, X.; Xu, Y.; Zhang, D.; Zhang, P.; Zhao, J.; et al. Identification of Potent Antimicrobial Peptides via a Machine-Learning Pipeline That Mines the Entire Space of Peptide Sequences. *Nat. Biomed. Eng.* **2023**, *7*, 797–810. [CrossRef]
22. Ma, Y.; Guo, Z.; Xia, B.; Zhang, Y.; Liu, X.; Yu, Y.; Tang, N.; Tong, X.; Wang, M.; Ye, X.; et al. Identification of Antimicrobial Peptides from the Human Gut Microbiome Using Deep Learning. *Nat. Biotechnol.* **2022**, *40*, 921–931. [CrossRef]
23. Xu, J.L.; He, J.; Wang, Z.C.; Wang, K.; Li, W.J.; Tang, S.K.; Li, S.P. *Rhodococcus qingshengii* sp. Nov., a Carbendazim-Degrading Bacterium. *Int. J. Syst. Evol. Microbiol.* **2007**, *57*, 2754. [CrossRef] [PubMed]
24. Lee, S.D.; Kim, I.S. *Rhodococcus spelaei* Sp. Nov., Isolated from a Cave, and Proposals That *Rhodococcus biphenylivorans* Is a Later Synonym of *Rhodococcus pyridinivorans*, *Rhodococcus qingshengii* and *Rhodococcus baikonurensis* Are Later Synonyms of *Rhodococcus erythropolis*, and *Rhodococcus percolatus* and *Rhodococcus imtechensis* Are Later Synonyms of *Rhodococcus opacus*. *Int. J. Syst. Evol. Microbiol.* **2021**, *71*, 004890.
25. Pettit, R.K. Small-Molecule Elicitation of Microbial Secondary Metabolites. *Microb. Biotechnol.* **2011**, *4*, 471–478. [CrossRef]
26. Kurosu, M.; Begari, E. Vitamin K2 in Electron Transport System: Are Enzymes Involved in Vitamin K2 Biosynthesis Promising Drug Targets? *Molecules* **2010**, *15*, 1531–1553. [CrossRef]
27. Kitagawa, W.; Tamura, T. A Quinoline Antibiotic from *Rhodococcus erythropolis* JCM 6824. *J. Antibiot.* **2008**, *61*, 680–682. [CrossRef]
28. Höfle, G.; Kunze, B. Biosynthesis of Aurachins A−L in *Stigmatella aurantiaca*: A Feeding Study. *J. Nat. Prod.* **2008**, *71*, 1843–1849. [CrossRef]
29. Katsuyama, Y.; Li, X.; Müller, R.; Nay, B. Chemically Unprecedented Biocatalytic (AuaG) Retro-[2,3]-Wittig Rearrangement: A New Insight into Aurachin B Biosynthesis. *ChemBioChem* **2014**, *15*, 2349–2352. [CrossRef]
30. Blin, K.; Shaw, S.; Augustijn, H.E.; Reitz, Z.L.; Biermann, F.; Alanjary, M.; Fetter, A.; Terlouw, B.R.; Metcalf, W.W.; Helfrich, E.J.N.; et al. antiSMASH 7.0: New and Improved Predictions for Detection, Regulation, Chemical Structures and Visualisation. *Nucleic Acids Res.* **2023**, *51*, W46–W50. [CrossRef] [PubMed]
31. Pritchard, L.; Glover, R.H.; Humphris, S.; Elphinstone, J.G.; Toth, I.K. Genomics and Taxonomy in Diagnostics for Food Security: Soft-Rotting Enterobacterial Plant Pathogens. *Anal. Methods* **2015**, *8*, 12–24. [CrossRef]
32. Team, R.C. R: A Language and Environment for Statistical Computing, Version 3.6; 2014. Available online: https://www.R-project.org (accessed on 15 May 2024).
33. Letunic, I.; Bork, P. Interactive Tree Of Life (iTOL) v4: Recent Updates and New Developments. *Nucleic Acids Res.* **2019**, *47*, W256–W259. [CrossRef]
34. Wei, B.; Hu, G.A.; Zhou, Z.Y.; Yu, W.C.; Du, A.Q.; Yang, C.L.; Yu, Y.L.; Chen, J.W.; Zhang, H.W.; Wu, Q.H.; et al. Global Analysis of the Biosynthetic Chemical Space of Marine Prokaryotes. *Microbiome* **2023**, *11*, 144. [CrossRef] [PubMed]
35. Navarro-Munoz, J.C.; Selem-Mojica, N.; Mullowney, M.W.; Kautsar, S.A.; Tryon, J.H.; Parkinson, E.; De Los Santos, E.L.C.; Yeong, M.; Cruz-Morales, P.; Abubucker, S.; et al. A Computational Framework to Explore Large-Scale Biosynthetic Diversity. *Nat. Chem. Biol.* **2020**, *16*, 60–68. [CrossRef]
36. Su, G.; Morris, J.H.; Demchak, B.; Bader, G.D. Biological Network Exploration with Cytoscape 3. *Curr. Protoc. Bioinforma.* **2014**, *47*, 8–13. [CrossRef]
37. Merwin, N.J.; Mousa, W.K.; Dejong, C.A.; Skinnider, M.A.; Cannon, M.J.; Li, H.; Dial, K.; Gunabalasingam, M.; Johnston, C.; Magarvey, N.A. DeepRiPP Integrates Multiomics Data to Automate Discovery of Novel Ribosomally Synthesized Natural Products. *Proc. Natl. Acad. Sci. USA* **2020**, *117*, 371–380. [CrossRef]
38. Chen, C.; Chen, H.; Zhang, Y.; Thomas, H.R.; Frank, M.H.; He, Y.; Xia, R. TBtools: An Integrative Toolkit Developed for Interactive Analyses of Big Biological Data. *Mol. Plant* **2020**, *13*, 1194–1202. [CrossRef] [PubMed]
39. Koren, S.; Walenz, B.P.; Berlin, K.; Miller, J.R.; Bergman, N.H.; Phillippy, A.M. Canu: Scalable and Accurate Long-Read Assembly via Adaptive k-Mer Weighting and Repeat Separation. *Genome Res.* **2017**, *27*, 722–736. [CrossRef] [PubMed]
40. Wick, R.R.; Judd, L.M.; Gorrie, C.L.; Holt, K.E. Unicycler: Resolving Bacterial Genome Assemblies from Short and Long Sequencing Reads. *PLoS Comput. Biol.* **2017**, *13*, e1005595. [CrossRef]
41. Adusumilli, R.; Mallick, P. Data Conversion with ProteoWizard msConvert. In *Proteomics: Methods and Protocols*; Comai, L., Katz, J.E., Mallick, P., Eds.; Springer: Berlin/Heidelberg, Germany, 2017; Volume 1550, pp. 339–368.
42. Pluskal, T.; Castillo, S.; Villar-Briones, A.; Orešič, M. MZmine 2: Modular Framework for Processing, Visualizing, and Analyzing Mass Spectrometry-Based Molecular Profile Data. *BMC Bioinform.* **2010**, *11*, 395. [CrossRef]

43. Nothias, L.-F.; Petras, D.; Schmid, R.; Duehrkop, K.; Rainer, J.; Sarvepalli, A.; Protsyuk, I.; Ernst, M.; Tsugawa, H.; Fleischauer, M.; et al. Feature-Based Molecular Networking in the GNPS Analysis Environment. *Nat. Methods* **2020**, *17*, 905–908. [CrossRef] [PubMed]
44. Mohimani, H.; Gurevich, A.; Shlemov, A.; Mikheenko, A.; Korobeynikov, A.; Cao, L.; Shcherbin, E.; Nothias, L.-F.; Dorrestein, P.C.; Pevzner, P.A. Dereplication of Microbial Metabolites through Database Search of Mass Spectra. *Nat. Commun.* **2018**, *9*, 4035. [CrossRef] [PubMed]

Disclaimer/Publisher's Note: The statements, opinions and data contained in all publications are solely those of the individual author(s) and contributor(s) and not of MDPI and/or the editor(s). MDPI and/or the editor(s) disclaim responsibility for any injury to people or property resulting from any ideas, methods, instructions or products referred to in the content.

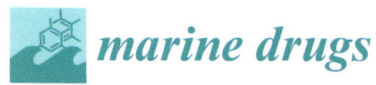 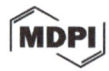

Article

Discovery of Prenyltransferase-Guided Hydroxyphenylacetic Acid Derivatives from Marine Fungus *Penicillium* sp. W21C371

Cancan Wang [†], Ye Fan [†], Chenjie Wang, Jing Tang, Yixian Qiu, Keren Xu, Yingjia Ding, Ying Liu, Youmin Ying * and Hong Wang *

College of Pharmaceutical Science & Collaborative Innovation Center of Yangtze River Delta Region Green Pharmaceuticals, Zhejiang University of Technology, Hangzhou 310014, China; cancanw1120@163.com (C.W.); m18767175381_1@163.com (Y.F.); 211123070063@zjut.edu.cn (C.W.); t_joyce@126.com (J.T.); 13588779931@163.com (Y.Q.); 201805150118@zjut.edu.cn (K.X.); 19857445690@163.com (Y.D.); 15844357993@163.com (Y.L.)
* Correspondence: ymying@zjut.edu.cn (Y.Y.); hongw@zjut.edu.cn (H.W.)
[†] These authors contributed equally to this work.

Abstract: Traditional isolation methods often lead to the rediscovery of known natural products. In contrast, genome mining strategies are considered effective for the continual discovery of new natural products. In this study, we discovered a unique prenyltransferase (PT) through genome mining, capable of catalyzing the transfer of a prenyl group to an aromatic nucleus to form C-C or C-O bonds. A pair of new hydroxyphenylacetic acid derivative enantiomers with prenyl units, (±)-peniprenydiol A (**1**), along with 16 known compounds (**2**–**17**), were isolated from a marine fungus, *Penicillium* sp. W21C371. The separation of **1** using chiral HPLC led to the isolation of the enantiomers **1a** and **1b**. Their structures were established on the basis of extensive spectroscopic analysis, including 1D, 2D NMR and HRESIMS. The absolute configurations of the new compounds were determined by a modified Mosher method. A plausible biosynthetic pathway for **1** was deduced, facilitated by PT catalysis. In the in vitro assay, **2** and **3** showed promising inhibitory activity against *Escherichia coli* β-glucuronidase (EcGUS), with IC_{50} values of 44.60 ± 0.84 μM and 21.60 ± 0.76 μM, respectively, compared to the positive control, D-saccharic acid 1,4-lactone hydrate (DSL). This study demonstrates the advantages of genome mining in the rational acquisition of new natural products.

Keywords: marine fungi; *Penicillium*; genome mining; phenylacetic acid; β-glucuronidase; bioactivity

Citation: Wang, C.; Fan, Y.; Wang, C.; Tang, J.; Qiu, Y.; Xu, K.; Ding, Y.; Liu, Y.; Ying, Y.; Wang, H. Discovery of Prenyltransferase-Guided Hydroxyphenylacetic Acid Derivatives from Marine Fungus *Penicillium* sp. W21C371. *Mar. Drugs* **2024**, *22*, 296. https://doi.org/10.3390/md22070296

Academic Editor: Zeinab Khalil

Received: 7 June 2024
Revised: 21 June 2024
Accepted: 24 June 2024
Published: 26 June 2024

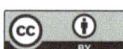

Copyright: © 2024 by the authors. Licensee MDPI, Basel, Switzerland. This article is an open access article distributed under the terms and conditions of the Creative Commons Attribution (CC BY) license (https://creativecommons.org/licenses/by/4.0/).

1. Introduction

The secondary metabolites produced by filamentous fungi are crucial sources of valuable pharmaceuticals and agrochemicals. *Penicillium*, one of the most common fungal genera, consists of more than 350 species with a worldwide distribution [1]. These fungi colonize a wide range of habitats, including conventional environments such as soil, vegetation, food, and indoor spaces, as well as extreme environments on Earth [2]. The diverse lifestyles and habitats of *Penicillium* species equip them with robust metabolic capabilities. Since the discovery of penicillin from *P. rubens* (often identified as *P. chrysogenum*), the fungi of the genus *Penicillium* have been extensively studied for their production of bioactive secondary metabolites [3]. Over the past several decades, many secondary metabolites with diverse structures and intriguing biological activity have been discovered from *Penicillium*, making it a promising reservoir of novel drug leads. However, the metabolic potential of *Penicillium* is reported to be underestimated and remains to be fully exploited, despite being one of the most well-studied fungal genera. In a recent large-scale genome-based study, Nielsen and co-workers conducted the first genus-wide analysis of the genomic diversity of 24 *Penicillium* species and identified 1317 putative biosynthetic gene clusters (BGCs), highlighting the potential of these species as sources of new antibiotics and other pharmaceuticals [4].

As the largest biome on Earth, the marine ecosystem boasts extraordinarily rich biodiversity due to its extreme physical and chemical conditions compared to the terrestrial ecosystems [5]. This vast biodiversity is partly demonstrated by the unique groups of marine microorganisms that produce a variety of secondary metabolites [6]. A significant number of fungi inhabit the marine environment, found in sea water, sediments, or living organisms such as sponges, corals, and algae. Among these, marine fungi of the genus *Penicillium* have garnered considerable attention as an important source of secondary metabolites, featuring novel structures and remarkable bioactive properties [7]. To date, more than 500 novel natural products have been isolated and characterized from marine *Penicillium* fungi, exhibiting benefits such as antibacterial [8–12], anti-inflammatory [13], enzyme inhibition, and cytotoxic properties [14,15].

Escherichia coli β-glucuronidase (EcGUS) is one of the most abundant bacterial β-glucuronidases, catalyzing the hydrolysis of glucuronide conjugates to produce the corresponding aglycones [16]. Anticancer drug irinotecan and anti-inflammatory drug indomethacin produce glucuronidated metabolites that are rapidly hydrolyzed by EcGUS, resulting in highly toxic aglycones. The accumulation of these aglycones in the intestine can lead to severe gastrointestinal adverse reactions, such as fatal diarrhea [17]. Consequently, targeting EcGUS has emerged as a crucial strategy to mitigate the adverse gastrointestinal effects associated with these drugs.

The genome mining technique for the discovery of natural products, which leverages genomic sequence data to identify previously uncharacterized compounds, has proven effective and efficient for over a decade [18]. With the rapid accumulation of genomic sequences from various organisms, genome mining methods have led to the identification of an increasing number of natural products [19]. Traditional approaches often result in the rediscovery of known compounds, whereas genome-based strategies are now seen as a promising solution for the continual discovery of novel natural products. Prenyltransferases (PTs) are capable of catalyzing the transfer of prenyl groups from various prenyl donors. These prenylated secondary metabolites, including indole alkaloids, flavonoids, coumarins, ketones, quinones, and naphthalenes, are widely found in terrestrial and marine organisms and exhibit various types of biological activity, such as cytotoxicity, antioxidation, and antimicrobial effects [20]. For example, XptB, a ketone prenyltransferase from *Aspergillus nidulans*, catalyzes the O-prenylation of 1,7-dihydroxy-6-methyl-8-hydroxymethylxanthone, resulting in the production of variecoxanthone A [21]. Additionally, *Streptomyces* sp. CNQ-509 produces the rare O-prenylated phenazines, marinophenazines A and B, through the catalytic action of the enzyme CnqPT1 [22]. In our study, we analyzed the genomic data of PTs from our lab and the NCBI public databases, generated a sequence similarity network (SSN) of PTs, and discovered a previously uncharacterized branch. Phylogenetic tree analysis revealed that this enzyme belongs to a distinct branch of PTs, highlighting its unique characteristics. The secondary metabolites produced were investigated under different culture conditions using PT-guided isolation. A pair of new *p*-hydroxyphenylacetic acid derivative enantiomers, (±)-peniprenydiol A (**1**), containing prenyl units, and 16 known compounds (**2–17**) were isolated from *Penicillium* sp. W21C371 (Figure 1). Their structures were determined using thorough NMR analysis and a modified Mosher method. A plausible biosynthetic pathway for **1** was deduced, facilitated by PT catalysis. Additionally, their EcGUS inhibition activity was evaluated.

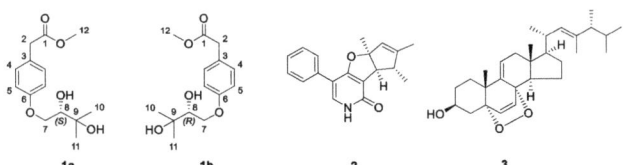

Figure 1. *Cont.*

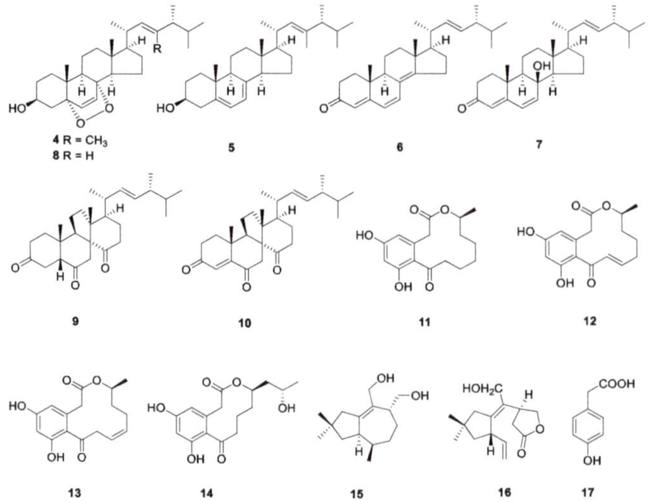

Figure 1. Chemical structures of compounds **1–17**.

2. Results

2.1. Bioinformatics Analysis and Phylogenetic Tree Construction of PTs

To explore PTs with different substrates, we conducted a comprehensive analysis of genomic data from our lab, the InterPro database, and the NCBI public database. Nearly 2000 prenyltransferases (PTs), including those from our lab and the InterPro database, were submitted to the Enzyme Function Initiative-Enzyme Similarity Tool (EFI-EST). Subsequently, an SSN of PTs was generated, where enzymes with similar functions clustered together. The SSN results showed that most known proteins clustered together (Figure 2A). A distinct evolutionary clade attracted our attention, as it did not cluster with any specific PTs, suggesting that this PT might be a novel enzyme catalyzing the transfer of prenyl units. In addition, 26 PTs were obtained from our lab and the NCBI public database, and phylogenetic trees were constructed using MEGA 7.0. The phylogenetic tree showed that the 26 PTs were divided into two large branches and five small branches. Among them, a unique small branch attracted our attention, suggesting that this enzyme may have structural novelty and the capability to catalyze the production of isoprenoids (Figure 2B). This unique PT originates from the marine fungus *Penicillium* sp. W21C371, which was sequenced in our laboratory. Comprehensive analysis indicates that this PT possesses distinctive properties, enabling it to catalyze the production of novel compounds. Therefore, further investigation into the secondary metabolites of *Penicillium* sp. W21C371 is warranted.

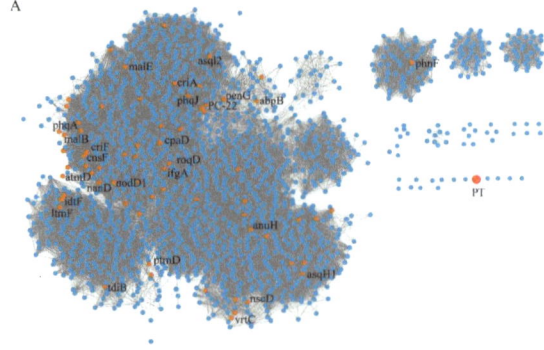

Figure 2. *Cont.*

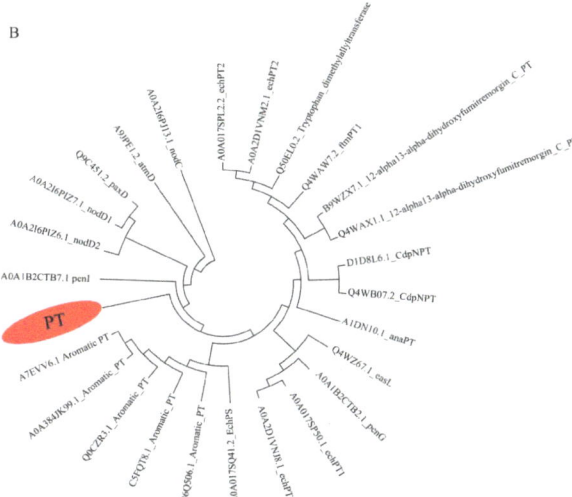

Figure 2. (**A**) Sequence similarity network (SSN) analysis of PTs and their homologous proteins (e-value: 10). (**B**) Phylogenetic tree analysis shows PTs and its homologues.

2.2. Structure Elucidation

Compound **1** (**1a**/**1b**) was obtained as a colorless oil. The molecular formula of **1** was determined as $C_{14}H_{20}O_5$ by HRESIMS (m/z 291.1186 [M + Na]$^+$, calcd. for $C_{14}H_{20}O_5Na^+$ 291.1203), indicating five degrees of unsaturation (Figures S14 and S15). The IR spectrum showed characteristic absorption bands for carbonyl (1732 cm^{-1}) and hydroxy (3361 cm^{-1}) groups (Figure S8). The ^{1}H NMR spectrum (Figure S2 and Table 1) displayed proton resonances attributable to two methyls at δ_H 1.22 (3H, s, H$_3$-10) and 1.24 (3H, s, H$_3$-11), one methoxy at δ_H 3.62 (3H, s, H$_3$-12), one oxygenated methine at δ_H 3.75 (dd, J = 7.8, 3.0 Hz, H-8), one oxygenated methylene at δ_H 3.92 (dd, J = 9.6, 7.8 Hz, H$_b$-7) and 4.26 (dd, J = 9.6, 3.0 Hz, H$_a$-7), and four aromatic protons at δ_H 6.90 (2H, d, J = 8.4 Hz, H-5 and 5′) and 7.19 (2H, d, J = 8.4 Hz, H-4 and 4′). The ^{13}C NMR, DEPT, and HSQC spectra (Figures S3–S5) revealed the presence of fourteen carbon resonances, including two methyls at δ_C 25.6 (C-11) and 26.7 (C-10); one methoxy at δ_C 51.9 (C-12); two methylenes at δ_C 40.4 (C-2) and 70.6 (C-7); four aromatic methines at δ_C 115.4 (C-5), 115.4 (C-5′), 131.1 (C-4), and 131.1 (C-4′); one oxygenated methine at δ_C 77.1 (C-8); and four non-protonated carbons (one oxygenated at δ_C 71.9 (C-9), two aromatic at δ_C 127.4 (C-3) and 159.2 (C-6), and one carbonyl at δ_C 172.6 (C-1)). The NMR data of **1** were similar to those of westerdijkin A, a hydroxyphenylacetic acid derivative from the deep-sea fungus *Aspergillus westerdijkiae* SCSIO 05233 [23]. Detailed comparative analyses revealed that the signals for the Δ^9 terminal double bond (δ_C 143.3 (C-9), δ_C 112.7 (C-10), δ_H 5.00 and 5.14 (H$_2$-10)) in westerdijkin A were replaced by the newly emerging signals assignable for one methyl (δ_H 1.22 (H$_3$-10) and δ_C 26.7 (C-10)) and one oxygenated quaternary carbon (δ_C 71.9 (C-9)) in **1**. The ^{1}H-^{1}H COSY plots (Figure S6) of H-4/H-5 and H-4′/H-5′, combined with the HMBC (Figure S7) correlations from H-4, H-4′, H-5, and H-5′ to C-6, and from H-5 and H-5′ to C-3, established the *para*-substituted benzene ring moiety in **1**. The HMBC correlations from H$_2$-2 to C-1, C-3, C-4, and C-4′, as well as from H$_3$-12 to C-1, suggested the presence of a methyl acetate residue that anchored at C-3 via C-2. In addition, the ^{1}H-^{1}H COSY plot of H$_2$-7 (δ_H 3.92 and 4.26)/H-8 (δ_H 3.75) and the HMBC correlations from H$_2$-7 (δ_H 3.92 and 4.26) and H-8 (δ_H 3.75) to the oxygenated quaternary carbon C-9 (δ_C 71.9) and from the two methyl singlets (δ_H 1.22 and 1.24) to C-8 (δ_C 77.1) and C-9 (δ_C 71.9), in combination with the molecular formula, constructed a 2,3-dihydroxyisopentane moiety that was linked to the benzene ring with an ether linkage between C-6 (δ_C 159.2) and C-7 (δ_C 70.6). The planar structure of **1** was thus established (Figure 3).

Table 1. ^{1}H (600 MHz) and ^{13}C NMR (150 MHz) data of **1** in Acetone-d_6 (δ_H in ppm, J in Hz).

Position	δ_C, Type	δ_H
1	172.6, C	-
2	40.4, CH$_2$	3.56, s
3	127.4, C	-
4	131.1, CH	7.19, d (8.4)
4'	131.1, CH	7.19, d (8.4)
5	115.4, CH	6.90, d (8.4)
5'	115.4, CH	6.90, d (8.4)
6	159.2, C	-
7	70.6, CH$_2$	3.92, dd, (9.6, 7.8) 4.26, dd, (9.6, 3.0)
8	77.1, CH	3.75, dd (7.8, 3.0)
9	71.9, C	
10	26.7, CH$_3$	1.22, s
11	25.6, CH$_3$	1.24, s
12	51.9, CH$_3$	3.62, s

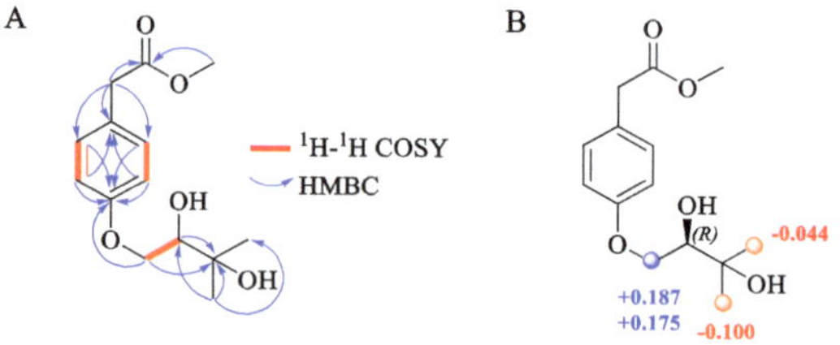

Figure 3. (**A**) Key ^{1}H-^{1}H COSY and HMBC correlations of (±)-peniprenydiol A (**1**). (**B**) $\Delta\delta = \delta_S - \delta_R$ values 171 in ppm obtained from the MTPA esters of **1b**.

Compound **1** was initially assumed to be optically pure based on its specific rotation ($[\alpha]_D^{20}$: +14 (c 0.1, MeOH)). Hence, a modified Mosher experiment was performed to determine the absolute configuration of C-8. Unexpectedly, when the (*R*)- and (*S*)-MTPA esters of **1** were subjected to HPLC analysis on a routine ODS C-18 column, two pairs of diastereoisomers were obtained ((*S*)-MTPA-**1a**/(*S*)-MTPA-**1b** and (*R*)-MTPA-**1a**/(*R*)-MTPA-**1b**), suggesting that **1** was probably a partially racemic mixture. This was confirmed by the chiral resolution of **1** on a Chiralpak AD-H column, which afforded a pair of enantiomers **1a** and **1b** in a ratio of ca. 3:7. According to the shielding/deshielding effects of MTPA, the $\Delta\delta_{H(S-R)}$ values indicated an 8*R* configuration for (+)-**1b** (Figure 3 and Figures S16 and S17 and Table S2). Thus, **1a** was deduced to be the enantiomer of **1b** based on their identical ^{1}H NMR and HRESIMS data (Supplementary Data, Figures S12–S15) and opposite specific rotations ($[\alpha]_D^{20}$: −32 (c 0.05, MeOH) for **1a** and $[\alpha]_D^{20}$: +36 (c 0.1, MeOH) for **1b**). Finally, (−)-**1a** and (+)-**1b** were named (−)-peniprenydiol A and (+)-peniprenydiol A, respectively.

Sixteen known compounds were identified as citridone A (**2**) [24], 5α,8α-epidioxy-23,24(*R*)-dimethylcholesta-6,9(11),22-trien-3β-ol (**3**) [23], 5α,8α-epidioxy-(23*E*,24*R*)-23-methylergosta-6,22-dien-3β-ol (**4**) [25], (22*E*)-23-methylergosta-5,7,22-trien-3β-ol (**5**) [26], ergosta-4,6,8(14),22-tetraen-3-one (**6**) [27], isocyathisterol (**7**) [28], ergosterol peroxide (**8**) [29], dankasterone B (**9**) [30], dankasterone (**10**) [31], curvularin (**11**) [32], 10,11-dedrocurvularin (**12**) [33], dehydrocurvularin (**13**) [34], sumalactone A (**14**) [35], morelsin D (**15**) [36], conocenolide A (**16**) [37], and *p*-hydroxy phenylacetic acid (**17**) [38] through the comparison of the spectroscopic data with those reported in the literature. The tremulane sesquiterpenoids, exemplified by morelsin D (**15**) and conocenolide A (**16**) in the present study, were obtained from Ascomycetes for the first time.

2.3. Plausible Biosynthetic Pathways of Peniprenydiol A

To investigate the connection between peniprenydiol A and its biosynthetic genes, we obtained the complete genome sequence of the marine fungus *Penicillium* sp. W21C371. The genome was analyzed and predicted using the online tool 2ndfind (https://biosyn.nih.go.jp/2ndfind/, accessed on 1 June 2024). Based on the analysis results, we propose that gene cluster A is responsible for the assembly and transport of peniprenydiol A. This gene cluster comprises multiple genes with diverse functions, including core genes, transporter proteins, regulatory proteins, tailoring enzymes, and genes of unknown function. Using peniprenydiol A as a case study to analyze its biosynthetic pathway, the core PyoF catalyzes the methylation reaction to produce **1c** [39]. This intermediate is then prenylated by the PyoR enzyme to form **1d** [40]. Finally, **1d** is converted into the final product through a non-enzymatic oxidation reaction (Figure 4).

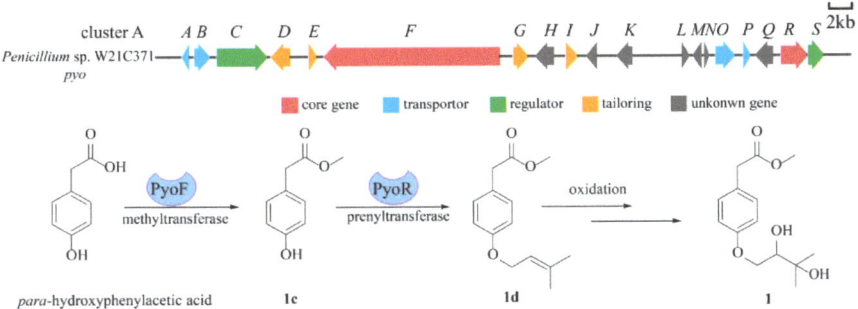

Figure 4. Proposed biosynthetic pathway for **1**.

2.4. EcGUS Inhibition Assay

All isolates **1–17** were evaluated for their in vitro inhibitory activity against EcGUS, a potential target for the treatment of drug-induced gastrointestinal disorders, employing D-saccharic acid 1,4-lactone (DSL) as the positive control. In the preliminary screening, compounds **2** and **3** showed relative inhibitory rates of over 60% at a concentration of 100 μM and were subjected to further evaluation. As a result (Table 2), **2** and **3** were found to significantly inhibit the activity of EcGUS in a dose-dependent manner, comparable to that of DSL. In view of the potent inhibitory activity of **2** and **3** against EcGUS, their kinetic mechanisms of inhibition were determined using Lineweaver–Burk plots (Figure 5 and Table S1). The inhibition constants of the enzyme K_i and the enzyme–substrate complex K_i' were obtained by secondary plots of "slope versus [I]" and "Y-intercept versus [I]", respectively. As shown in Figure 5, the data lines of **2** intersected in the X axis. Meanwhile, the V_{max} value decreased with the increased concentration of **2**, while the K_m value did not change. This suggested that **2** was a non-competitive inhibitor of EcGUS that bound with EcGUS and/or the EcGUS–substrate complex at a site other than the active site. The intersection of the data lines of **3** in the third quadrant demonstrated that **3** inhibited EcGUS in a mixed-type manner, which was verified by the changed K_m and V_{max} values with the increased concentration of **3**. As a mixed-type inhibitor of EcGUS, **3** was supposed to bind either the free EcGUS or the EcGUS–substrate complex. The inhibition constant K_i (89.04 μM) for **3** was larger than K_i' (48.80 μM), implying that it bound more easily and tightly to the EcGUS–substrate complex than the free EcGUS. To the best of our knowledge, **2** and **3** represent the first citridone and ergosterol derivatives with potent EcGUS-inhibitory activity. However, **2** and **3** were obtained in limited amount in the present study, preventing the in vivo evaluation of their EcGUS inhibition activity. The optimization of the fermentation and separation processes with the aim of increasing the yields of **2** and **3** is underway, which may help to accumulate greater amounts of the two compounds for further in-depth pharmacological studies.

Table 2. Inhibitory activity of **2** and **3** against EcUGS.

Compound	IC$_{50}$ (µM)
2	44.60 ± 0.84
3	21.60 ± 0.76
DSL	47.94 ± 0.89

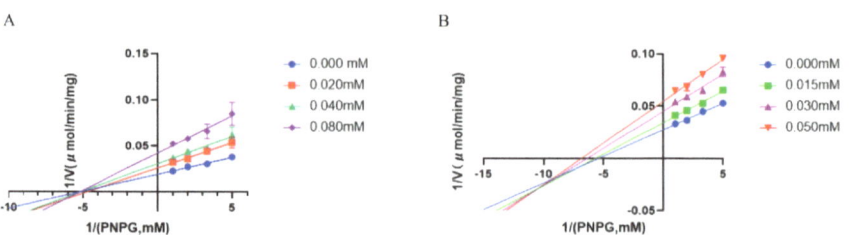

Figure 5. Lineweaver–Burk plots of (**A**) **2**, (**B**) **3** against DSL. All data are expressed as mean ± SD of triplicate reactions.

3. Materials and Methods

3.1. General Experimental Procedures

Optical rotations were obtained with a Rudolph Research Autopol III automatic polarimeter. IR spectra were recorded on a Thermo Nicolet 6700 FT-IR microscope instrument (FT-IR microscope transmission) in KBr pellets. UV spectra were measured on a TU-1900 spectrometer (Persee, Beijing, China). Meanwhile, 1D and 2D-NMR spectra were obtained at 600 MHz for ^{1}H and 150 MHz for ^{13}C on a Bruker Avance 600 spectrometer, with solvent peaks used as references. HRESIMS data were measured on an Agilent-6210-LC/TOF mass spectrometer (Agilent Technologies, Inc., Santa Clara, CA, USA). EcGUS-inhibitory activity was measured spectrophotometrically using a SpectraMax Plus 384 microplate reader (Molecular Devices, San Jose, CA, USA). Column chromatography (CC) was performed on silica gel (SiO$_2$; 200–300 mesh; Qingdao Marine Chemical Co., Ltd.), ODS C-18 gel (50 mm; YMC Co., Ltd., Kyoto, Japan), and MCI CHP20P gel (75–150 µm, Tokyo, Japan). Semi-preparative HPLC was performed on an Cosmosil 5C18-MS-II column (5 µm, 250 × 10 mm) with a Shimadzu LC-20AT system eluting with methanol/water or acetonitrile/water at a flow rate of 3 mL/min. Chiral separation was performed on a Chiralpak AD-H column (5 µm, 4.6 × 250 mm). Thin layer chromatography (TLC) was performed on precoated silica gel GF254 plates (Qingdao Marine Chemical Co., Ltd., Qingdao, China) and visualized by UV light and/or spraying with 10% H$_2$SO$_4$ in 95% EtOH, followed by heating. All solvents used were of analytical grade and obtained from commercially available sources. All reagents used for biological evaluation were obtained from Sigma-Aldrich (St. Louis, MO, USA).

3.2. Fungal Material

The fungus *Penicillium* sp. W21C371 was isolated from a seawater sample collected at Marceau Trench in 2017. It has been deposited in the China Typical Culture Preservation Centre, Wuhan University, Wuhan, China, with the deposit number of CCTCC NO: M2022063. For the identification of the fungus, the genomic DNA was extracted using the Trelief® Hi-Pure Plant Genomic DNA Kit (Tsingke, Beijing, China), according to the manufacturer's instructions. The primers for the internal transcribed spacer 1 (ITS1) and 4 (ITS4) regions were TCCGTAGGTGAACCTGCGG (5′→3′) and TCCTCCGCTTATTGATATGC (5′→3′), respectively. The PCR amplification of the extracted DNA was performed in a 50 µL reaction mixture consisting of 1 µL gDNA template, 2 µL each of the forward and reverse primers, and 45 µL of Tsingke 1× TSE101 golden mix. The thermocycler was programed with the following PCR conditions: initial denaturation at 98 °C for 2 min, followed by 35 cycles of denaturation at 98 °C for 10 s, annealing at 55 °C for 10 s, and extension at 72 °C for 15 s, with a final extension at 72 °C for 5 min. Upon the completion of amplification, the PCR products were analyzed using gel electrophoresis with a 1% agarose gel (1 g of agarose in 100 mL of Tris buffer) stained with ethidium bromide. Sequencing was carried out by Sanger's method [41] on a 3730xl DNA Analyzer (Thermo Fisher Scientific, Waltham, MA, USA) at Beijing Tsingke Biotech Co., Ltd. (Beijing, China). The ITS sequence was deposited in GeneBank under Accession No. PP733993.

3.3. Bioinformatics Analysis and Phylogenetic Tree Construction of PTs

The sequences of PTs were obtained from our lab, the InterPro database, and the NCBI database. Sequence similarity networks (SSNs) were constructed using the Enzyme Function Initiative (EFI; accessed at https://efi.igb.illinois.edu/, accessed on 1 June 2024) [42]. Cytoscape 3.5.1 was employed for network visualization. Multiple sequence alignments were performed using MUSCLE. Phylogenetic trees were constructed using the maximum likelihood method in MEGA6 and visualized using the Interactive Tree of Life (ITOL, http://itol.embl.de/, accessed on 1 June 2024).

3.4. Fermentation and Extraction

The fungus was cultured on potato dextrose agar (PDA) plates for 5 days at 28 °C. The spores were washed with 10 mL sterile water containing 2% tween 80 and aseptically inoculated into 45 conical flasks (1000 mL) containing rice medium (rice 100 g, distilled water 135 mL, sterilized at 121 °C for 20 min and cooled). The conical flasks were kept at 28 °C. After culturing for 20 days, the collected cultures were mashed and soaked in 95% ethanol for 4 days at room temperature and filtered (repeated 3 times). The filtrate was condensed in a vacuum to give a crude extract (550 g), which was suspended in distilled water (1.5 L) and partitioned with EtOAc (1.5 L) 3 times. The EtOAc layer was combined and concentrated in a vacuum to yield an EtOAc-soluble extract (64 g).

3.5. Isolation and Purification

The EtOAc-soluble extract (64 g) was subjected to MCI CHP20P CC eluting with a gradient of MeOH-H_2O (20:80→100:0, v/v) to offer six fractions (Fr. A–F). Fr. B (2.26 g) was fractionated by silica gel CC eluting with a gradient of CH_2Cl_2-MeOH (60:1→40:1, v/v) to give five sub-fractions (Fr. B1–B5). Fr. B1 was separated by semi-preparative HPLC eluting with MeOH/H_2O (35:65, v/v) to give **1** (21.1 mg, t_R = 10.5 min). Fr. B2 was subjected to semi-preparative HPLC eluting with CH_3CN-H_2O (45:55, v/v) to afford **13** (1 mg, t_R = 11.5 min). Fr. C (8.56 g) was subjected to silica gel CC eluting with a gradient of CH_2Cl_2-MeOH (40:1→5:1, v/v) to give three sub-fractions (Fr. C1–C3). Fr. C2 was separated by semi-preparative HPLC eluting with MeOH/H_2O (40:60, v/v) to yield **14** (2 mg, t_R = 16.5 min) and **17** (6.5 mg, t_R = 14.5 min). Fr. D (14.7 g) was subjected to silica gel CC eluting with a gradient of CH_2Cl_2-MeOH (50:1→30:1, v/v) to give **11** (1.5 g) and four sub-fractions (Fr. D1–D4). Fr. D1 was chromatographed over ODS C-18 gel eluting with a gradient of MeOH-H_2O (60:40→80:20, v/v) to furnish **12** (37.7 mg), **15** (19.5 mg), and **16** (5.4 g). The purification of Fr. E (12.5 g) by silica gel CC eluting with a gradient of CH_2Cl_2-MeOH (50:1→20:1, v/v) yielded four sub-fractions (Fr. E1-Fr. E4). Fr. E2 was subjected to silica gel CC eluting with a gradient of MeOH-H_2O (80:20→90:10, v/v) to afford **9** (17 mg). Moreover, **2** (15.4 mg) was obtained from Fr. E4 by silica gel CC eluting with a gradient of MeOH-H_2O (80:20→90:10, v/v). Fr. F (12.5 g) was first separated on a silica gel column eluting with a gradient of CH_2Cl_2-MeOH (50:1→20:1, v/v) to yield four sub-fractions (Fr. F1–F4). Fr. F1 was subjected to ODS C-18 CC and eluted with a gradient of MeOH-H_2O (75:25→100:0, v/v) to offer **6** (10 mg). Fr. F2 was separated on an ODS C-18 column eluting with a gradient of MeOH-H_2O (80:20→100:0, v/v) to furnish **5** (55.0 mg), **4** (4 mg), and **7** (15.3 mg). Fr. F3 was purified by semi-preparative HPLC eluting with MeOH-H_2O (95:5, v/v) to give **10** (3 mg, t_R = 15.5 min). Fr. F4 was separated by semi-preparative HPLC eluting with MeOH/H_2O (95:5, v/v) to furnish **3** (1.7 mg, t_R = 10.0 min) and **8** (15.2 mg, t_R = 12.0 min). Finally, **1** (5.0 mg) was separated by chiral HPLC eluting with isopropanol/n-hexane

(18:82, v/v) at a flow rate of 1 mL/min to yield **1a** (0.8 mg, t_R = 16.7 min) and **1b** (3.2 mg, t_R = 22.0 min) (Figure S11).

3.6. Spectroscopic Data

Peniprenydiol A (**1**), colorless oil, $[\alpha]_D^{20}$: +14 (c 0.1, MeOH), IR (KBr) (Figure S8): 3361, 2921, 2850, 1732, 1659, 1632, 1612, 1584, 1513, 1462, 1435, 1297, 1245, 1157, 1094, 1030, 805 cm^{-1}. UV λ_{max} (MeOH) nm (log ε): 207 (3.91) (Figure S10); HR-ESI-MS m/z: 291.1186 [M + Na]$^+$ (calcd. for $C_{14}H_{20}O_5Na^+$, 291.1203). For ^{1}H- and ^{13}C-NMR data, see Table 1.

(−)-Peniprenydiol A (**1a**), colorless oil, $[\alpha]_D^{20}$: −32 (c 0.05, MeOH), HR-ESI-MS m/z 291.1202 [M + Na]$^+$ (calcd. for $C_{14}H_{20}O_5Na^+$, 291.1203). For ^{1}H-NMR data, see Figure S12.

(+)-Peniprenydiol A (**1b**), colorless oil, $[\alpha]_D^{20}$: +36 (c 0.1, MeOH), HR-ESI-MS m/z 291.1202 [M + Na]$^+$ (calcd. for $C_{14}H_{20}O_5Na^+$, 291.1203). For ^{1}H-NMR data, see Figure S13.

3.7. Preparation of (R)- and (S)-MTPA Esters of **1b**

Compound **1** (1 mg, 3.73 μmol) was dissolved in 0.5 mL of anhydrous pyridine-d$_5$, and (S)-MTPA chloride (5 μL, 26.5 μmol) was added under N$_2$. The mixture was allowed to react for 36 h at room temperature. Further purification of the (R)-MTPA ester of **1** using semi-preparative HPLC with an ODS C18 column afforded the (R)-MTPA esters of **1a** and **1b**. The (S)-MTPA esters of **1a** and **1b** were prepared with (R)-MTPA chloride and were purified in the same manner [43].

3.8. Bioassay

The EcGUS inhibition assay was performed according to the method previously reported, employing DSL as the positive control [44]. The results are presented as means ± SD for three independent experiments.

4. Discussion

With the rapid development of bioinformatics, genome mining strategies have been widely applied to discover new natural products. By combining SSN analysis and phylogenetic tree construction, we can identify enzymes and genes with potential new functions. Using this approach, we discovered a unique PT that can transfer an isopropyl group to an aromatic nucleus, forming C-C or C-O bonds. Utilizing PT-guided separation techniques, we isolated a pair of novel hydroxyphenylacetic acid derivative enantiomers with prenyl units, (±)-peniprenydiol A, from the rice extracts of *Penicillium* sp. W21C371. The structure was formed through a crucial step involving PT catalysis, based on the known structure of p-hydroxy phenylacetic acid. In natural product studies, these compounds can appear in different enantiomeric forms. One form is a racemate, an equal mixture of two enantiomers, while the other form consists of non-racemic enantiomers in an unequal mixture. Currently, researchers focus more on racemic natural products, while non-racemic enantiomers are largely overlooked. This is because the optical purity of new natural products is rarely reported upon publication. It is usually assumed that when new chiral natural products exhibit optical activity, they are also optically pure. We measured the optical rotation of **1** [$\alpha]_D^{20}$: +14 (c 0.1, MeOH) and considered it optically pure. Subsequently, using a modified Mosher method to determine the configuration of its 8-OH group, we found that the compound exists as non-racemic enantiomers in unequal proportions. This compound was separated by chiral chromatography to obtain a pair of non-racemic enantiomers, (−)-**1** and (+)-**1**.

Citridone A (**2**), featuring a unique phenyl-R-furopyridone skeleton (6-6/5/5 ring system), belongs to the citridone family of fungal pyridines and was first isolated by Ōmura and co-workers from *Penicillium* sp. FKI-1938. It was identified as a potentiator of miconazole against *Candida albicans* [45]. Additionally, it could inhibit the biosynthesis of staphyloxanthin, a key virulence factor in methicillin-resistant *Staphylococcus aureus* (MRSA), rendering it a promising antibiotic lead with a new mode of action [46]. As a result, citridone A (**2**) has drawn attention from both chemists and biochemists. The total synthesis of citridone A (**2**) was accomplished in 2011 [47], while the biosynthetic pathway was unveiled in 2020 [48]. Compounds **3**–**10** are derivatives of ergosterol, a representative fungisterol that is a component of the fungal cell membrane and determines the fluidity, permeability, and activity of membrane-associated proteins in fungi [49]. Compounds **3**–**5** are notable in this series of fungal sterols for harboring an additional C-23 methyl group, which was proposed to be formed by *S*-adenosyl-*L*-methine (SAM) [50]. Preliminary structure–activity relationship studies suggest that both the C-23 methyl group and $\Delta^{9(11)}$ double bond play important roles in retaining the EcGUS-inhibitory activity, as seen in the activity of **3**, **4**, and **8**. To the best of our knowledge, **2** and **3** represent the first citridone and ergosterol derivatives with potent EcGUS-inhibitory activity. Morelsin D (**15**) and conocenolide A (**16**) are tremulane sesquiterpenoids that have been only reported from Basidiomycetes so far. It is worth noting that our work represents the first report of tremulane sesquiterpenoids from Ascomycetes. The well-established genetic manipulation systems in Ascomycetes, particularly within the genus *Penicillium*, may facilitate biosynthetic studies and the metabolic engineering of this type of sesquiterpenoid.

5. Conclusions

In summary, we conducted a comprehensive genome mining analysis using genomic data from our lab, the InterPro database, and the publicly available NCBI database. Through this analysis, we identified a unique PT capable of catalyzing the transfer of a prenyl group to an aromatic nucleus, forming C-C or C-O bonds. From the marine fungus *Penicillium* sp. W21C371, a pair of novel hydroxyphenylacetic acid derivative enantiomers, (±)-peniprenydiol A (**1**) with prenyl units, along with sixteen known compounds **2**–**17**, were isolated through PT-guided isolation. The plausible biosynthetic pathways of compound **1** were deduced. This study also marks the first time that tremulane sesquiterpenoids, exemplified by morelsin D (**15**) and conocenolide A (**16**), have been obtained from Ascomycetes. Additionally, compounds **2** and **3** were identified as potent EcGUS inhibitors for the first time, exhibiting non-competitive and mixed-type inhibition, respectively.

Supplementary Materials: The following supporting information can be downloaded at: https://www.mdpi.com/article/10.3390/md22070296/s1, Table S1: Inhibition kinetics of **2** and **3** against EcGUS; Table S2: Selected ^{1}H (600 MHz) NMR data of **1b** and its MTPA esters in Pyridine-d_5 (δ_H in ppm, *J* in Hz); Table S3: Putative functions of selected genes from peniprenydiol A gene cluster. Figure S1: HPLC-DAD chromatogram of twenty-one extracts of *Penicillium* sp. W21C371; Figure S2: ^{1}H NMR spectrum of **1** in Acetone-d_6 (600 MHz); Figure S3: ^{13}C NMR spectrum of **1** in Acetone-d_6 (150 MHz); Figure S4: DEPT spectrum of **1** in Acetone-d_6; Figure S5: HSQC spectrum of **1** in Acetone-d_6; Figure S6: ^{1}H-^{1}H COSY spectrum of **1** in Acetone-d_6; Figure S7: HMBC spectrum of **1** in Acetone-d_6; Figure S8: The IR spectrum of **1**; Figure S9: The HRESIMS spectroscopic data of **1**; Figure S10: UV spectrum of **1**; Figure S11: Chiral HPLC separation profile of **1a**/**1b**; Figure S12: ^{1}H NMR spectrum of **1a** in Pyridine-d_5 (600 MHz); Figure S13: ^{1}H NMR spectrum of **1b** in Pyridine-d_5 (600 MHz); Figure S14: The HRESIMS spectrum of compound **1a**; Figure S15: The HRESIMS spectrum of compound **1b**; Figure S16: ^{1}H NMR spectrum of (*R*)-MTPA ester of **1b** in Pyridine-d_5 (600 MHz); Figure S17: ^{1}H NMR spectrum of (*S*)-MTPA ester of **1b** in Pyridine-d_5 (600 MHz).

Author Contributions: Conceptualization, project administration, and funding acquisition, Y.Y. and H.W.; methodology, C.W. (Cancan Wang) and Y.F.; software, J.T. and Y.Q.; formal analysis, K.X. and Y.D.; investigation, C.W. (Chenjie Wang) and Y.L.; resources, C.W. (Cancan Wang); data curation, Y.Y.; writing—original draft preparation, C.W. (Cancan Wang) and Y.F.; writing—review and editing, Y.Y. and H.W. All authors have read and agreed to the published version of the manuscript.

Funding: This research was funded by the National Key Research and Development Program of China (No. 2022YFC2804205 and 2022YFC2804104), the Natural Foundation of Zhejiang Province (LGF21H300003), the National Natural Science Foundation of China (No. 42276137), and the Key Research and Development Program of Zhejiang Province (No. 2021C03084).

Institutional Review Board Statement: Not applicable.

Data Availability Statement: Data are contained within the article or Supplementary Materials.

Conflicts of Interest: The authors declare no conflicts of interest.

References

1. Perrone, G.; Susca, A. *Penicillium* species and their associated mycotoxins. *Methods Mol. Biol.* **2017**, *1542*, 107–119.
2. Petersen, C.; Sørensen, T.; Nielsen, M.R.; Sondergaard, T.E.; Sørensen, J.L.; Fitzpatrick, D.A.; Frisvad, J.C.; Nielsen, K.L. Comparative genomic study of the *Penicillium* genus elucidates a diverse pangenome and 15 lateral gene transfer events. *IMA Fungus* **2023**, *14*, 3. [CrossRef]
3. Houbraken, J.; Frisvad, J.C.; Samson, R.A. Fleming's penicillin producing strain is not *Penicillium chrysogenum* but *P. rubens*. *IMA Fungus* **2011**, *2*, 87–95. [CrossRef]
4. Nielsen, J.C.; Grijseels, S.; Prigent, S.; Ji, B.; Dainat, J.; Nielsen, K.F.; Frisvad, J.C.; Workman, M.; Nielsen, J. Global analysis of biosynthetic gene clusters reveals vast potential of secondary metabolite production in *Penicillium* species. *Nat. Microbiol.* **2017**, *2*, 17044–17053. [CrossRef]
5. Shu, W.S.; Huang, L.N. Microbial diversity in extreme environments. *Nat. Rev. Microbiol.* **2022**, *20*, 219–235. [CrossRef]
6. König, G.M.; Kehraus, S.; Seibert, S.F.; Abdel-Lateff, A.; Müller, D. Natural products from marine organisms and their associated microbes. *Chembiochem.* **2006**, *7*, 229–238. [CrossRef]
7. Ma, H.G.; Liu, Q.; Zhu, G.L.; Liu, H.S.; Zhu, W.M. Marine natural products sourced from marine-derived *Penicillium* fungi. *J. Asian Nat. Prod. Res.* **2016**, *18*, 92–115. [CrossRef]
8. Liu, S.; Su, M.; Song, S.J.; Jung, J.H. Marine-derived *Penicillium* species as producers of cytotoxic metabolites. *Mar. Drugs* **2017**, *15*, 329. [CrossRef]
9. Yang, X.; Liu, J.; Mei, J.; Jiang, R.; Tu, S.; Deng, H.; Liu, J.; Yang, S.; Li, J. Origins, structures, and bioactivities of secondary metabolites from marine-derived *Penicillium* fungi. *Mini-Rev. Med. Chem.* **2021**, *21*, 2000–2019. [CrossRef]
10. Hu, X.Y.; Li, X.M.; Yang, S.Q.; Liu, H.; Meng, L.H.; Wang, B.G. Three new sesquiterpenoids from the algal-derived fungus *Penicillium chermesinum* EN-480. *Mar. Drugs* **2020**, *18*, 194. [CrossRef]
11. Shah, M.; Sun, C.; Sun, Z.; Zhang, G.; Che, Q.; Gu, Q.; Zhu, T.; Li, D. Antibacterial polyketides from antarctica sponge-derived fungus *Penicillium* sp. HDN151272. *Mar. Drugs* **2020**, *18*, 71. [CrossRef]
12. Chen, J.; Wang, W.; Hu, X.; Yue, Y.; Lu, X.; Wang, C.; Wei, B.; Zhang, H.; Wang, H. Medium-sized peptides from microbial sources with potential for antibacterial drug development. *Nat. Prod. Rep.* 2024; ahead of print. [CrossRef]
13. Li, F.L.; Sun, W.G.; Zhang, S.T.; Gao, W.X.; Lin, S.; Yang, B.Y.; Chai, C.W.; Li, H.Q.; Wang, J.P.; Hu, Z.X.; et al. New cyclopiane diterpenes with anti-inflammatory activity from the sea sediment-derived fungus *Penicillium* sp. TJ403-2. *Chin. Chem. Lett.* **2020**, *31*, 197–201. [CrossRef]
14. Dai, L.T.; Yang, L.; Kong, F.D.; Ma, Q.Y.; Xie, Q.Y.; Dai, H.F.; Yu, Z.F.; Zhao, Y.X. Cytotoxic indole-diterpenoids from the marine-derived fungus *Penicillium* sp. KFD28. *Mar. Drugs* **2021**, *19*, 613. [CrossRef]
15. Pang, X.; Zhou, X.; Lin, X.; Yang, B.; Tian, X.; Wang, J.; Xu, S.; Liu, Y. Structurally various sorbicillinoids from the deep-sea sediment derived fungus *Penicillium* sp. SCSIO06871. *Bioorg. Chem.* **2021**, *107*, 104600. [CrossRef]
16. Wang, P.; Jia, Y.; Wu, R.; Chen, Z.; Yan, R. Human gut bacterial β-glucuronidase inhibition: An emerging approach to manage medication therapy. *Biochem. Pharmacol.* **2021**, *190*, 114566. [CrossRef]
17. Chen, S.; Yueh, M.F.; Bigo, C.; Barbier, O.; Wang, K.; Karin, M.; Nguyen, N.; Tukey, R.H. Intestinal glucuronidation protects against chemotherapy-induced toxicity by irinotecan (CPT-11). *Proc. Natl. Acad. Sci. USA* **2013**, *110*, 19143–19148. [CrossRef]
18. Bauman, K.D.; Butler, K.S.; Moore, B.S.; Chekan, J.R. Genome mining methods to discover bioactive natural products. *Nat. Prod. Rep.* **2021**, *38*, 2100–2129. [CrossRef]
19. Chevrette, M.G.; Gavrilidou, A.; Mantri, S.; Selem-Mojica, N.; Ziemert, N.; Barona-Gómez, F. The confluence of big data and evolutionary genome mining for the discovery of natural products. *Nat. Prod. Rep.* **2021**, *38*, 2024–2040. [CrossRef]
20. Fredimoses, M.; Zhou, X.; Ai, W.; Tian, X.; Yang, B.; Lin, X.; Xian, J.Y.; Liu, Y. Westerdijkin A, a new hydroxyphenylacetic acid derivative from deep sea fungus *Aspergillus westerdijkiae* SCSIO 05233. *Nat. Prod. Res.* **2015**, *29*, 158–162. [CrossRef]
21. Pockrandt, D.; Ludwig, L.; Fan, A.; König, G.M.; Li, S.M. New insights into the biosynthesis of prenylated xanthones: Xptb from *Aspergillus nidulans* catalyses an O-prenylation of xanthones. *ChemBioChem* **2012**, *13*, 2764–2771. [CrossRef]
22. Zeyhle, P.; Bauer, J.S.; Steimle, M.; Leipoldt, F.; Rösch, M.; Kalinowski, J.; Gross, H.; Heide, L. A membrane-bound prenyltransferase catalyzes the O-Prenylation of 1,6-dihydroxyphenazine in the marine bacterium *Streptomyces* sp. CNQ-509. *ChemBioChem* **2014**, *15*, 2385–2392. [CrossRef]
23. Wang, F.; Fang, Y.; Zhang, M.; Lin, A.; Zhu, T.; Gu, Q.; Zhu, W. Six new ergosterols from the marine-derived fungus *Rhizopus* sp. *Steroids* **2008**, *73*, 19–26. [CrossRef]
24. Fukuda, T.; Tomoda, H.; Omura, S. Citridones, new potentiators of antifungal miconazole activity, produced by *Penicillium* sp. FKH938. II. Structure elucidation. *J. Antibiot.* **2005**, *58*, 315–321. [CrossRef]
25. Yaoita, Y.; Amemiya, K.; Ohnuma, H.; Furumura, K.; Masaki, A.; Matsuki, T.; Kikuchi, M. Sterol constituents from five edible mushrooms. *Chem. Pharm. Bull.* **1998**, *46*, 944–950. [CrossRef]
26. Ohnuma, N.; Amemiya, K.; Kakuda, R.; Yaoita, Y.; Machida, K.; Kikuchi, M. Sterol constituents from two edible mushrooms, *Lentinula edodes* and *Tricholoma matsutake*. *Chem. Pharm. Bull.* **2000**, *48*, 749–751. [CrossRef]

27. Lee, W.Y.; Park, Y.; Ahn, J.K.; Park, S. Cytotoxic activity of ergosta-4,6,8(14),22-tetraen-3-one from the sclerotia of *Polyporus umbellatus*. *Bull. Korean Chem. Soc.* **2005**, *26*, 1464–1466.
28. Liu, X.H.; Miao, F.P.; Liang, X.R. Ergosteroid derivatives from an algicolous strain of *Aspergillus ustus*. *Nat. Prod. Res.* **2014**, *28*, 1182–1186. [CrossRef]
29. Wang, X.H.; Hou, Y.Z.; Pan, X.H.; Wang, Q. Sterol compounds and their anti-complementary activities of *Cordia dichotoma*. *Chem. Nat. Compd.* **2020**, *56*, 759–760. [CrossRef]
30. Amagata, T.; Tanaka, M.; Yamada, T.; Doi, M.; Minoura, K.; Ohishi, H.; Yamori, T.; Numata, A. Variation in cytostatic constituents of a sponge-derived *Gymnascella dankaliensis* by manipulating the carbon source. *J. Nat. Prod.* **2007**, *70*, 1731–1740. [CrossRef]
31. Amagata, T.; Doi, M.; Tohgo, M.; Minoura, K.; Numata, A. Dankasterone, a new class of cytotoxic steroid produced by a *Gymnascella* species from a marine sponge. *Chem. Commun.* **1999**, *30*, 1321–1322. [CrossRef]
32. Ghisalberti, E.; Hockless, D.; Rowland, C. Structural study of curvularin, a cell division inhibitor. *Aust. J. Chem.* **1993**, *46*, 571–577. [CrossRef]
33. Zhao, L.; Zhang, H. Isolation of Secondary. Metabolites of 9F series marine fungi and their bioactivities against *Pyricularia oryzae*. *Nat. Prod. Res. Dev.* **2005**, *17*, 677–680.
34. Kusano, M.; Nakagami, K.; Fujioka, S.; Kawano, T.; Shimada, A.; Kimura, Y. βγ-dehydrocurvularin and related compounds as nematicides of *Pratylenchus penetrans* from the fungus *Aspergillus* sp. *Biosci. Biotechnol. Biochem.* **2003**, *67*, 1413–1416. [CrossRef]
35. Wu, Y.H.; Zhang, Z.H.; Zhong, Y.; Huang, J.J.; Li, X.X.; Jiang, J.Y.; Deng, Y.Y.; Zhang, L.H.; He, F. Sumalactones A–D, four new curvularin-type macrolides from a marine deep sea fungus *Penicillium sumatrense*. *RSC Adv.* **2017**, *7*, 40015–40019. [CrossRef]
36. Yang, C.; Meng, Q.; Zhang, Y.; Hu, Y.; Xiao, S.J.; Zhang, Y.Q.; Ju, J.H.; Fu, S.B. Morelsins A–F, six sesquiterpenoids from the liquid culture of *Morchella importuna*. *Tetrahedron* **2020**, *76*, 131356. [CrossRef]
37. Liu, D.Z.; Wang, F.; Liu, J.K. Sesquiterpenes from cultures of the basidiomycete *Conocybe siliginea*. *J. Nat. Prod.* **2007**, *70*, 1503–1506. [CrossRef]
38. Wu, B.; Wu, L.J.; Zhang, L. Studies on the antibacterial chemical components of *Senecio cannabifolius less* (I). *J. Shenyang Pharm. Univ.* **2004**, *21*, 341–345. (In Chinese)
39. Ward, L.C.; McCue, H.V.; Carnell, A.J. Carboxyl methyltransferases: Natural functions and potential applications in industrial biotechnology. *ChemCatChem* **2021**, *13*, 121–128. [CrossRef]
40. Munakata, R.; Olry, A.; Takemura, T.; Tatsumi, K.; Ichino, T.; Villard, C.; Kageyama, J.; Kurata, T.; Nakayasu, M.; Jacob, F.; et al. Parallel evolution of UbiA superfamily proteins into aromatic O-prenyltransferases in plants. *Proc. Natl. Acad. Sci. USA* **2021**, *118*, e2022294118. [CrossRef]
41. Sanger, F.; Nicklen, S.; Coulson, A.R. DNA sequencing with chain-terminating inhibitors. *Proc. Natl. Acad. Sci. USA* **1977**, *74*, 5463–5467. [CrossRef]
42. Oberg, N.; Zallot, R.; John, A. EFI-EST, EFI-GNT, and EFI-CGFP: Enzyme Function Initiative (EFI) web resource for genomic enzymology tools. *J. Mol. Biol.* **2023**, *435*, 168018. [CrossRef]
43. Hoye, T.R.; Jeffrey, C.S.; Shao, F. Mosher ester analysis for the determination of absolute configuration of stereogenic (chiral) carbinol carbons. *Nat. Protoc.* **2007**, *2*, 2451–2458. [CrossRef]
44. Zhou, T.S.; Wei, B.; He, M.; Li, Y.S.; Wang, Y.K.; Wang, S.J.; Chen, J.W.; Zhang, H.W.; Cui, Z.N.; Wang, H. Thiazolidin-2-cyanamides derivatives as novel potent *Escherichia coli* β-glucuronidase inhibitors and their structure–inhibitory activity relationships. *J. Enzyme Inhib. Med. Chem.* **2020**, *35*, 1736–1742. [CrossRef]
45. Fukuda, T.; Hasegawa, Y.; Sakabe, Y.; Tomoda, H.; Omura, S. Citrinamides, new potentiators of antifungal miconazole activity, produced by *Penicillium* sp. FKI-1938. *J. Antibiot.* **2008**, *61*, 550–555. [CrossRef]
46. Fukuda, T.; Shimoyama, K.; Nagamitsu, T.; Tomoda, H. Synthesis and biological activity of citridone A and its derivatives. *J. Antibiot.* **2014**, *67*, 445–450. [CrossRef]
47. Zhang, Z.; Qiao, T.; Watanabe, K.; Tang, Y. Concise biosynthesis of phenylfuropyridones in fungi. *Angew. Chem. Int. Ed.* **2020**, *59*, 19889–19893. [CrossRef]
48. Miyagawa, T.; Nagai, K.; Yamada, A.; Sugihara, Y.; Fukuda, T.; Fukuda, T.; Uchida, R.; Tomoda, H.; Omura, S.; Nagamitsu, T. Total synthesis of citridone A. *Org. Lett.* **2011**, *13*, 1158–1161. [CrossRef]
49. Ermakova, E.; Zuev, Y. Effect of ergosterol on the fungal membrane properties. All-atom and coarse-grained molecular dynamics study. *Chem. Phys. Lipids* **2017**, *209*, 45–53. [CrossRef]
50. Nes, W.D. Enzyme mechanisms for sterol C-methylations. *Phytochemistry* **2003**, *64*, 75–95. [CrossRef]

Disclaimer/Publisher's Note: The statements, opinions and data contained in all publications are solely those of the individual author(s) and contributor(s) and not of MDPI and/or the editor(s). MDPI and/or the editor(s) disclaim responsibility for any injury to people or property resulting from any ideas, methods, instructions or products referred to in the content.

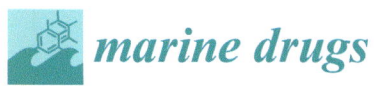 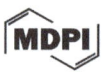

Article

Meroterpenoids from Marine Sponge *Hyrtios* sp. and Their Anticancer Activity against Human Colorectal Cancer Cells

Jie Wang [1,*,†], Yue-Lu Yan [1,†], Xin-Yi Yu [1], Jia-Yan Pan [1], Xin-Lian Liu [1], Li-Li Hong [2,*] and Bin Wang [1,*]

[1] Zhejiang Provincial Engineering Technology Research Center of Marine Biomedical Products, School of Food and Pharmacy, Zhejiang Ocean University, Zhoushan 316022, China; yyuelu03@163.com (Y.-L.Y.); 17355410304@163.com (X.-Y.Y.); pjy2388@163.com (J.-Y.P.); lxl19960817@163.com (X.-L.L.)
[2] Research Center for Marine Drugs, Department of Pharmacy, Ren Ji Hospital, School of Medicine, Shanghai Jiao Tong University, Shanghai 200127, China
* Correspondence: 011103@zjou.edu.cn (J.W.); hongll0792@sjtu.edu.cn (L.-L.H.); wangbin@zjou.edu.cn (B.W.)
† These authors contributed equally to this work.

Abstract: Two new meroterpenoids, hyrtamide A (**1**) and hyrfarnediol A (**2**), along with two known ones, 3-farnesyl-4-hydroxybenzoic acid methyl ester (**3**) and dictyoceratin C (**4**), were isolated from a South China Sea sponge *Hyrtios* sp. Their structures were elucidated by NMR and MS data. Compounds **2**–**4** exhibited weak cytotoxicity against human colorectal cancer cells (HCT-116), showing IC$_{50}$ values of 41.6, 45.0, and 37.3 μM, respectively. Furthermore, compounds **3** and **4** significantly suppressed the invasion of HCT-116 cells while also downregulating the expression of vascular endothelial growth factor receptor 1 (VEGFR-1) and vimentin proteins, which are key markers associated with angiogenesis and epithelial–mesenchymal transition (EMT). Our findings suggest that compounds **3** and **4** may exert their anti-invasive effects on tumor cells by inhibiting the expression of VEGFR-1 and impeding the process of EMT.

Keywords: marine sponge; *Hyrtios* sp.; meroterpenoids; invasion; VEGFR-1; colorectal cancer

Citation: Wang, J.; Yan, Y.-L.; Yu, X.-Y.; Pan, J.-Y.; Liu, X.-L.; Hong, L.-L.; Wang, B. Meroterpenoids from Marine Sponge *Hyrtios* sp. and Their Anticancer Activity against Human Colorectal Cancer Cells. *Mar. Drugs* **2024**, *22*, 183. https://doi.org/10.3390/md22040183

Academic Editors: Hong Wang, Huawei Zhang and Bin Wei

Received: 8 April 2024
Revised: 16 April 2024
Accepted: 17 April 2024
Published: 19 April 2024

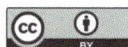

Copyright: © 2024 by the authors. Licensee MDPI, Basel, Switzerland. This article is an open access article distributed under the terms and conditions of the Creative Commons Attribution (CC BY) license (https://creativecommons.org/licenses/by/4.0/).

1. Introduction

Colorectal cancer (CRC) ranks as the third most prevalent malignancy globally and represents the second leading cause of cancer-related mortality, with an annual incidence of 1.9 million cases and over 0.9 million deaths worldwide [1]. Over 90% of cancer deaths are caused by metastasis of cancer cells [2], making the treatment of metastatic colorectal cancer (mCRC) a significant clinical challenge at present. The surgical prognosis for patients with colorectal cancer is intricately linked to the tumor-node-metastasis (TNM) staging system; patients with stage I–III have five-year survival rates of approximately 90%, 75%, and 50%, respectively. In contrast, those with stage IV disease have a five-year survival rate of less than 5%. Furthermore, a considerable proportion of patients diagnosed with stage II and III colorectal cancer, ranging from 29% to 60%, still experience local recurrence or distant metastases after undergoing surgery [3]. Consequently, addressing tumor metastasis emerges as an urgent imperative in the therapeutic management of colorectal cancer.

Vascular endothelial growth factor receptor (VEGFR), a pivotal regulator of angiogenesis and vascular permeability [4], plays an indispensable role in various biological processes including tumor neovascularization, invasion of tumor cells, and metastasis [5,6]. The VEGFR family primarily comprises three subtypes: namely, VEGFR-1, VEGFR-2, and VEGFR-3 [7]. VEGFR-1, a VEGF receptor with high affinity, exerts specific effects on endothelial cells [8]. In addition to its involvement in tumor vasculature, the activation of VEGFR-1 present in tumor cells through ligand interaction has the potential to stimulate cellular chemotaxis and infiltration into the surrounding extracellular matrix [9]. Colorectal cancer exhibited the presence of VEGFR-1, and its interaction with ligands augmented the migratory and invasive potential of tumor cells [8,9]. Additionally, activation of VEGFR-1 promotes epithelial–mesenchymal transition (EMT), suggesting that VEGFR-1 may initiate EMT to facilitate tumor metastasis [10].

Meroterpenoids are composed of terpenoid units (mevalonic acid pathway) and non-terpenoid units (including polyketide pathways, amino acid pathways, shikimic acid pathways, and other biosynthetic pathways) [11]. The structural and biological diversity of meroterpenoids is attributed to the diverse terpenoid units (including chain length, cyclization, rearrangement, etc.), intricate non-terpenoid moieties, and various modes of molecular aggregation [12,13]. Marine sponges, being a significant reservoir of natural marine products [14], exhibit an annual average production of over 200 novel compounds [15], with a notable abundance in meroterpenoids which display various biological activities, such as anti-tumor [16], anti-inflammation [17], anti-microbial [18], anti-oxidant [19], anti-leishmanial [20] and enzyme inhibitory [21] activities. Meroterpenoids from marine sponges exert anti-tumor effects by arresting the cell cycle progression, inducing apoptosis, suppressing tumor angiogenesis, and inhibiting invasion and metastasis [22,23].

The marine sponges belonging to the *Hyrtios* genus have demonstrated their potential as a valuable reservoir of novel and biologically active compounds, such as alkaloids, meroterpenoids, and sesterterpenes, and many of them exhibit significant anti-tumor activity [24]. In our ongoing efforts to explore novel and bioactive compounds derived from marine sponges [25–27], two new meroterpenoids, hyrtamide A (**1**) and hyrfarnediol A (**2**), as well as two previously reported meroterpenoids, 3-farnesyl-4-hydroxybenzoic acid methyl ester (**3**) [28] and dictyoceratin C (**4**) [29] (Figure 1), were discovered in a marine sponge *Hyrtios* sp. Herein, we discuss the isolation, structural analysis, and cytotoxicity of these meroterpenoids, as well as the anti-invasion effects on colorectal cancer HCT-116 cells of compounds **3** and **4**.

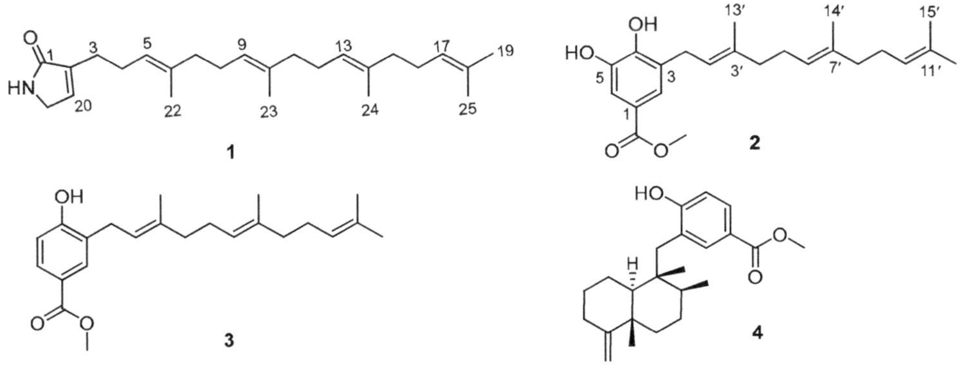

Figure 1. Structures of compounds **1–4**.

2. Results

2.1. Structural Determination

Compound **1** was yielded as a yellowish oil. The molecular formula of **1** was determined as $C_{25}H_{39}NO$ based on the HRESIMS ion peak at m/z 392.2914 [M + Na]$^+$ (calculated for $C_{25}H_{39}NONa$, 392.2929), with seven degrees of unsaturation (Figure S1). The ^{1}H NMR data (Table 1, Figure S3) showed five methyls at δ_H 1.60 (br s, H-22, 23, 24, 25) and 1.68 (s, H-19), eight methylenes at δ_H 1.98 (m, H-7, 11, 15), 2.06 (m, H-8, 12, 16), 2.26 (q, J = 7.0 Hz, H-4), and 2.33 (t, J = 7.0 Hz, H-3), one N-methylene at δ_H 3.91 (t, J = 1.5 Hz, H-21), and five olefinic protons at δ_H 6.73 (q, J = 1.5 Hz, H-20), 5.15 (t, J = 7.0 Hz, H-5) and 5.11 (m, H-9, 13, 17). The ^{13}C NMR and DEPT135 spectra (Table 1, Figure S4) exhibited 25 carbon signals, including five methyl carbons [δ_C 16.2 (C-23, 24), 16.3 (C-22), 17.9 (C-25), 25.9 (C-19)], eight methylene carbons [δ_C 25.8 (C-3), 26.1 (C-4), 26.9 (C-12, 16), 27.0 (C-8), 39.9 (C-7, 11, 15)], one N-methylene carbon δ_C 46.6 (C-21), five methine carbons [δ_C 124.6 (C-17), 124.4 (C-9, 13), 123.5 (C-5), 137.7 (C-20)], five quaternary carbons [δ_C 131.5 (C-18), 135.1

(C-14), 135.2 (C-10), 136.3 (C-6), 139.7 (C-2)], and one carbonyl carbon δ_C 175.3 (C-1). The COSY correlation of H-20/H-21, combined with HMBC correlations from H-20 (δ_H 6.73) to C-1 (δ_C 175.3), C-2 (δ_C 139.7), and C-21 (δ_C 46.6), from H-21 (δ_H 3.91) to C-1 (δ_C 175.3) and C-2 (δ_C 139.7), and from H-3 (δ_H 2.33) to C-1 (δ_C 175.3), C-2 (δ_C 139.7), and C-20 (δ_C 137.7), led to the identification of a 3-en-α-pyrrolidone fragment (Figures 2, S6 and S7). The geranylgeranyl fragment was determined by COSY correlations of H-3/H-4/H-5, H-7/H-8/H-9, H-11/H-12/H-13, and H-15/H-16/H-17 and HMBC correlations from H-3 (δ_H 2.33) to C-5 (δ_C 123.5), from H-4 (δ_H 2.26) to C-2 (δ_C 139.7), C-5 (δ_C 123.5), and C-6 (δ_C 136.3), from H-5 (δ_H 5.15) to C-7 (δ_C 39.9) and C-22 (δ_C 16.3), from H-7, 11, 15 (δ_H 1.98) to C-5 (δ_C 123.5), C-9, 13 (δ_C 124.4), C-17 (δ_C 124.6), C-22 (δ_C 16.3) and C-23, 24 (δ_C 16.2), from H-9, 13, 17 (δ_H 5.11) to C-7, 11, 15 (δ_C 39.9), C-19 (δ_C 25.9) and C-23, 24 (δ_C 16.2), from H-19 (δ_H 1.68) to C-25 (δ_C 17.9), C-17 (δ_C 124.6) and C-18 (δ_C 131.5), and the methylene carbon C-3 was located at C-2 on the 3-en-α-pyrrolidone fragment which was demonstrated by the HMBC correlations from H-3 (δ_H 2.33) to C-1 (δ_C 175.3), C-2 (δ_C 139.7), and C-20 (δ_C 137.7), and the chemical shift of C-2 (δ_C 139.7, quaternary carbon). Therefore, the planar structure of compound **1** was obtained. The NOESY correlations (Figure S8) of H-4/H-22, H-5/H-7, H-8/H-23, H-9/H-11, H-12/H-24, and H-13/H-15, and the shielded chemical shifts of C-22 (δ_C 16.3), C-23 (δ_C 16.2), and C-24 (δ_C 16.2) suggested that $\Delta^{5,6}$, $\Delta^{9,10}$, and $\Delta^{13,14}$ double bonds were both E. Compound **1** was named hyrtamide A.

Table 1. ^{1}H and ^{13}C NMR data of compounds **1** and **2** in CDCl$_3$.

Position	1 (600 and 150 MHz)		Position	2 (400 and 100 MHz)	
	δ_C, Type	δ_H, Mult. (J in Hz)		δ_C, Type	δ_H, Mult. (J in Hz)
1	175.3, C		1	122.3, C	
2	139.7, C		2	124.0, CH	7.44, br s
3	25.8, CH$_2$	2.33, t (7.0)	3	127.3, C	
4	26.1, CH$_2$	2.26, q (7.0)	4	147.0, C	
5	123.5, CH	5.15, t (7.0)	5	146.7, C	
6	136.3, C		6	114.7, CH	7.46, br s
7	39.9, CH$_2$	1.98, m	1′	29.6, CH$_2$	3.40, d, (6.4)
8	27.0, CH$_2$	2.06, m	2′	121.3, CH	5.34, m
9	124.4, CH	5.11, m	3′	139.3, C	
10	135.2, C		4′	39.9, CH$_2$	2.11, m; 1.97, m
11	39.9, CH$_2$	1.98, m	5′	26.9, CH$_2$	2.04, m; 1.97, m
12	26.9, CH$_2$	2.06, m	6′	123.8, CH	5.10, m
13	124.4, CH	5.11, m	7′	135.9, C	
14	135.1, C		8′	39.9, CH$_2$	2.11, m; 1.97, m
15	39.9, CH$_2$	1.98, m	9′	26.6, CH$_2$	2.11, m
16	26.9, CH$_2$	2.06, m	10′	124.5, CH	5.10, m
17	124.6, CH	5.11, m	11′	131.6, C	
18	131.5, C		12′	25.9, CH$_3$	1.68, s
19	25.9, CH$_3$	1.68, s	13′	16.5, CH$_3$	1.79, s
20	137.7, CH	6.73, q (1.5)	14′	16.3, CH$_3$	1.60, s
21	46.6, CH$_2$	3.91, t (1.5)	15′	17.9, CH$_3$	1.60, s
22	16.3, CH$_3$	1.60, s	1-C=O	167.4, C	
23	16.2, CH$_3$	1.60, s	-OCH$_3$	52.2, CH$_3$	3.87, s
24	16.2, CH$_3$	1.60, s			
25	17.9, CH$_3$	1.60, s			

Compound **2** was a yellowish powder, and exhibited a positive HRESIMS ion peak at m/z 373.2377 [M + H]$^+$ (calculated for C$_{23}$H$_{33}$O$_4$, 373.2379), indicating its molecular formula as C$_{23}$H$_{32}$O$_4$, corresponding to eight degrees of unsaturation (Figure S9). The ^{1}H and ^{13}C NMR data (Table 1, Figures S11 and S12) were characterized by the presence of two aromatic methines at δ_H 7.46 (br s, H-6)/δ_C 114.7 and δ_H 7.44 (br s, H-2)/δ_C 124.0, suggesting the two aromatic protons were in the meta position. Further examination of the ^{1}H and ^{13}C NMR data of **2** revealed the presence of three olefinic methines [δ_H 5.10 (m,

H-6′, 10′) and 5.34 (m, H-2′); δ_C 123.8, 124.5, and 121.3], an oxygenated methyl [δ_H 3.87 (s), δ_C 52.2], and four methyls [δ_H 1.60 (br s, H-14′, 15′), 1.58 (s, H-12′), and 1.79 (s, H-13′); δ_C 16.3, 17.9, 25.9, and 16.5]. The HMBC correlations (Figures 3 and S14) from H-2 (δ_H 7.44) to 1-C=O (δ_C 167.4), C-4 (δ_C 147.0), and C-6 (δ_C 114.7), from H-6 (δ_H 7.46) to 1-C=O (δ_C 167.4) and C-5 (δ_C 146.7), and from -OCH$_3$ (δ_H 3.87) to 1-C=O (δ_C 167.4) indicated the presence of a 4,5-dihydroxybenzoic acid methyl ester. The COSY correlations (Figure S15) of H-1′/H-2′, H-5′/H-6′, and H-9′/H-10′, combined with HMBC correlations from H-1′ (δ_H 3.40) to C-3′ (δ_C 139.3), from H-4′ (δ_H 2.11, 1.97) to C-3′ (δ_C 139.3) and C-6′ (δ_C 123.8), from H-8′ (δ_H 2.11, 1.97) to C-6′ (δ_C 123.8) and C-9′ (δ_C 26.6), from H-15′ (δ_H 1.60) to C-10′ (δ_C 124.5) and C-12′ (δ_C 25.9), from H-14′ (δ_H 1.60) to C-6′ (δ_C 123.8) and C-8′ (δ_C 39.9), from H-13′ (δ_H 1.79) to C-2′ (δ_C 121.3) and C-4′ (δ_C 39.9) indicated the presence of a farnesyl fragment. The HMBC correlations from H-1′ (δ_H 3.40) to C-2 (δ_C 124.0), C-3 (δ_C 127.3), and C-4 (δ_C 147.0) revealed that the farnesyl moiety was attached to C-3 of the benzene ring. E-configurations of the $\Delta^{2',3'}$ and $\Delta^{6',7'}$ double bonds in the farnesyl fragment of **2** were confirmed based on the NOESY interactions (Figure S16) of H-2′/H-4′, H-6′/H-8′, H-1′/H-13′, and H-5′/H-14′, and the shielded chemical shifts of C-13′ (δ_C 16.5) and C-14′ (δ_C 16.3). Consequently, the structure of **2** was assigned as 3-farnesyl-4,5-dihydroxybenzoic acid methyl ester and named hyrfarnediol A.

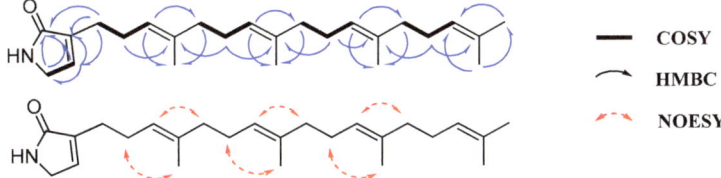

Figure 2. The key COSY, HMBC, and NOESY correlations of compound **1**.

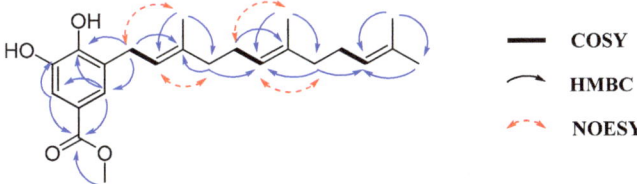

Figure 3. The key COSY, HMBC, and NOESY correlations of compound **2**.

The two known meroterpenoids, 3-farnesyl-4-hydroxybenzoic acid methyl ester (**3**) [28] and dictyoceratin C (**4**) [29], were identified by comparing their NMR and MS data (Figures S17–S22) with the values reported in the existing literature.

2.2. Bioactive Assay

2.2.1. Cytotoxicity of Compounds **1**–**4** against HCT-116 Cells

Colorectal cancer stands as one of the most frequently diagnosed malignant neoplasms within the gastrointestinal tract. The World Health Organization's statistics place CRC as the third most common type of cancer globally, characterized by its high incidence and mortality rates, along with a significant propensity for metastasis [30]. Numerous meroterpenoids have been identified to exhibit potent inhibitory effects on HCT-116 cells—a cell line derived from human colorectal carcinoma [23]. In view of this, we assessed the cytotoxic effect against HCT-116 cells of compounds **1**–**4** utilizing the MTT assay method (Table 2). Compounds **2**–**4** showed weak cytotoxicity towards HCT-116 cells, with IC$_{50}$ values of 41.6, 45.0, and 37.3 μM, respectively; however, compound **1** failed to manifest any inhibitory effect even at a concentration level of up to 54 μM. Nevertheless, owing to the insufficient quantity of compound **2** for subsequent activity analyses, we opted to proceed with cell invasion experiments using compounds **3** and **4**.

Table 2. Cytotoxic activities of compounds **2**–**4** against HCT-116.

Compound	IC$_{50}$ (µM)
2	41.6 ± 3.8
3	45.0 ± 3.0
4	37.3 ± 3.3
Doxorubicin	3.8 ± 0.1

2.2.2. Anti-Invasive Activity of **3** and **4** in HCT-116 Cells

More than 90% of cancer deaths result from the metastasis of cancer cells [2]. Invasion takes place at an early stage of the metastatic process and represents a pivotal step in this progression [31,32]. Many meroterpenoids demonstrated significant anti-invasive activity, including sponge-derived terpene quinones/phenols strongylophorine-26 and avinosol [33,34]. To evaluate the impact of compounds **3** and **4** on HCT-116 cell invasiveness, we employed Transwell assays. The results demonstrated that at concentrations of 3, 9, and 27 µM, there were notable decreases in cell invasion capabilities in a dose-dependent manner (Figure 4).

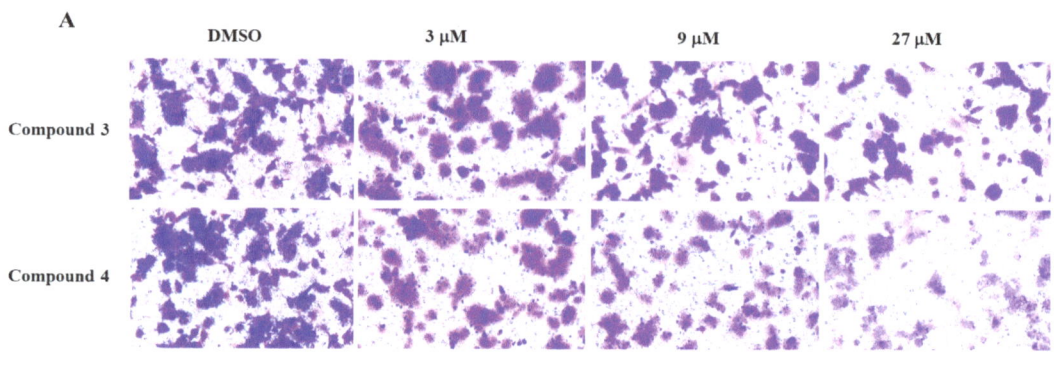

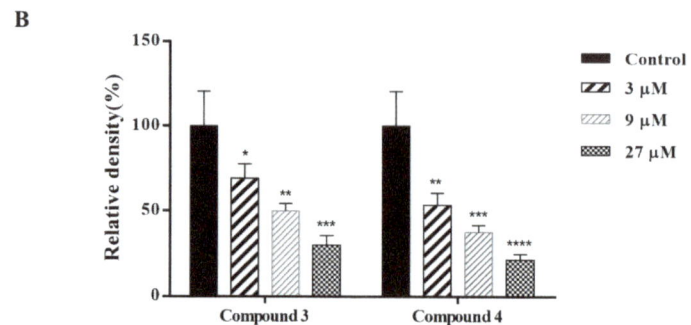

Figure 4. The inhibiting effects of compounds **3** and **4** on the invasion activity of HCT 116 cells. (**A**) Representative images in the invasion assay; (**B**) Relative percentage of invaded cells. Data are presented as the mean ± standard deviation (n = 3). * p < 0.05, ** p < 0.01, *** p < 0.001, **** p < 0.0001.

2.2.3. Effects of **3** and **4** on Expressions of VEGFR-1 and Vimentin

To elucidate the underlying mechanisms responsible for the inhibitory effects of compounds **3** and **4** on cell invasion in HCT-116 cells, proteins associated with EMT and metastasis were analyzed. VEGFR-1 is one of the VEGF receptors, which in tumor cells can be activated by its ligands (such as VEGF-B and PlGF) to significantly increase the invasion capabilities of the tumor cells [9]. This receptor is also closely associated with the process of EMT, which is linked to metastasis [10]. Tumor cells undergoing EMT exhibit alterations in relevant molecular biomarkers [35]. Vimentin serves as a critical biomarker for EMT, which is typically expressed in mesenchymal cells. Its expression levels become upregulated during the process of cancer metastasis [36]. During EMT, vimentin undergoes reorganization and mediates signaling pathways, all the while providing structural support to various cellular organelles due to its unique viscoelastic properties [36]. Moreover, it facilitates cell migration through the formation of cellular protrusions, reduction in cell adhesion, and enhancement of migratory capacity [36]. Additionally, vimentin modulates DNA repair pathways to facilitate EMT and confer cellular resilience against diverse stresses encountered during the process of cancer invasion [36]. Overall, vimentin appears to play a crucial role in mediating metastasis through EMT processes [36].

In this study, the effects of compounds **3** and **4** on the expression of migration-related proteins VEGFR-1 and vimentin in HCT-116 cells were examined using Western blot analysis at concentrations of 3, 9, and 27 μM (Figure 5). Experimental results indicated that compounds **3** and **4** significantly downregulated the expression of VEGFR-1 and vimentin in a concentration-dependent manner, indicating that compounds **3** and **4** may inhibit the expression of VEGFR-1, thereby impeding the EMT process.

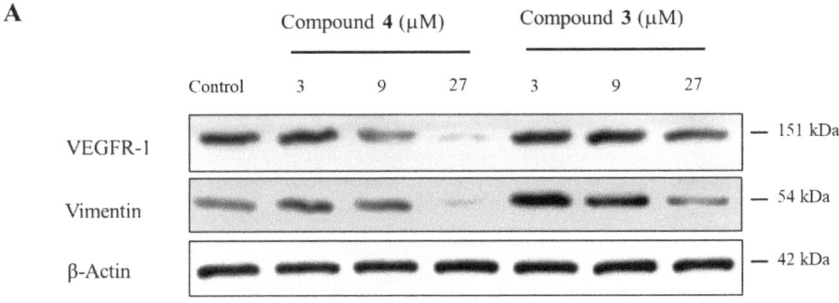

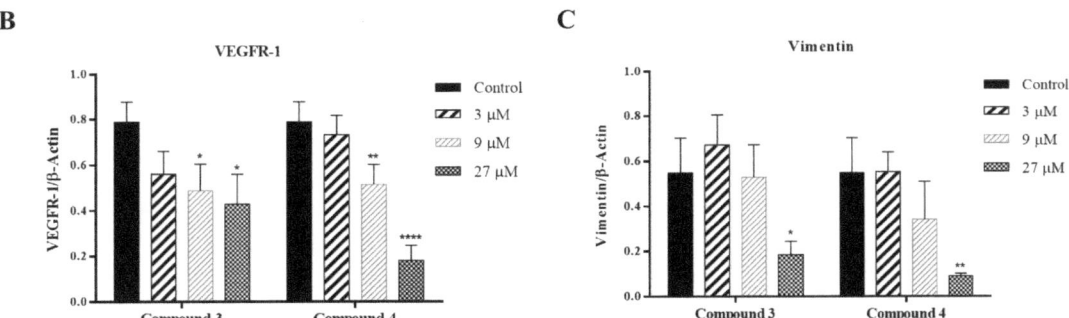

Figure 5. The effects of compounds **3** and **4** on the protein levels of VEGFR-1 and vimentin in HCT 116 cells. (**A**) Western blot analysis of VEGFR-1 and vimentin, β-actin was used as the internal control; (**B**) Relative protein level of VEGFR-1 against β-actin; (**C**) Relative protein level of vimentin against β-actin. Data are presented as the mean ± standard deviation (n = 3). * $p < 0.05$, ** $p < 0.01$, **** $p < 0.0001$.

3. Discussion

A meroditerpenoid, hyrtamide A (**1**), and three sesquiterpene phenols, hyrfarnediol A (**2**), 3-farnesyl-4-hydroxybenzoic acid methyl ester (**3**) and dictyoceratin C (**4**) were isolated from a marine sponge *Hyrtios* sp. In the cytotoxicity assay, compounds **2**–**4** demonstrated weak cytotoxic activity, while no activity was observed for hyrtamide A (**1**), which suggests that the presence of the phenol fragment in compounds **2**–**4** may play a vital role in cytotoxicity. Compounds **3** and **4** exhibited anti-invasive effects, in contrast to previously reported sesquiterpene phenols/quinones, such as avarol, avarone, and ilimaquinone which did not show any anti-invasive activity [33,34]. Through structural comparison, we hypothesize that the phenolic hydroxyl and methyl ester groups present in compounds **3** and **4** may serve as the active functional groups responsible for their anti-invasive activity.

Compounds **3** and **4** downregulated the expression of VEGFR-1 and vimentin proteins. Several reported phenols and sesquiterpene quinones inhibited VEGFR expression [37–40]. We consider that hydroxyl groups play an important role in inhibiting VEGFR expression. Additionally, in compounds **3** and **4**, the methyl ester group may also play an indispensable role. Most naturally derived VEGFR inhibitors primarily target VEGFR-2 and VEGFR-3; however, there are only few compounds known to inhibit VEGFR-1 [37–40]. VEGFR-1 is closely related to angiogenesis promotion along with evidence suggesting its involvement in inducing EMT to facilitate tumor cell invasion [10]. Compounds **3** and **4** inhibited the expression of VEGFR-1 protein and suppressed vimentin simultaneously. Thus, we propose that compounds **3** and **4** likely inhibit EMT by suppressing the expression of VEGFR-1, thereby restraining HCT-116 cells invasion.

4. Materials and Methods

4.1. General Experimental Procedures

The NMR experiments were conducted on Bruker Avance DRX-600 and Bruker AMX-400 MHz NMR spectrometers (Bruker BioSpin, Bremen, Germany) in CDCl$_3$ (δ_H 7.26, δ_C 77.16). HRESIMS spectra were recorded on an Agilent 6230 TOF mass spectrometer (Agilent Technologies, Santa Clara, CA, USA). MPLC was carried out on an Interchim PuriFlash 450 instrument (Interchim, Montlucon, France). TLC was carried out on silica gel HSGF$_{254}$ plates (Yantai Jiangyou Silica Gel Limited Company, Yantai, China). Column chromatography was conducted using Sephadex LH-20 (18−110 µm, Pharmacia Co., London, UK) and ODS C$_{18}$ (15 µm, Santai Technologies, Inc., Changzhou, China). HPLC was performed using a Waters 1525 equipped with a Waters 2998 PDA detector (Waters, Milford, CT, USA). A C$_{18}$ column (YMC-Pack Pro, 250 × 10 mm, 5 µm, YMC, Kyoto, Japan) was used for RP HPLC.

4.2. Sponge Material

The marine sponge sample was collected from the vicinity of Yongxing Island in the South China Sea in May 2013. The species was previously identified and described as a *Hyrtios* sp. [29]. A voucher specimen (no. 1312) is deposited at Research Center for Marine Drugs, Department of Pharmacy, Ren Ji Hospital, School of Medicine, Shanghai Jiao Tong University.

4.3. Extraction and Isolation

The sponge *Hyrtios* sp. (0.2 kg, dry weight) was subjected to a triple extraction with 95% EtOH to produce an ethanolic extract. This extract underwent partitioning between petroleum ether and a 90% methanol–water mixture at equal ratios. The methanol–water fraction was then diluted to 60% with water and further partitioned using CH$_2$Cl$_2$, resulting in a CH$_2$Cl$_2$ extract weighing 1.3 g. The CH$_2$Cl$_2$ extract was separated using a Sephadex LH-20 column with CH$_2$Cl$_2$/MeOH (1:1), resulting in the isolation of three fractions (A–C). Fraction B (0.86 g) was subjected to MPLC (MeOH/H$_2$O, 50–100%) and yielded six fractions (B1–B6).

Purification of subfraction B4 via RP HPLC (MeOH/H$_2$O, 80%) afforded two compounds: dictyoceratin C (**4**, t_R = 85 min, 29.0 mg) and 3-farnesyl-4-hydroxybenzoic acid methyl ester (**3**, t_R = 102 min, 13.3 mg). Similarly, subfraction B5 when processed through RP HPLC (MeCN/H$_2$O, 80%) produced hyrfarnediol A (**2**, t_R = 48 min, 2.6 mg). Hyrtamide A (**1**, t_R = 70 min, 3.0 mg) was purified from subfraction B6 utilizing RP HPLC (MeCN/H$_2$O, 85%).

4.4. Compound Characteristics

Hyrtamide A (**1**): Yellowish oil; UV (DAD from MeOH/H$_2$O) λ_{max} 221 nm; ^{1}H and ^{13}C NMR (600/150 MHz, CDCl$_3$) data, as shown in Table 1; HRESIMS m/z 392.2914 [M + Na]$^+$ (calcd. for C$_{25}$H$_{39}$NONa, 392.2929).

Hyrfarnediol A (**2**): Yellowish powder; UV (DAD from MeOH/H$_2$O) λ_{max} 199 and 268 nm; ^{1}H and ^{13}C NMR (400/100 MHz, CDCl$_3$) data, as shown in Table 1; HRESIMS m/z 373.2377 [M + H]$^+$ (calcd. for C$_{23}$H$_{33}$O$_4$, 373.2379).

4.5. Cytotoxicity Test

The HCT-116 cell line, sourced from Shanghai Institute of Biochemistry and Cell Biology, Chinese Academy of Sciences (Shanghai, China), was cultured at 37 °C with 5% CO$_2$ in McCoy's 5A medium (Procell, Wuhan, China). The HCT-116 cells were seeded at a concentration of 1×10^4 cells/well and incubated for 24 h. The cell line was treated with test compounds (at concentrations of 10.0, 20.0, 40.0, and 80.0 µM) and the positive control (doxorubicin, at concentrations of 1.0, 2.0, 4.0, and 8.0 µM) for 48 h. Then, they were co-incubated with MTT solution (20 µL, Sinopharm Chemical Reagent Co., Ltd., Shanghai, China) at 37 °C for 4 h. The absorbance was quantified at a wavelength of 490 nm using a microplate reader (Synergy, BioTek Instruments, Inc., Winooski, VT, USA). The cytotoxicity assays were performed with at least three replicates [41].

4.6. Invasion Assay

The HCT-116 cells were harvested and suspended in a medium without serum at a concentration of approximately 1×10^6 cells/mL. The upper compartment of a transwell chamber, pre-coated with Matrigel (BD Biosciences, Franklin Lakes, NJ, USA), was then seeded with these cells. The lower chamber was filled with a medium containing 20% FBS (Genom, Hangzhou, China) and various concentrations of compounds **3** and **4** (with DMSO as the control). The cells were treated with 4% paraformaldehyde (Biosharp, Hefei, China) and fixed for 24 h. The non-invasive cells located on the outermost layer of the membrane were removed lightly using a sterile cotton swab. The membrane-bound cells were subjected to crystal violet staining for 10 min, followed by three rounds of washing with PBS (Genom, Hangzhou, China), and the captured images were observed under an inverted microscope (Olympus, Tokyo, Japan).

4.7. Western Blot

After treating HCT-116 cells with DMSO or different concentrations of compounds **3** and **4** for 24 h, the cells were rinsed with PBS that had been pre-cooled, followed by lysis using 150 µL of lysis buffer. The samples were incubated on ice for 30 min and vigorously shaken to ensure complete cell lysis. Subsequently, centrifugation was performed at 12,000 rpm and 4 °C for 15 min. The supernatant was collected for protein concentration analysis. SDS-PAGE electrophoresis was performed, followed by protein transfer onto a PVDF membrane. The membrane was subsequently blocked with 5% skimmed milk powder for 1 h prior to overnight incubation at 4 °C with primary antibodies against VEGFR-1 and vimentin (Abcam, Cambridge, UK). Following five rounds of TBST washing, secondary antibodies (1:3000, Elabscience, Wuhan, China) were added and incubated at 25 °C for 2 h. Then, blot bands were visualized with an ECL reagent (Bio-Rad, Hercules, CA, USA) and were quantified by densitometry using ImageJ 1.51j software (NIH, Bethesda, Rockville, MD, USA). The results were normalized using β-actin (Abcam, Cambridge, UK) as an internal control [42].

4.8. Statistical Analysis

All the data were obtained in three independent replicates, and analyzed with Graphpad Prism 6 software (Graphpad Software, San Diego, CA, USA) and represented as mean ± standard deviation. A p-value less than 0.05 was deemed to have statistical significance.

5. Conclusions

In summary, four meroterpenoids were isolated from a marine sponge *Hyrtios* sp., including two new compounds hyrtamide A (**1**) and hyrfarnediol A (**2**), and two known ones, 3-farnesyl-4-hydroxybenzoic acid methyl ester (**3**) and dictyoceratin C (**4**). Compounds **2**–**4** exhibited weak cytotoxic activities. Compounds **3** and **4** significantly inhibited the invasion of HCT-116 cells and notably suppressed the expression of VEGFR-1 and vimentin (a biomarker of EMT), suggesting that they may inhibit tumor cell metastasis by preventing the EMT process through downregulation of VEGFR-1 expression. The mechanisms behind the anti-metastatic effects of compounds **3** and **4** require further investigation.

Supplementary Materials: The following supporting information can be downloaded at: https://www.mdpi.com/article/10.3390/md22040183/s1, Figures S1–S16: HRESIMS, UV, ^{1}H and ^{13}C NMR, HSQC, HMBC, COSY, and ROESY spectra of hyrtamide A (**1**) and hyrfarnediol A (**2**). Figures S17–S22: ESI-MS, ^{1}H and ^{13}C NMR spectra of 3-farnesyl-4-hydroxybenzoic acid methyl ester (**3**) and dictyoceratin C (**4**).

Author Contributions: Conceptualization, J.W. and Y.-L.Y.; methodology, J.W. and Y.-L.Y.; formal analysis, J.W. and J.-Y.P.; investigation, Y.-L.Y. and X.-L.L.; resources, J.W. and B.W.; data curation, Y.-L.Y. and X.-Y.Y.; writing—original draft preparation, J.W. and Y.-L.Y.; writing—review and editing, L.-L.H. and B.W.; visualization, Y.-L.Y. and X.-Y.Y.; supervision, J.W. and L.-L.H.; project administration, B.W.; funding acquisition, J.W. All authors have read and agreed to the published version of the manuscript.

Funding: This research was funded by Zhejiang Provincial Natural Science Foundation of China (No. LQ23H300005).

Institutional Review Board Statement: Not applicable.

Data Availability Statement: The data presented in this study can be accessed in the Supplementary Materials; further inquiries can be directed to the corresponding author.

Acknowledgments: We are grateful to Yizhen Yan of Research Center for Marine Drugs, Department of Pharmacy, Ren Ji Hospital, School of Medicine, Shanghai Jiao Tong University for his invaluable technical support. To commemorate him and express our gratitude for all the assistance he has provided, this article is dedicated to him with the utmost respect.

Conflicts of Interest: The authors declare no conflicts of interest.

References

1. Brenner, H.; Heisser, T.; Cardoso, R.; Hoffmeister, M. Reduction in colorectal cancer incidence by screening endoscopy. *Nat. Rev. Gastroenterol. Hepatol.* **2024**, *21*, 125–133. [CrossRef] [PubMed]
2. Brenner, H.; Kloor, M.; Pox, C.P. Colorectal cancer. *Lancet* **2014**, *383*, 1490–1502. [CrossRef] [PubMed]
3. Ganesh, K.; Massagué, J. Targeting metastatic cancer. *Nat. Med.* **2021**, *27*, 34–44. [CrossRef] [PubMed]
4. Zeng, J.; Deng, Q.; Chen, Z.; Yan, S.; Dong, Q.; Zhang, Y.; Cui, Y.; Li, L.; He, Y.; Shi, J. Recent development of VEGFR small molecule inhibitors as anticancer agents: A patent review (2021–2023). *Bioorg. Chem.* **2024**, *146*, 107278. [CrossRef] [PubMed]
5. Hiratsuka, S.; Nakao, K.; Nakamura, K.; Katsuki, M.; Maru, Y.; Shibuya, M. Membrane fixation of vascular endothelial growth factor receptor 1 ligand-binding domain is important for vasculogenesis and angiogenesis in mice. *Mol. Cell Biol.* **2005**, *25*, 346–354. [CrossRef] [PubMed]
6. Bae, D.G.; Kim, T.D.; Li, G.; Yoon, W.H.; Chae, C.B. Anti-flt1 peptide, a vascular endothelial growth factor receptor 1-specific hexapeptide, inhibits tumor growth and metastasis. *Clin. Cancer Res.* **2005**, *11*, 2651–2661. [CrossRef] [PubMed]
7. Karaman, S.; Paavonsalo, S.; Heinolainen, K.; Lackman, M.H.; Ranta, A.; Hemanthakumar, K.A.; Kubota, Y.; Alitalo, K. Interplay of vascular endothelial growth factor receptors in organ-specific vessel maintenance. *J. Exp. Med.* **2022**, *219*, e20210565. [CrossRef] [PubMed]

8. Fan, F.; Wey, J.S.; McCarty, M.F.; Belcheva, A.; Liu, W.; Bauer, T.W.; Somcio, R.J.; Wu, Y.; Hooper, A.; Hicklin, D.J.; et al. Expression and function of vascular endothelial growth factor receptor-1 on human colorectal cancer cells. *Oncogene* **2005**, *24*, 2647–2653. [CrossRef] [PubMed]
9. Ceci, C.; Atzori, M.G.; Lacal, P.M.; Graziani, G. Role of VEGFs/VEGFR-1 signaling and its inhibition in modulating tumor invasion: Experimental evidence in different metastatic cancer models. *Int. J. Mol. Sci.* **2020**, *21*, 1388. [CrossRef] [PubMed]
10. Yang, A.D.; Camp, E.R.; Fan, F.; Shen, L.; Gray, M.J.; Liu, W.; Somcio, R.; Bauer, T.W.; Wu, Y.; Hicklin, D.J.; et al. Vascular endothelial growth factor receptor-1 activation mediates epithelial to mesenchymal transition in human pancreatic carcinoma cells. *Cancer Res.* **2006**, *66*, 46–51. [CrossRef]
11. Jiang, M.; Wu, Z.; Liu, L.; Chen, S. The chemistry and biology of fungal meroterpenoids (2009–2019). *Org. Biomol. Chem.* **2021**, *19*, 1644–1704. [CrossRef] [PubMed]
12. Fuloria, N.K.; Raheja, R.K.; Shah, K.H.; Oza, M.J.; Kulkarni, Y.A.; Subramaniyan, V.; Sekar, M.; Fuloria, S. Biological activities of meroterpenoids isolated from different sources. *Front. Pharmacol.* **2022**, *13*, 830103. [CrossRef]
13. Nazir, M.; Saleem, M.; Tousif, M.I.; Anwar, M.A.; Surup, F.; Ali, I.; Wang, D.; Mamadalieva, N.Z.; Alshammari, E.; Ashour, M.L.; et al. Meroterpenoids: A comprehensive update insight on structural diversity and biology. *Biomolecules* **2021**, *11*, 957. [CrossRef]
14. Hong, L.L.; Ding, Y.F.; Zhang, W.; Lin, H.W. Chemical and biological diversity of new natural products from marine sponges: A review (2009–2018). *Mar. Life. Sci. Technol.* **2022**, *4*, 356–372. [CrossRef] [PubMed]
15. Carroll, A.R.; Copp, B.R.; Grkovic, T.; Keyzers, R.A.; Prinsep, M.R. Marine natural products. *Nat. Prod. Rep.* **2024**, *41*, 162–207. [CrossRef]
16. Kim, C.K.; Woo, J.K.; Kim, S.H.; Cho, E.; Lee, Y.J.; Lee, H.S.; Sim, C.J.; Oh, K.B.; Shin, J. Meroterpenoids from a tropical *Dysidea* sp. sponge. *J. Nat. Prod.* **2015**, *78*, 2814–2821. [CrossRef] [PubMed]
17. Gui, Y.H.; Jiao, W.H.; Zhou, M.; Zhang, Y.; Zeng, D.Q.; Zhu, H.R.; Liu, K.C.; Sun, F.; Chen, H.F.; Lin, H.W. Septosones A-C, in vivo anti-inflammatory meroterpenoids with rearranged carbon skeletons from the marine sponge *Dysidea septosa*. *Org. Lett.* **2019**, *21*, 767–770. [CrossRef]
18. Nguyen, H.M.; Ito, T.; Kurimoto, S.; Ogawa, M.; Win, N.N.; Hung, V.Q.; Nguyen, H.T.; Kubota, T.; Kobayashi, J.; Morita, H. New merosesquiterpenes from a Vietnamese marine sponge of *Spongia* sp. and their biological activities. *Bioorg. Med. Chem. Lett.* **2017**, *27*, 3043–3047. [CrossRef]
19. Hagiwara, K.; Hernandez, J.E.G.; Harper, M.K.; Carroll, A.; Motti, C.A.; Awaya, J.; Nguyen, H.Y.; Wright, A.D. Puupehenol, a potent antioxidant antimicrobial meroterpenoid from a Hawaiian deep-water *Dactylospongia* sp. sponge. *J. Nat. Prod.* **2015**, *78*, 325–329. [CrossRef]
20. Gray, C.A.; Lira, S.P.; Silva, M.; Pimenta, E.F.; Thiemann, O.H.; Oliva, G.; Hajdu, E.; Andersen, R.J.; Berlinck, R.G.S. Sulfated meroterpenoids from the Brazilian sponge *Callyspongia* sp. are inhibitors of the antileishmaniasis target adenosine phosphoribosyl transferase. *J. Org. Chem.* **2007**, *72*, 1062. [CrossRef]
21. Jiao, W.H.; Cheng, B.H.; Shi, G.H.; Chen, G.D.; Gu, B.B.; Zhou, Y.J.; Hong, L.L.; Yang, F.; Liu, Z.Q.; Qiu, S.Q. Dysivillosins A–D: Unusual anti-allergic meroterpenoids from the marine sponge *Dysidea villosa*. *Sci. Rep.* **2017**, *7*, 8947. [CrossRef] [PubMed]
22. Gordaliza, M. Cytotoxic terpene quinones from marine sponges. *Mar. Drugs* **2010**, *8*, 2849–2870. [CrossRef] [PubMed]
23. Han, N.; Li, J.; Li, X. Natural marine products: Anti-colorectal cancer in vitro and in vivo. *Mar. Drugs* **2022**, *20*, 349. [CrossRef] [PubMed]
24. Shady, N.H.; El-Hossary, E.M.; Fouad, M.A.; Gulder, T.A.M.; Kamel, M.S.; Abdelmohsen, U.R. Bioactive natural products of marine sponges from the genus *Hyrtios*. *Molecules* **2017**, *22*, 781. [CrossRef] [PubMed]
25. Wang, J.; Mu, F.R.; Jiao, W.H.; Huang, J.; Hong, L.L.; Yang, F.; Xu, Y.; Wang, S.P.; Sun, F.; Lin, H.W. Meroterpenoids with protein tyrosine phosphatase 1B inhibitory activity from a *Hyrtios* sp. marine sponge. *J. Nat. Prod.* **2017**, *80*, 2509–2514. [CrossRef] [PubMed]
26. Wang, J.; Liu, L.; Hong, L.L.; Zhan, K.X.; Lin, Z.J.; Jiao, W.H.; Lin, H.W. New bisabolane-type phenolic sesquiterpenoids from the marine sponge *Plakortis simplex*. *Chin. J. Nat. Med.* **2021**, *19*, 626–631. [CrossRef] [PubMed]
27. Fan, D.X.; Luo, X.C.; Ding, Y.F.; Liu, L.Y.; Wang, X.; Pan, J.Y.; Ji, Y.Y.; Wang, J.; Li, C.; Hong, L.L.; et al. Isolation and absolute configuration of alkylpyridine alkaloids from the marine sponge *Hippospongia lachne*. *Phytochemistry* **2024**, *220*, 114017. [CrossRef] [PubMed]
28. Maxwell, A.; Rampersad, D. Prenylated 4-hydroxybenzoic acid derivatives from *Piper marginatum*. *J. Nat. Prod.* **1988**, *51*, 370–373. [CrossRef]
29. Kwak, J.H.; Schmitz, F.J.; Kelly, M. Sesquiterpene quinols/quinones from the Micronesian sponge *Petrosaspongia metachromia*. *J. Nat. Prod.* **2000**, *63*, 1153–1156. [CrossRef] [PubMed]
30. Tauriello, D.V.F.; Batlle, E. Targeting the microenvironment in advanced colorectal cancer. *Trends Cancer* **2016**, *2*, 495–504. [CrossRef]
31. Majidpoor, J.; Mortezaee, K. Steps in metastasis: An updated review. *Med. Oncol.* **2021**, *38*, 3. [CrossRef] [PubMed]
32. Kim, Y.H.; Choi, Y.W.; Lee, J.; Soh, E.Y.; Kim, J.; Park, T.J. Senescent tumor cells lead the collective invasion in thyroid cancer. *Nat. Commun.* **2017**, *8*, 15208. [CrossRef] [PubMed]

33. Warabi, K.; McHardy, L.M.; Matainaho, L.; Soest, R.V.; Roskelley, C.D.; Roberge, M.; Andersen, R.J. Strongylophorine-26, a new meroditerpenoid isolated from the marine sponge *Petrosia (Strongylophora) corticata* that exhibits anti-invasion activity. *J. Nat. Prod.* **2004**, *67*, 1387–1389. [CrossRef] [PubMed]
34. Diaz-Marrero, A.R.; Austin, P.; van Soest, R.; Matainaho, T.; Roskelley, C.D.; Roberge, M.; Andersen, R.J. Avinosol, a meroterpenoid-nucleoside conjugate with antiinvasion activity isolated from the marine sponge *Dysidea* sp. *Org. Lett.* **2006**, *8*, 3749–3752. [CrossRef] [PubMed]
35. Dongre, A.; Weinberg, R.A. New insights into the mechanisms of epithelial–mesenchymal transition and implications for cancer. *Nat. Rev. Mol. Cell. Biol.* **2019**, *20*, 69–84. [CrossRef] [PubMed]
36. Usman, S.; Waseem, N.H.; Nguyen, T.K.N.; Mohsin, S.; Jamal, A.; Teh, M.-T.; Waseem, A. Vimentin is at the heart of epithelial mesenchymal transition (EMT) mediated metastasis. *Cancers* **2021**, *13*, 4985. [CrossRef] [PubMed]
37. Nathan, J.; Ramachandran, A. Efficacy of marine biomolecules on angiogenesis by targeting hypoxia inducible factor/vascular endothelial growth factor signaling in zebrafish model. *J. Biochem. Mol. Toxicol.* **2022**, *36*, e22954. [CrossRef] [PubMed]
38. Nandi, S.; Dey, R.; Samadder, A.; Saxena, A.; Saxena, A.K. Natural sourced inhibitors of EGFR, PDGFR, FGFR and VEGFR mediated signaling pathways as potential anticancer agents. *Curr. Med. Chem.* **2022**, *29*, 212–223. [CrossRef] [PubMed]
39. Stahl, P.; Kissau, L.; Mazitschek, R.; Huwe, A.; Furet, P.; Giannis, A.; Waldmann, H. Total synthesis and biological evaluation of the nakijiquinones. *J. Am. Chem. Soc.* **2001**, *123*, 11586–11593. [CrossRef] [PubMed]
40. Wang, Y.; Duan, M.; Zhao, L.; Ma, P. Guajadial inhibits NSCLC growth and migration following activation of the VEGF receptor-2. *Fitoterapia* **2018**, *129*, 73–77. [CrossRef]
41. Ge, M.-X.; Chen, R.-P.; Zhang, L.; Wang, Y.-M.; Chi, C.-F.; Wang, B. Novel Ca-chelating peptides from protein hydrolysate of Antarctic krill (*Euphausia superba*): Preparation, characterization, and calcium absorption efficiency in Caco-2 cell monolayer model. *Mar. Drugs* **2023**, *21*, 579. [CrossRef] [PubMed]
42. Zheng, S.-L.; Wang, Y.-M.; Chi, C.-F.; Wang, B. Chemical characterization of honeysuckle polyphenols and their alleviating function on ultraviolet B-damaged HaCaT cells by modulating the Nrf2/NF-κB signaling pathways. *Antioxidants* **2024**, *13*, 294. [CrossRef] [PubMed]

Disclaimer/Publisher's Note: The statements, opinions and data contained in all publications are solely those of the individual author(s) and contributor(s) and not of MDPI and/or the editor(s). MDPI and/or the editor(s) disclaim responsibility for any injury to people or property resulting from any ideas, methods, instructions or products referred to in the content.

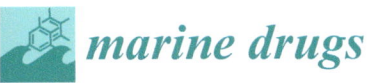

Article

Marine-Fungus-Derived Natural Compound 4-Hydroxyphenylacetic Acid Induces Autophagy to Exert Antithrombotic Effects in Zebrafish

Shaoshuai Xin [1,†], Mengqi Zhang [2,†], Peihai Li [1], Lizhen Wang [1], Xuanming Zhang [1], Shanshan Zhang [1], Zhenqiang Mu [3], Houwen Lin [4], Xiaobin Li [1,*] and Kechun Liu [1,*]

1. Biology Institute, Qilu University of Technology (Shandong Academy of Sciences), Jinan 250103, China; qiluxss@163.com (S.X.); liph@sdas.org (P.L.); wlzh1106@126.com (L.W.); zhangmx@sdas.org (X.Z.); zhangss@sdas.org (S.Z.)
2. Key Laboratory of Novel Food Resources Processing, Ministry of Agriculture and Rural Affairs, Key Laboratory of Agro-Products Processing Technology of Shandong Province, Institute of Agro-Food Science and Technology, Shandong Academy of Agricultural Sciences, 23788 Gongye North Road, Jinan 250100, China; mengqi139@126.com
3. Chongqing Key Laboratory of High Active Traditional Chinese Medicine Delivery System & Chongqing Engineering Research Center of Pharmaceutical Sciences, Chongqing Medical and Pharmaceutical College, Chongqing 410331, China; 10976@cqmpc.edu.cn
4. Research Center for Marine Drugs, State Key Laboratory of Oncogenes and Related Genes, Department of Pharmacy, School of Medicine, Shanghai Jiao Tong University, Shanghai 200127, China; franklin67@126.com

* Correspondence: lixb@sdas.org (X.L.); hliukch@sdas.org (K.L.); Tel./Fax: +86-531-82605352 (X.L.); +86-531-82605331 (K.L.)
† These authors contributed equally to this work.

Abstract: Marine natural products are important sources of novel drugs. In this study, we isolated 4-hydroxyphenylacetic acid (HPA) from the marine-derived fungus *Emericellopsis maritima* Y39–2. The antithrombotic activity and mechanism of HPA were reported for the first time. Using a zebrafish model, we found that HPA had a strong antithrombotic activity because it can significantly increase cardiac erythrocytes, blood flow velocity, and heart rate, reduce caudal thrombus, and reverse the inflammatory response caused by Arachidonic Acid (AA). Further transcriptome analysis and qRT–PCR validation demonstrated that HPA may regulate autophagy by inhibiting the PI3K/AKT/mTOR signaling pathway to exert antithrombotic effects.

Keywords: marine-derived fungus; 4-hydroxyphenylacetic acid; antithrombotic; autophagy

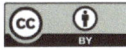

1. Introduction

Thrombus can lead to acute myocardial infarction, ischemic heart disease, valvular heart disease, peripheral vascular disease, and other cardiovascular diseases (CVDs), and approximately 20 million people die of cardiovascular disease each year [1,2]. Due to aging, changing lifestyles, and population expansion, the burden of thrombotic disorders on health care systems is increasing [3]. Existing studies suggest that signaling pathways, such as the NF-κB, Toll's-like receptor, MAPK, mTOR, PI3K, and autophagy pathways, are associated with thrombosis [4–7]. Acetylsalicylic acid (ASA), warfarin, and heparin are currently the most widely used antithrombotic medications; nonetheless, they have side effects, including bleeding and drug resistance [8,9]. Therefore, there is an urgent need for new antithrombotic drugs that are safer and more reliable than existing drugs.

Natural products are important sources for the discovery of antithrombotic drugs. The oligotrophic environment, low temperature, high salinity, high pressure, and low oxygen content found in the ocean allow organisms to have special metabolic adaptation mechanisms and produce novel structures and a variety of biological activities [10]. Marine fungi are a rich source of natural products [11]. The fungal genus *Emericellopsis* (Hypocreales,

Sordariomycetes, Ascomycota) has been found to comprise 27 species, including 23 species and 4 varieties [12]. In recent years, a significant amount of secondary metabolites, such as peptides, terpenes, peptaibols, alkaloids, and flavonoids, have been isolated from *Emericellopsis* sp. [12–14]. To date, research on the bioactivities of secondary metabolites from *Emericellopsis* sp. has focused on their anti-inflammatory, antibacterial, and antitumor activities [12,13,15–18], but few studies have investigated their antithrombotic activity.

The zebrafish is a small vertebrate tropical water fish that has become a widely used model organism for screening natural active compounds [19,20]. The zebrafish model has the characteristics of high throughput and high connotation and has become an important link between cell and mammalian models in drug screening and evaluation systems. The thrombus formation mechanism of zebrafish is similar to that of humans, whose thrombocytes express the platelet glycoproteins GPIIb/IIIa and GPIb and have both endogenous and exogenous clotting pathways [21]. Experiments have shown that the efficacy of some antithrombotic drugs commonly used in the clinic on zebrafish is similar to that in mammals [22], indicating the reliability of screening antithrombotic drugs in zebrafish models. At the protein level, the homology of key parts of zebrafish and humans is nearly 100%, so zebrafish is also very suitable for the study of signaling pathways and the screening of targeted drugs [23]. AA and phenyl hydrazine (PHZ) are commonly used to construct zebrafish thrombus models for screening and mechanistic studies of antithrombotic active ingredients [24,25].

Previously, using a zebrafish model, we examined the antithrombotic activity of extracts from small-scale fermentations of eleven different strains of marine-derived fungus. The results showed that extracts from the marine-derived fungus *Emericellopsis maritima* Y39–2 have antithrombotic activity. In this study, we focused on isolating biologically active natural products from Y39–2, and the metabolite 4-hydroxyphenylacetic acid (HPA) (Figure 1) was separated and shown to have significant antithrombotic activity. Mechanistic investigations revealed that HPA can inhibit the mTOR signaling pathway to activate autophagy, thus playing an antithrombotic role.

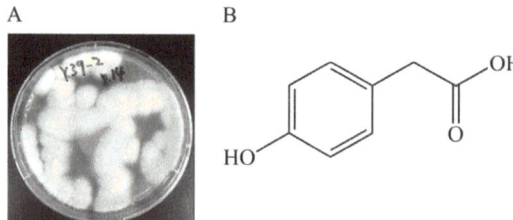

Figure 1. (**A**) The marine-derived fungus *Emericellopsis maritima* Y39–2. (**B**) Structure of the HPA.

HPA is a phenolic compound that was first isolated from the pathogen *Hypochnus sasakii* [26] and subsequently found in the fungi *Oidiodendron* sp. [27] and *Neofusicoccum parvum* [28], the brown alga *Undaria* [29], colonic microorganisms [30], the Chinese herb *Aster tataricus* [31], and human saliva [32]. This compound has a wide range of effects, such as attenuating sepsis-induced acute kidney injury [30], preventing acute acetaminophen-induced liver injury [33], reducing inflammation and edema in lung injury [31], and regulating growth [29,34], anxiolytic [35], antioxidative [36], antimicrobial [37,38], and nematicidal activity [27]. This is the first time that the antithrombotic activity and mechanism of HPA have been explored. The results obtained in this study broaden the resources of potential antithrombotic agents and lay the foundation for developing new antifungal drugs.

2. Results
2.1. Safe Concentration of HPA for Zebrafish

We treated larvae 72 h post-fertilization (hpf) with different concentrations of HPA for 6 h. The results are shown in Figure 2. At 6 h post-exposure (hpe), no mortality was detected in zebrafish larvae that were exposed to 0 to 657.2 µM HPA. When the HPA treatment concentration was increased from 1314.5 to 3943.5 µM, the mortality rate of zebrafish larvae increased sharply from 6.67% to 100%. The lethality curves were plotted based on the mortality of zebrafish larvae, and the 1% lethal concentration (LC_1) for HPA was calculated to be 914.6 µM. No malformations were observed in any of the HPA treatment groups. Based on the test results, concentrations of 82.2, 164.3, 328.6, and 657.2 µM were selected for the evaluation of the antithrombotic activity of HPA.

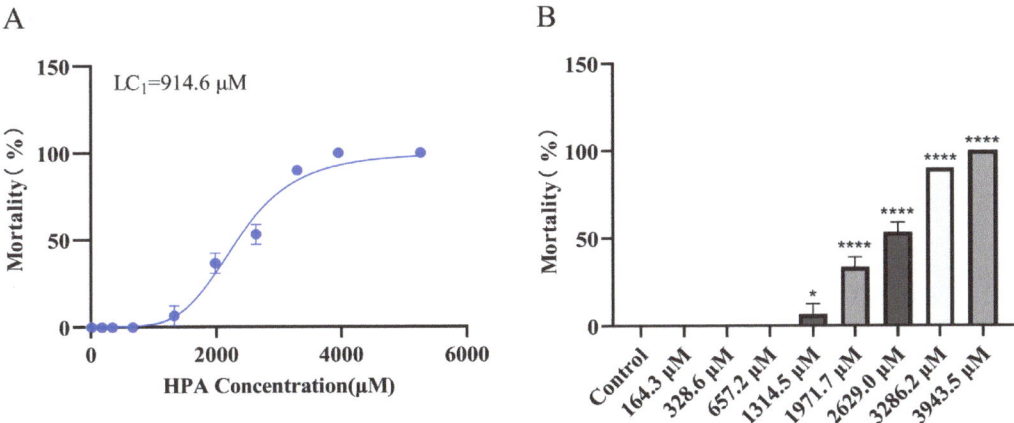

Figure 2. Observation of 72 hpf zebrafish larvae exposed to HPA for 6 h. (**A**) Mortality curve and (**B**) mortality rate at 6 hpe. The data are presented as the means ± SEMs; **** $p < 0.0001$ and * $p < 0.05$ compared to the control group.

2.2. Antithrombotic Activity of HPA

As shown in Figure 3, the area and staining intensity of caudal thrombus in zebrafish in the model group were obviously greater than those in the control group, indicating that AA can significantly induce caudal thrombus formation. The ASA group and all of the HPA treatment groups showed notable reductions in the area and staining intensity of caudal thrombus in a concentration-dependent manner when the HPA concentration ranged from 82.2 µM to 328.6 µM.

The cardiac erythrocyte staining results are shown in Figure 4. Compared with the blank control group, AA significantly reduced the staining area and the staining intensity of zebrafish cardiac erythrocytes. After HPA exposure at concentrations of 164.3 and 328.6 µM, the area and intensity of cardiac erythrocyte staining significantly increased, which indicated strong antithrombotic activity. Combined with the results of the zebrafish caudal thrombus assay, the area and staining intensity of caudal thrombus was inversely proportional to the area and intensity of zebrafish caudal thrombus staining, which is consistent with previous research [24,25].

The number of migrating inflammatory cells in each group is shown in Figure 5. We counted the number of macrophages that migrated to the lateral line after the zebrafish cloaca, i.e., the number of green fluorescent dots in the red dashed area of Figure 5A. AA caused a significant increase in the number of migrating inflammatory cells. Like in the ASA group, at concentrations ranging from 82.2 to 657.2 µM, HPA markedly reduced the migration of inflammatory cells in zebrafish and reversed the inflammatory response caused by AA.

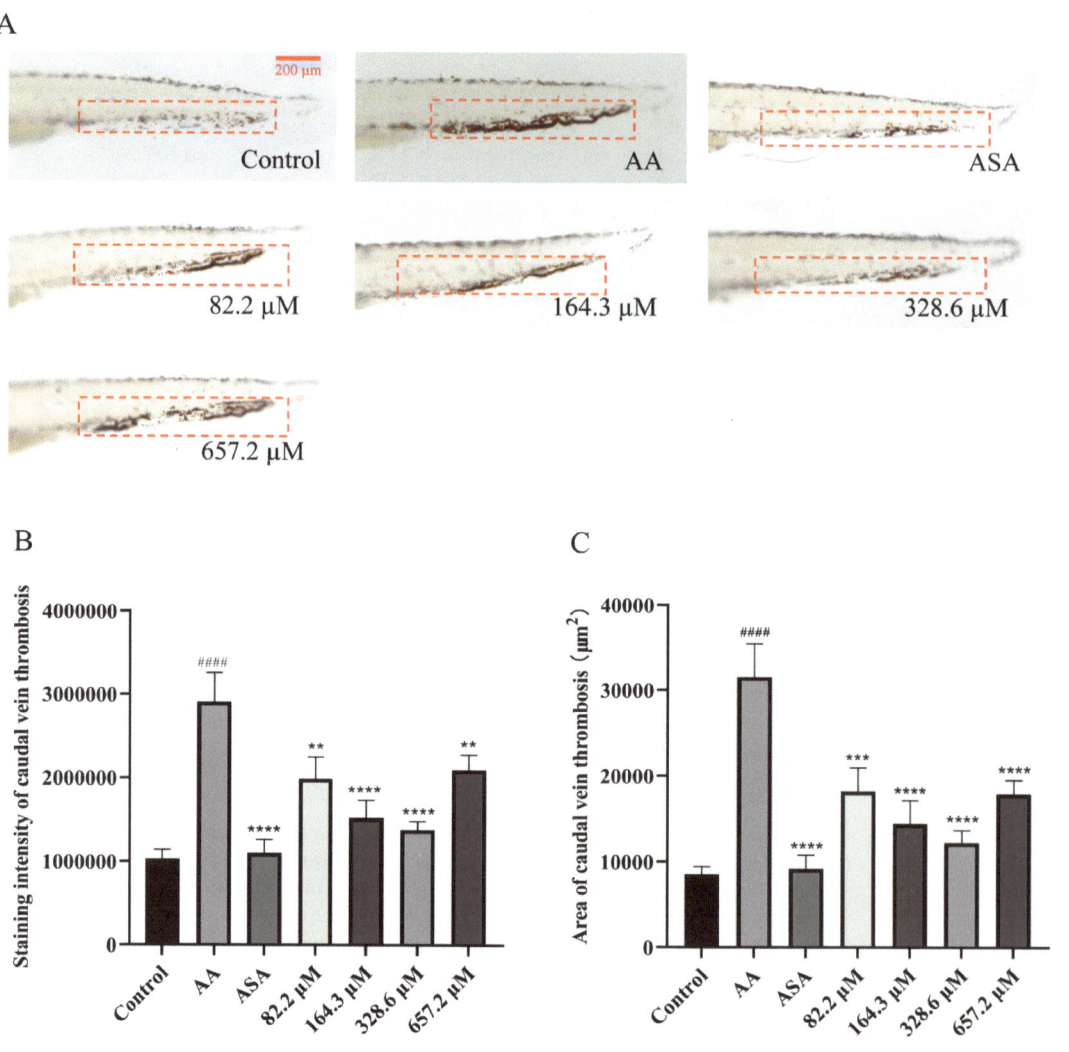

Figure 3. Reduction of caudal thrombus in zebrafish treated with HPA. (**A**) Typical images of caudal thrombus staining in zebrafish. Quantitative analysis of (**B**) the intensity and (**C**) the area of caudal thrombus staining. The data are presented as the means ± SEMs; #### $p < 0.0001$ compared to the control group; **** $p < 0.0001$, *** $p < 0.001$, and ** $p < 0.01$ compared to the AA group.

We analyzed the blood flow velocity and counted the heart rate in one minute for each group of zebrafish (Figure 6). Zebrafish in the AA group showed a massive reduction in blood flow velocity and heart rate. Compared with those in the AA group, the blood flow velocity and heart rate of zebrafish in the HPA groups exposed to 164.3, 328.6, and 657.2 μM were clearly greater than those in the AA group. However, zebrafish blood flow velocity and heart rate were lower at an HPA concentration of 657.2 μM than at an HPA concentration of 164.3 and 328.6μM; this suggests an atypical dose effect for the action of HPA.

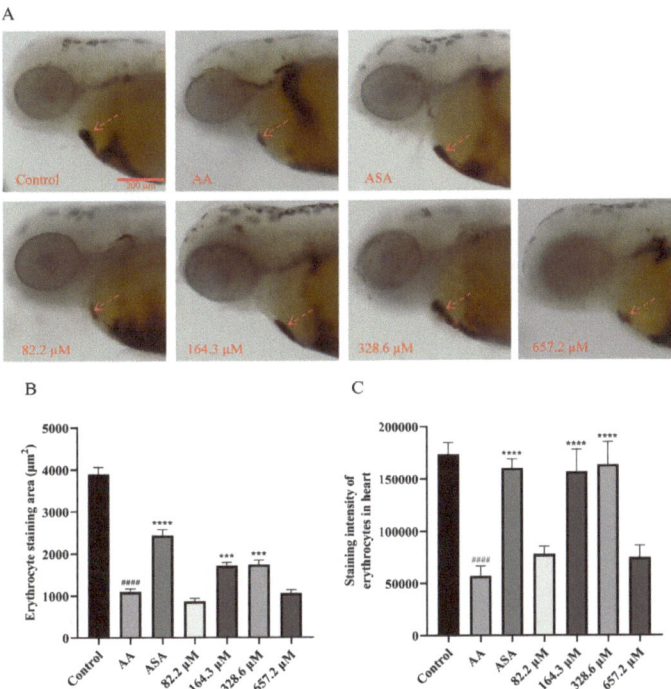

Figure 4. Increase in cardiac erythrocytes in zebrafish treated with HPA. (**A**) Typical images of erythrocyte staining in zebrafish heart (shaded areas are indicated by arrows). Quantitative analysis of (**B**) the area and (**C**) the intensity of cardiac erythrocyte staining. The data are presented as the means ± SEMs; #### $p < 0.0001$ compared to the control group; **** $p < 0.0001$ and *** $p < 0.001$ compared to the AA group.

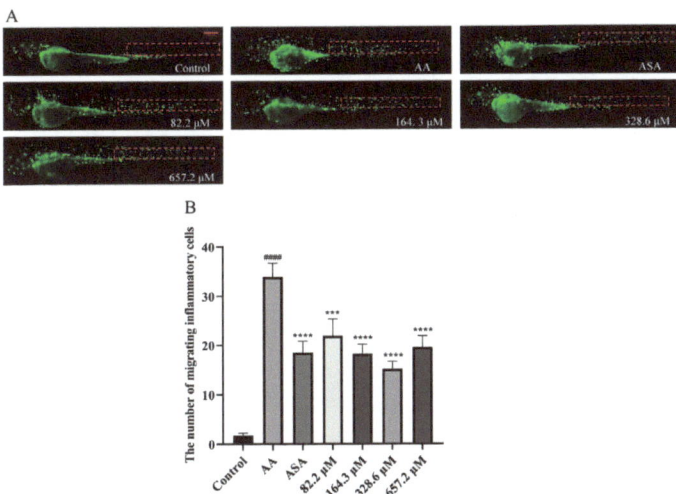

Figure 5. Reduction in the AA-induced inflammatory response in zebrafish treated with HPA. (**A**) Typical images of inflammatory cell migration in zebrafish from all groups. (**B**) Quantitative evaluation of the quantity of migrating inflammatory cells. The data are presented as the means ± SEMs; #### $p < 0.0001$ compared to the control group; **** $p < 0.0001$ and *** $p < 0.001$ compared to the AA group.

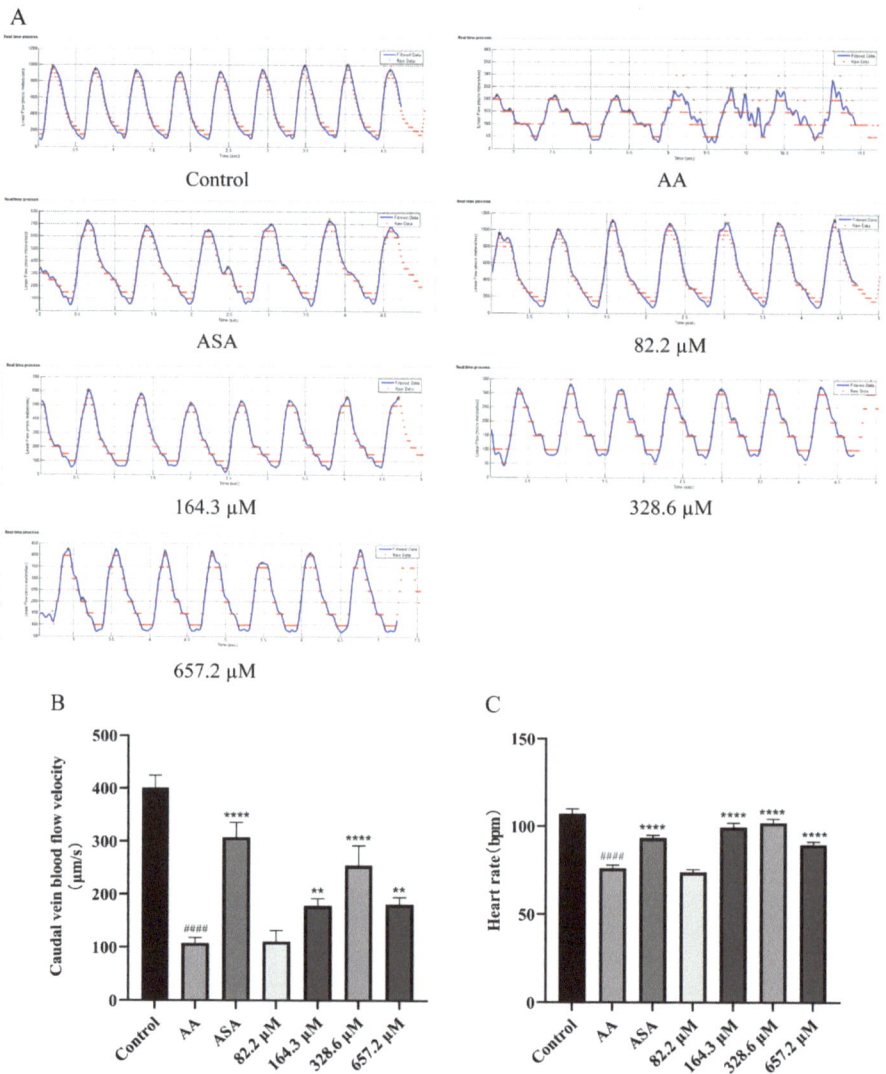

Figure 6. Improvement in caudal blood flow velocity and heart rate in zebrafish treated with HPA. (**A**) Blood flow dynamics of the caudal vein in zebrafish. Quantitative analysis of (**B**) the caudal blood flow velocity and (**C**) the heart rate in one minute. The data are presented as the means ± SEMs; #### $p < 0.0001$ compared to the control group; **** $p < 0.0001$ and ** $p < 0.01$ compared to the AA group.

2.3. Functional Classification and Annotation of The Transcriptome

Figure 7 displays the distributions of the differentially expressed genes (DEGs). In the AA group, 5090 significant DEGs were found compared to those in the control group, comprising 2572 upregulated and 2518 downregulated genes. In contrast to the AA group, the HPA group exhibited 2641 differentially expressed genes (DEGs), comprising 1452 upregulated and 1189 downregulated genes. There were 1035 DEGs coexpressed in the two comparison combinations (AA vs. control and HPA vs. AA), of which 101 DEGs were upregulated in the combination of AA vs. control and downregulated in the combination of HPA vs. AA, and 90 DEGs were downregulated in the combination of AA vs. control and upregulated in the combination of HPA vs. AA. In brief, the expression of 191 DEGs showed opposite trends in the two comparisons above.

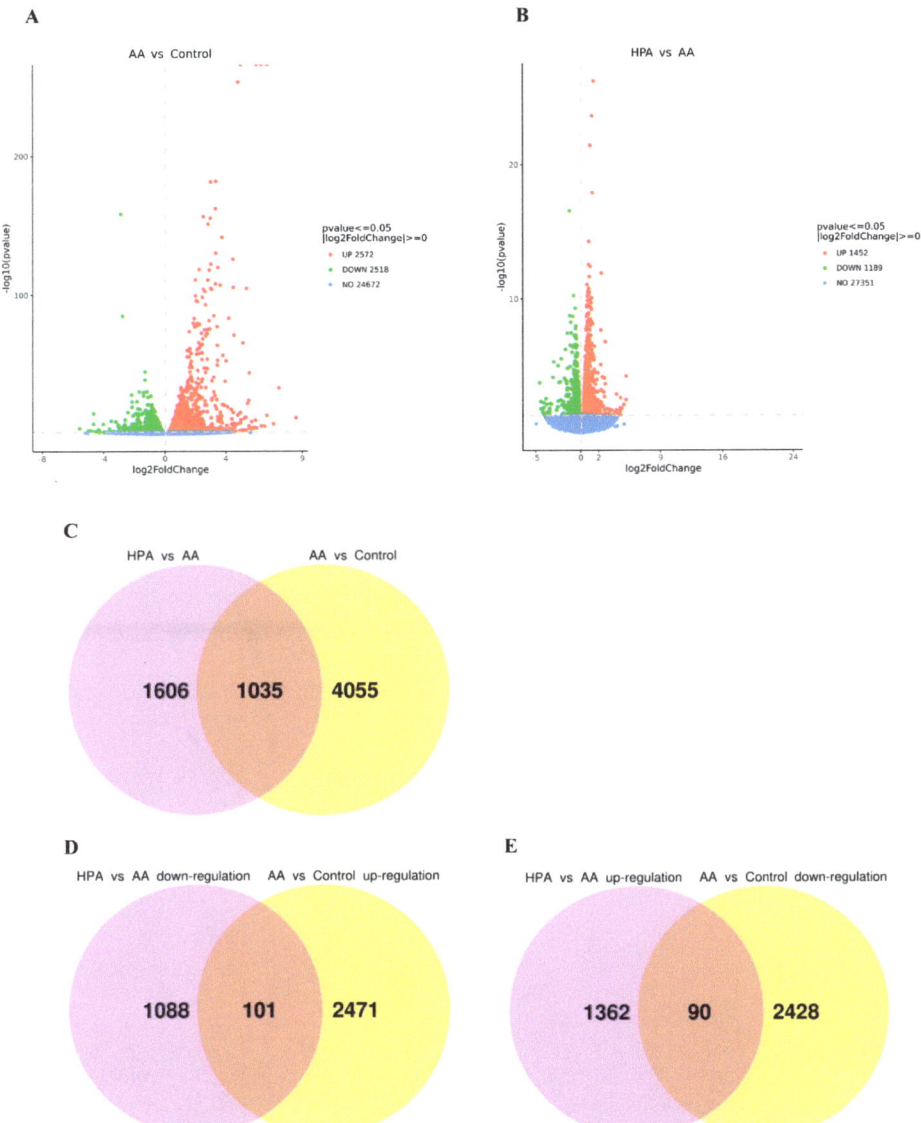

Figure 7. Differentially expressed genes (DEGs) in zebrafish. (**A**,**B**) Volcano plots for DEGs of AA vs. control and HPA vs. AA. (**C**) Venn plot for the DEGs of AA vs. control and HPA vs. AA. (**D**) Venn plot of the DEGs downregulated in the HPA group vs. the AA group and upregulated in the AA group vs. the control group. (**E**) Venn plot of the DEGs upregulated in the HPA group vs. the AA group and downregulated in the AA group vs. the control group.

According to the Gene Ontology (GO) enrichment analysis of the 191 DEGs, the 30 most significant terms are shown in Figure 8. These significant DEGs were enriched in many gene functions, such as negative regulation of transcription, notochord development, trans-Golgi network transport vesicle membrane, RNA polymerase binding, and transcriptional activator activity.

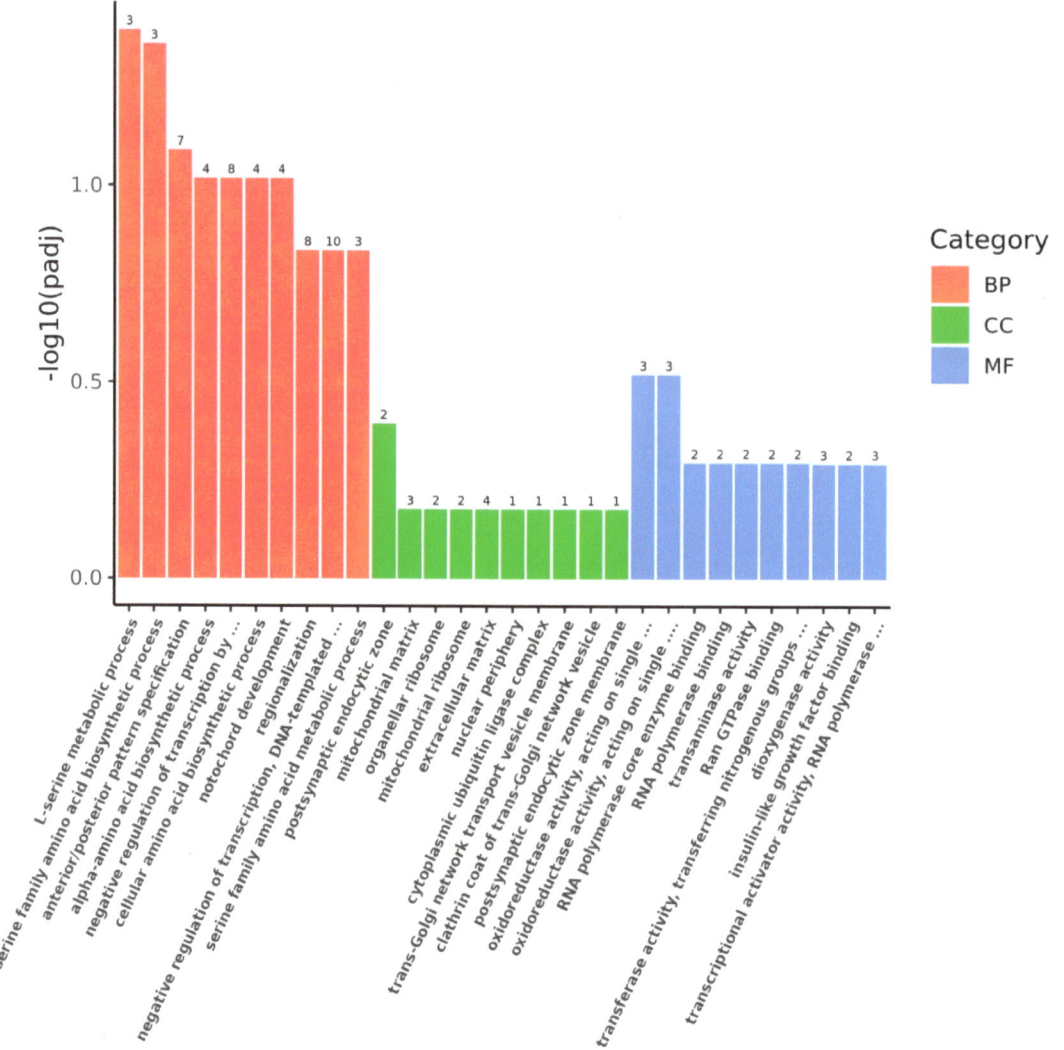

Figure 8. GO enrichment analysis results of 191 DEGs obtained from screening. BP in red: biological processes, CC in green: cellular composition, MF in blue: molecular function.

The Kyoto Encyclopedia of Genes and Genomes (KEGG) enrichment analysis of the 191 DEGs revealed the 20 most significant pathways. As shown in Figure 9, these DEGs were primarily concentrated in pathways associated with metabolism, including biosynthesis of amino acids, glycine, serine and threonine metabolism, carbon metabolism, cysteine and methionine metabolism, glutathione metabolism, insulin signaling pathway, alanine, aspartate, glutamate metabolism, taurine and hypotaurine metabolism, one carbon pool by folate, 2-oxocarboxylic acid metabolism, lysine degradation, and arginine biosynthesis. Additionally, the apelin signaling pathway, aminoacyl-tRNA biosynthesis pathway, erbB signaling pathway, cofactor biosynthesis pathway, autophagy pathway, mTOR signaling pathway, notch signaling pathway, and adipocytokine signaling pathway were among the top 20 enriched factors.

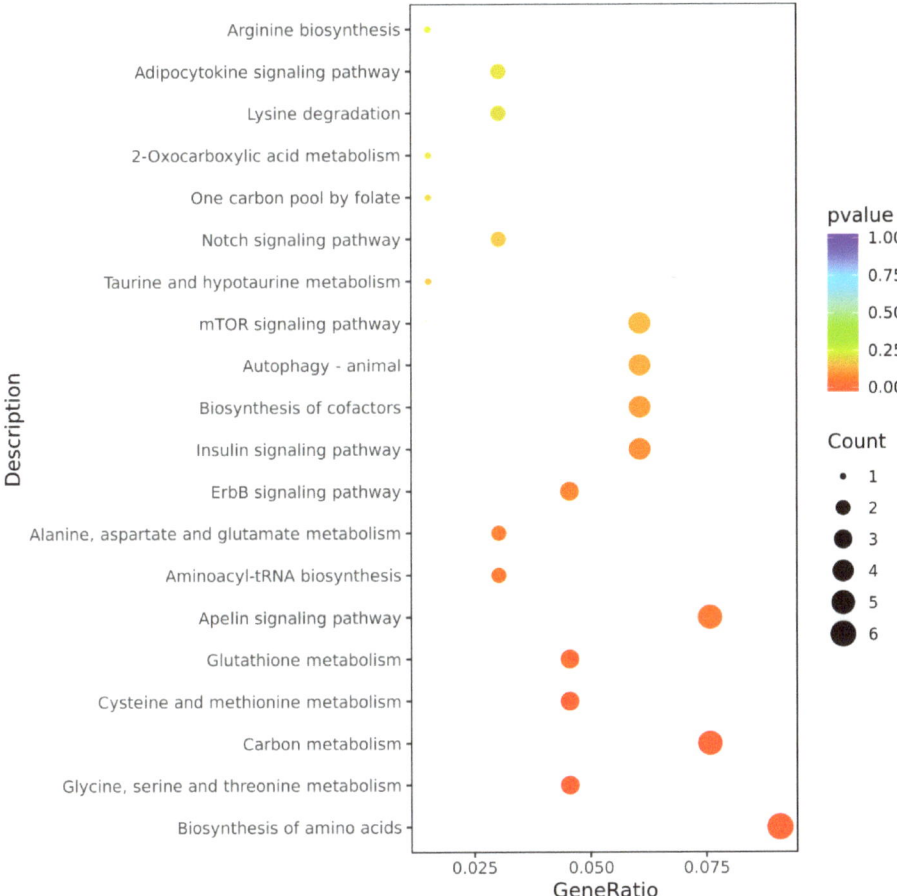

Figure 9. KEGG enrichment analysis results of 191 DEGs obtained from screening.

2.4. qRT–PCR Analysis

To confirm the results of the transcriptome analysis, genes in the mTOR and autophagy signaling pathways were selected for qRT–PCR. As shown in Figure 10A, compared to those in the control group, AA significantly increased the expression of the *pik3r1*, *pik3r3b*, *akt1*, and *mtor* genes in the PI3K/AKT/mTOR signaling pathway. After incubation with HPA, the expression levels of these genes decreased. For the autophagy signaling pathway, the results showed (Figure 10B) that AA treatment downregulated the expression levels of *ulk1b*, *eif2ak3*, *becn1*, and *ambra1a* in zebrafish, while HPA treatment upregulated their expression levels. Therefore, the mechanism of HPA antithrombotic activity involved the downregulation of *pik3r1*, *pik3r3b*, *akt1*, and *mtor* and the upregulation of *ulk1b*, *eif2ak3*, *becn1*, and *ambra1a*.

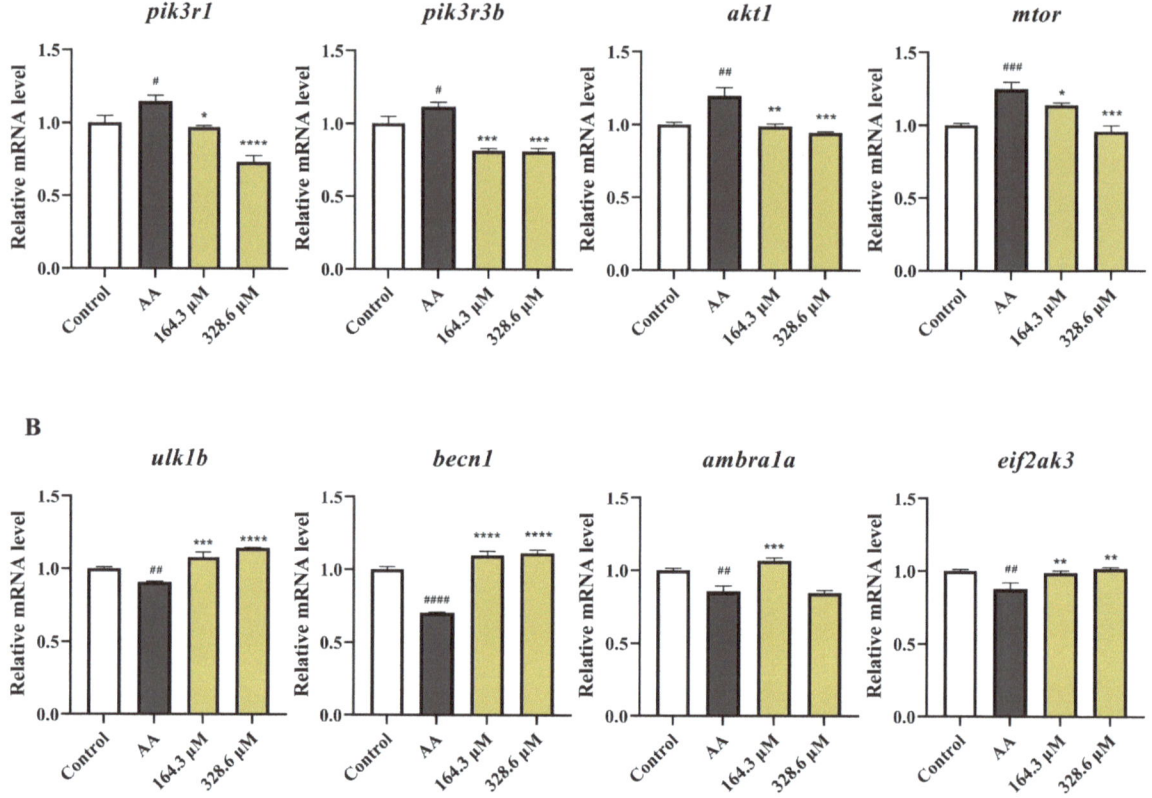

Figure 10. The results of qRT–PCR analysis. Quantitative analysis of the mRNA expression levels of genes associated with (**A**) the PI3K/AKT/mTOR signaling pathway and (**B**) the autophagy signaling pathway. The data are presented as the means ± SEMs; #### $p < 0.0001$, ### $p < 0.001$, ## $p < 0.01$, and # $p < 0.05$ compared to the control group; **** $p < 0.0001$, *** $p < 0.001$, ** $p < 0.01$, and * $p < 0.05$ compared to the AA group.

3. Discussion

Thrombosis is a major cause of morbidity and mortality worldwide, and safe and reliable antithrombotic drugs are urgently needed [39,40]. Marine natural products are promising drug sources, and many natural products with antithrombotic activity have been isolated from marine sources [41,42]. In the zebrafish model, AA can be used to induce experimental thrombosis [43,44]. In this paper, AA-induced zebrafish of the AB lineage were used as a model to assess the antithrombotic effect of HPA. To determine the safe concentration of HPA for use in zebrafish for the evaluation of antithrombotic activity, we conducted an HPA safety concentration test and obtained an LC_1 of 914.6 μM for HPA.

Thrombosis can prevent blood from returning to the heart and reduce the number of cardiac erythrocytes [45], which was consistent with the results of the AA-treated group, suggesting that AA induces thrombosis. HPA dramatically reduced the caudal thrombus area and restored the volume of blood returned to the heart. Thrombosis can slow blood flow [46] and lower the heart rate. In this study, we found that the blood flow velocity and heart rate were significantly greater in the HPA group than in the AA group. Thrombosis can trigger an immune response, which in turn is accompanied by inflammation [47]. Our experiments also indicated that the number of migrating inflammatory cells significantly increased in the AA-treated group and then obviously decreased in the HPA-treated group.

The results of the bioassay protocols indicated an atypical dose effect for the antithrombotic activity of HPA. Based on the results of the caudal thrombus assay, we can confirm that HPA with a concentration of 82.2–328.6 μM has antithrombotic activity in a dose-dependent manner. In the other assay, we found that when the concentration of HPA was 82.2 μM, there was no significant difference in the cardiac erythrocyte, caudal blood flow velocity, or heart rate assay compared with that in the AA group. This may be due to the limited antithrombotic effect of HPA at 82.2 μM, which leads to the insignificance of these indicators. In addition, the antithrombotic activity was lower in the 657.2 μM HPA-treated group than in the 328.6 μM HPA-treated group, which may be due to excessive autophagy. In contrast to appropriately enhanced autophagy, excessive autophagy can cause cell death [48], while macrophage autophagic death releases inflammatory factors and triggers the inflammatory response [49], and autophagic death of smooth muscle cells and vascular endothelial cells reduces plaque stability and promotes thrombosis [50].

According to transcriptome analysis and qRT–PCR validation, HPA exerts its antithrombotic effects by inhibiting the PI3K/AKT/mTOR signaling pathway and enhancing autophagy. Previous studies have shown that platelet activation and aggregation are the pathological basis of thrombosis and that the rupture or erosion of atherosclerotic plaques triggers platelet aggregation, leading to local coagulation activation and thrombosis [51,52]. The PI3K/AKT/mTOR signaling pathway plays an important role in the thrombosis process [53]. Inhibition of the PI3K/AKT pathway can depress platelet activation and adhesion, thereby suppressing thrombosis [54–56], and mTOR is phosphorylated at Ser^{2448} by the PI3K/Akt signaling pathway and plays a key role in platelet aggregation [57]. In this study, HPA significantly downregulated the mRNA expression levels of *pik3r1*, *pik3r3b*, *akt1*, and *mtor*, suggesting that HPA inhibits the PI3K/AKT/mTOR signaling pathway. In addition, the inhibition of the PI3K/AKT/mTOR pathway can induce autophagy [58], and appropriately enhancing autophagy in macrophages can suppress the formation and development of atherosclerotic plaques, promote plaque stabilization, and prevent plaque rupture, thus inhibiting thrombosis [7,52,59,60]. The *ulk1b* gene plays an important role in autophagy and as downstream genes of *ulk1b*, *becn1*, and *ambra1a* can participate in the process of autophagic membrane segregation [61,62], and *eif2ak3* can induce autophagy [63]. In our study, the mRNA expression levels of *ulk1b*, *eif2ak3*, *becn1*, and *ambra1a* were upregulated by 164.3 and 328.6 μM HPA, suggesting that HPA can induce autophagy.

4. Experimental Methods

4.1. General Experimental Procedures

Images were observed and captured with an SZX16 fluorescence microscope, a DP2-BSW image acquisition system (Olympus, Tokyo, Japan), and an AXIO-V16 fluorescence microscope (Zeiss, Oberkochen, Germany). An HPG280-BX Illumination Incubator (Donglian Electronic Technology Development Co., Ltd., Harbin, China) was used for zebrafish culture after drug administration. A zebrafish culture system (ESEN Technology Development Co., Ltd., Beijing, China) was used to cultivate the zebrafish. NMR spectra were recorded on a Bruker Avance spectrometer (Bruker, Billerica, MA, USA) operating at 400 (^{1}H) and 100 (^{13}C) MHz with TMS as an internal standard. ESI-MS data were acquired on an Agilent 6210 ESI/TOF mass spectrometer (Agilent, Santa Clara, CA, USA).

4.2. Fungal Material

After isolating the fungus from a sea water sample taken in 2013 from the Indian Ocean (88°59′51″ E, 2°59′54″ S), we identified it as *Emericellopsis maritima* (GenBank: MH871998.1) through ITS sequence analysis and rDNA amplification. The strain was placed at the Institute of Biology Institute of the Shandong Academy of Sciences' Drug Screening Research Laboratory.

4.3. Fermentation, Extraction, and Isolation

The fermentation media consisted of 50 g of rice and 75 mL of sea water in 500 mL Erlenmeyer flasks, and the strains were cultured in 40 bottles of fermentation media for 60 days at room temperature. All of the fermented material was extracted twice with ethyl acetate and a mixture of dichloromethane:methanol (1:1). Then, the extract was concentrated under reduced pressure, dispersed with water, and extracted with an equal volume of ethyl acetate 4 times to obtain the ethyl acetate phase, which was further concentrated under reduced pressure to obtain the crude extract. Through silica gel column chromatography (CC) and elution with petroleum ether:ethyl acetate (100:0–0:100), the crude extract was separated into 7 fractions, Frs. 1–7. Fr. 6 was subjected to silica CC and then purified using HPLC using 30% MeOH–H_2O to give the compound HPA.

Compound HPA: White crystal powder, ESI-MS *m/z*: 151 [M − H]$^-$. ^{13}C NMR (100 MHZ, CD_3OD) δ_C: 175.0 (C-8), 156.0 (C-4), 129.9 (C-2, 6), 125.6 (C-1), 114.8 (C-3, 5), 39.9 (C-7); ^{1}H NMR (400 MHZ, CD_3OD) δ_H: 7.09 (2H, d, J = 8.8 Hz, H-2, 6), 6.72 (2H, d, J = 8.8 Hz, H-3, 5), 3.47 (2H, s, H-7). The above data are consistent with literature reports [64].

4.4. Safety Concentration Test

We selected healthy zebrafish larvae at 72 hpf under a stereoscopic microscope, transferred them to 24-well plates (ten larvae per well), and treated them for 6 h with different concentrations of HPA (0, 164.3, 328.6, 657.2, 1314.5, 1971.7, 2629.0, 3286.2, 3943.5, or 5258.0 µM). All treatments were performed in triplicate, and the number of subjects per condition was 30. Zebrafish were observed and imaged on a camera using an Olympus microscope, and the mortality rate of the zebrafish in each group was determined. The lethal curve was plotted using GraphPad Prism 9.0 (GraphPad Software, Inc., San Diego, CA, USA) with the HPA concentration and mortality rate as the horizontal and vertical coordinates, respectively, and then the LC_1 was calculated through Nonlinear regression (curve fit).

4.5. Bioassay Protocols

4.5.1. Zebrafish Maintenance

The zebrafish (*Danio rerio*) strains used in this experiment were the AB wild-type and *Tg (zlyz:EGFP)* transgenic lines. Male and female zebrafish were maintained separately at 28.0 °C ± 0.5 °C in an automatic circulating aquarium with a 14/10 h light/dark photoperiod. The embryos were obtained from natural spawning. After fertilization, the eggs were collected, cleaned, and sterilized with methylene blue solution and then placed in zebrafish embryo culture water supplemented with 5.0 mM of NaCl, 0.17 mM of KCl, 0.4 mM of $CaCl_2$, and 0.16 mM of $MgSO_4$ in a constant temperature light incubator at 28.0 °C ± 0.5 °C. The culture water was changed every 24 h.

4.5.2. Chemical Treatment

Healthy zebrafish larvae were chosen at 72 h post-fertilization (hpf) and placed into 24-well plates (ten larvae per well). The plants were randomly divided into 7 groups: a blank control group (fresh fish farming water), a thrombus model group (80 µM AA), a positive control group (80 µM AA + 125.0 µM ASA), and groups treated with different concentrations of HPA (80 µM AA + 82.2, 164.3, 328.6, or 657.2 µM HPA). After treatment with ASA and HPA for 6 h, the solution was aspirated, then the blank control group was treated with fish farming water, and all other groups were treated with 80 µM AA. The plates were incubated at 28 ± 0.5 °C for 1 h. All treatments were performed in triplicate, and the number of subjects per condition was 30.

4.5.3. Caudal Thrombus Assay

At the end of drug treatment, the solution was pipetted out, and then the zebrafish larvae were stained with 1.0 mg/mL of O-dianisidine dye liquor for 10 min in the dark.

After washing with zebrafish culture solution three times, each zebrafish was fixed with 4% paraformaldehyde, and then the caudal thrombi of the zebrafish were observed and photographed under a Zeiss fluorescence microscope. The stained area and intensity of the caudal thrombus in the zebrafish were measured and calculated using Image-Pro Plus 5.0 software (Media Cybernetics, Inc., Bethesda, MD, USA).

4.5.4. Cardiac Erythrocyte Assay

After staining, rinsing, and fixation (as described in Section 4.5.3), each zebrafish was observed and photographed under a Zeiss fluorescence microscope. The thrombus density was quantified according to the stained area, and the intensity of erythrocytes in the heart was analyzed using Image-Pro Plus 5.0 software.

4.5.5. Caudal Blood Flow Velocity and Heart Rate Assay

After drug treatment, each group of zebrafish was washed three times with zebrafish culture water and then observed with an Olympus fluorescence inverted microscope. The heart rates of the zebrafish were obtained, and a video of blood flow for 15 s was recorded from the postcloacal vessels of the zebrafish using the blood flow system Zebralab (ViewPoint, Lyon, France). Analysis of blood flow velocity was then performed using MicroZebraLab BloodFlow 3.4.6 software (ViewPoint, Lyon, France).

4.5.6. Inflammatory Cell Assay

The transgenic zebrafish *Tg (zlyz:EGFP)* with green fluorescent protein (EGFP)-labeled macrophages was selected for this experiment. After drug treatment, images of the caudal inflammatory cells in the zebrafish were recorded under an Olympus inverted fluorescence microscope. The number of caudal inflammatory cells that migrated to the tail notochord and above was counted.

4.6. Transcriptome Analysis

At 72 hpf, normal zebrafish larvae were selected and transferred to 6-well plates. The blank control group (fresh fish farming water), thrombus model group (80 µM AA), and HPA group (80 µM AA + 164.3 or 328.6 µM HPA) were randomly divided, with 50 larvae in each group. Drug treatment for each group followed the same strategy as described in Section 4.5.2. All treatments were carried out in triplicate. TRIzol reagent was used to extract total RNA from the zebrafish. An Agilent 2100 Bioanalyzer (Agilent Technologies, Santa Clara, CA, USA) was used to assess the integrity of the RNA. The raw material for the RNA sample preparations was total RNA. Briefly, poly-T oligo-attached magnetic beads were used to separate mRNA from the total RNA. Divalent cations were used to carry out fragmentation in First Strand Synthesis Reaction Buffer (5X) at a high temperature, and then the libraries were established using the NEB common library building method [65]. Next, Novogene Co., Ltd. (Beijing, China) carried out transcriptome sequencing and analysis.

DESeq2 (version 1.20.0) software (Novogene Co., Ltd., Tianjin, China) was used to carry out differential expression analyses between the two comparison combinations (AA vs. control and HPA vs. AA). A model based on the negative binomial distribution was used to identify DEGs in the gene expression data. P values less than 0.05 indicated significantly differentially expressed genes, which were chosen for further examination. Gene Ontology (GO) and Kyoto Encyclopedia of Genes and Genomes (KEGG) pathway analyses were used to examine the statistical enrichment of DEGs.

4.7. qRT–PCR Assay

Based on the results of the transcriptome analysis, 7 key DEGs were selected for further qRT–PCR analyses. The names and sequences of the primers used are shown in Table 1. Sample treatment and collection were the same as those described in Section 4.6, and total RNA was extracted from the samples with an RNA extraction kit (Vazyme, Nanjing, China). cDNA was obtained through reverse transcription of total RNA with a reverse transcription kit (Vazyme, Nanjing, China). The qRT–PCR system for each well in the 8-tube strip consisted of 2 µL of cDNA (10 ng/µL), 0.4 µL of forward primer, 0.4 µL of reverse primer, 7.2 µL of ddH$_2$O, and 10 µL of SYBR qPCR master mix (Vazyme, Nanjing, China). qRT–PCR was performed in a LightCyler 96 system (Roche, Basel, Switzerland), and the reaction conditions were 30 s at 95 °C, followed by 40 cycles of 95 °C for 15 s and 60 °C for 30 s. β-actin expression levels were used as a normalization control for the expression of other genes. The qRT–PCR data were analyzed using the comparative threshold cycle method ($2^{-\Delta\Delta Ct}$) to calculate the relative expression of each group of genes.

Table 1. The sequences of primers.

Gene Name	Forward Primer (5′→3′)	Reverse Primer (5′→3′)
β-actin	ACCACGGCCGAAAGAGAAAT	GATACCGCAAGATTCCATACCC
pik3r1	TTCAGACATCAGCCCACAAGTT	GCCTGACTGTCACTCCATTCG
pik3r3b	TGACACCAGTAAACGGCAATG	TGTTTCCACCTTTCCTTAGCG
akt1	GTGAAGGAGAAAGCAACAGGCA	ATGACTTCAGAGCCGTCAGGAA
mtor	ACGCTGCACGCACTGATTC	AGAGTCAAATGGTCATAGTCAGGG
ulk1b	GTGCCTTCGCAGTGGTTTT	TGCTGTAGGAATACTCGGATGGT
eif2ak3	AACCGTCTGGAGACACCGAT	TGCTGAGGCTTGAGGATACCA
becn1	AGATGGCGTGGCTCGAAAAT	GCACTCCTCACAAAGTGGGT
ambra1a	ACGCACTCATCCGTCAATAGG	TTCACCGACGCATTACTGATTTC

4.8. Statistical Analysis

Software called GraphPad Prism 9.0 was used to process the statistical analysis. All of the experimental data are shown as mean ± SEM. The comparison between groups was performed using One-Way ANOVA and Dunnett's t-test. At p values less than 0.05, the differences between the groups were considered significant.

5. Conclusions

To summarize, 4-hydroxyphenylacetic acid was isolated from the marine fungus *Emericellopsis maritima* Y39–2, and its antithrombotic activity was determined using a zebrafish model. HPA significantly improved AA-induced thrombus in zebrafish. Specifically, it can increase cardiac erythrocytes, blood flow velocity, and heart rate in zebrafish, reduce caudal thrombus, and reverse the inflammatory response caused by AA. Further research showed that HPA exerted its antithrombotic effect by inhibiting the PI3K/AKT/mTOR signaling pathway and inducing autophagy.

Author Contributions: S.X. performed the bioassays and mechanism studies of the compound and wrote the manuscript. M.Z. performed isolation and structure determination of the compound. P.L. and L.W. performed the fermentation of the fungus and extraction of the culture broths. X.Z. and S.Z. revised the manuscript. Z.M. and H.L. designed the study. X.L. and K.L. supervised the bioassays and revised the manuscript. All authors have read and agreed to the published version of the manuscript.

Funding: This work was supported by the National Key R&D Program of China (2022YFC2804100), the Shandong Provincial Natural Science Foundation (ZR2021ZD29 and ZR2022MH240), the Taishan Scholar Project from Shandong Province to Houwen Lin (ts20190950), and the Jinan Talent Project for University (202228035).

Institutional Review Board Statement: The experiments were performed in accordance with standard ethical guidelines. The procedures were approved by the Ethics Committee of the Biology Institute of Shandong Academy of Science (SWS20240225).

Data Availability Statement: The data presented in this study are available on request from the corresponding author.

Conflicts of Interest: The authors declare no conflicts of interest.

References

1. Barzkar, N.; Jahromi, S.T.; Vianello, F. Marine microbial fibrinolytic enzymes: An overview of source, production, biochemical properties and thrombolytic activity. *Mar. Drugs* **2022**, *20*, 46. [CrossRef] [PubMed]
2. Heron, M. Deaths: Leading causes for 2019. *Natl. Vital Stat. Rep.* **2021**, *70*, 1–114. [PubMed]
3. Roth, G.A.; Mensah, G.A.; Johnson, C.O.; Addolorato, G.; Ammirati, E.; Baddour, L.M.; Barengo, N.C.; Beaton, A.Z.; Benjamin, E.J.; Benziger, C.P.; et al. GBD-NHLBI-JACC global burden of cardiovascular diseases writing group. Global burden of cardiovascular diseases and risk factors, 1990–2019: Update from the GBD 2019 Study. *J. Am. Coll. Cardiol.* **2020**, *76*, 2982–3021. [CrossRef] [PubMed]
4. Wang, Z.; Fang, C.; Yao, M.; Wu, D.; Chen, M.; Guo, T.; Mo, J. Research progress of NF-κB signaling pathway and thrombosis. *Front. Immunol.* **2023**, *14*, 1257988. [CrossRef] [PubMed]
5. Gu, Y.N.; Xie, C.Y. Advancing investigate of deep vein thrombosis for inflammation and signaling pathway. *Chin. J. Immunol.* **2020**, *36*, 113–118.
6. Su, X.L.; Su, W.; Wang, Y.; Wang, Y.H.; Ming, X.; Kong, Y. The pyrrolidinoindoline alkaloid Psm2 inhibits platelet aggregation and thrombus formation by affecting PI3K/Akt signaling. *Acta Pharmacol. Sin.* **2016**, *37*, 1208–1217. [CrossRef] [PubMed]
7. Mu, F.; Jiang, Y.; Ao, F.; Wu, H.; You, Q.; Chen, Z. RapaLink-1 plays an antithrombotic role in antiphospholipid syndrome by improving autophagy both in vivo and vitro. *Biochem. Biophys. Res. Commun.* **2020**, *525*, 384–391. [CrossRef] [PubMed]
8. Nakanishi, M.; Oota, E.; Soeda, T.; Masumo, K.; Tomita, Y.; Kato, T.; Imanishi, T. Emergency cardiac surgery and heparin resistance in a patient with essential thrombocythemia. *JA Clin. Rep.* **2016**, *2*, 35. [CrossRef] [PubMed]
9. Stupnisek, M.; Franjic, S.; Drmic, D.; Hrelec, M.; Kolenc, D.; Radic, B.; Bojic, D.; Vcev, A.; Seiwerth, S.; Sikiric, P. Pentadecapeptide BPC 157 reduces bleeding time and thrombocytopenia after amputation in rats treated with heparin, warfarin or aspirin. *Thromb. Res.* **2012**, *129*, 652–659. [CrossRef]
10. Barbosa, F.; Pinto, E.; Kijjoa, A.; Pinto, M.; Sousa, E. Targeting antimicrobial drug resistance with marine natural products. *Int. J. Antimicrob. Agents* **2020**, *56*, 106005. [CrossRef]
11. Ma, H.G.; Liu, Q.; Zhu, G.L.; Liu, H.S.; Zhu, W.M. Marine natural products sourced from marine-derived *Penicillium* fungi. *J. Asian Nat. Prod. Res.* **2016**, *18*, 92–115. [CrossRef]
12. Kuvarina, A.E.; Gavryushina, I.A.; Sykonnikov, M.A.; Efimenko, T.A.; Markelova, N.N.; Bilanenko, E.N.; Bondarenko, S.A.; Kokaeva, L.Y.; Timofeeva, A.V.; Serebryakova, M.V.; et al. Exploring peptaibol's profile, antifungal, and antitumor activity of Emericellipsin A of *Emericellopsis* Species from Soda and Saline Soils. *Molecules* **2022**, *27*, 1736. [CrossRef] [PubMed]
13. Agrawal, S.; Saha, S. The genus *Simplicillium* and *Emericellopsis*: A review of phytochemistry and pharmacology. *Biotechnol. Appl. Biochem.* **2022**, *69*, 2229–2239. [CrossRef] [PubMed]
14. Shao, S.R.; Yang, B.; Li, H.M.; Fu, C.Y.; Liu, Y.H.; Li, Y.Q. Research about the secondary metabolites of soft coral-derivedepiphytic fungus *Emericellopsis* sp. SCSIO41202 from the South China Sea. *Acta Med. Sin.* **2022**, *35*, 7–12.
15. Inostroza, A.; Lara, L.; Paz, C.; Perez, A.; Galleguillos, F.; Hernandez, V.; Becerra, J.; González-Rocha, G.; Silva, M. Antibiotic activity of Emerimicin IV isolated from *Emericellopsis minima* from Talcahuano Bay, Chile. *Nat. Prod. Res.* **2018**, *32*, 1361–1364. [CrossRef]
16. Baranova, A.A.; Georgieva, M.L.; Bilanenko, E.N.; Andreev, Y.A.; Rogozhin, E.A.; Sadykova, V.S. Antimicrobial potential of alkalophilic micromycetes *Emericellopsis alkalina*. *Appl. Biochem. Microbiol.* **2017**, *53*, 703–710. [CrossRef]
17. Kuvarina, A.E.; Gavryushina, I.A.; Kulko, A.B.; Ivanov, I.A.; Rogozhin, E.A.; Georgieva, M.L.; Sadykova, V.S. The Emericellipsins A-E from an alkalophilic fungus *Emericellopsis alkalina* show potent activity against multidrug-resistant pathogenic fungi. *J. Fungi* **2021**, *7*, 153. [CrossRef] [PubMed]
18. Abraúl, M.; Alves, A.; Hilário, S.; Melo, T.; Conde, T.; Domingues, M.R.; Rey, F. Evaluation of lipid extracts from the marine fungi *Emericellopsis cladophorae* and *Zalerion maritima* as a source of anti-Inflammatory, antioxidant and antibacterial compounds. *Mar. Drugs* **2023**, *21*, 199. [CrossRef] [PubMed]
19. Santoriello, C.; Zon, L.I. Hooked! Modeling human disease in zebrafish. *J. Clin. Investig.* **2012**, *122*, 2337–2343. [CrossRef] [PubMed]
20. Zon, L.I.; Peterson, R.T. In vivo drug discovery in the zebrafish. *Nat. Rev. Drug Discov.* **2005**, *4*, 35–44. [CrossRef]
21. Chico, T.J.; Ingham, P.W.; Crossman, D.C. Modeling cardiovascular disease in the zebrafish. *Trends Cardiovasc. Med.* **2008**, *18*, 150–155. [PubMed]
22. Zhu, X.Y.; Liu, H.C.; Guo, S.Y.; Xia, B.; Song, R.S.; Lao, Q.C.; Xuan, Y.X.; Li, C.Q. A zebrafish thrombosis model for assessing antithrombotic drugs. *Zebrafish* **2016**, *13*, 335–344. [CrossRef]
23. Howe, K.; Clark, M.D.; Torroja, C.F.; Torrance, J.; Berthelot, C.; Muffato, M.; Collins, J.E.; Humphray, S.; McLaren, K.; Matthews, L.; et al. The zebrafish reference genome sequence and its relationship to the human genome. *Nature* **2013**, *496*, 498–503. [CrossRef] [PubMed]
24. Xu, N.; Li, M.C.; Li, Y.Y.; Yan, H.Y.; Han, L.W.; Huang, X.; Li, S.W.; Wang, P.; Shi, Y.P.; Wang, L.; et al. Screening of antithrombotic active Fractions and chemical constituents in Sparganii Rhizoma based on zebrafish model. *Chin. J. Hosp. Pharm.* **2019**, *39*, 1439–1443.
25. Zhang, Y.; Zhu, X.Y.; Guo, S.Y.; Li, C.Q. Phenylhydrazine-induced modelling of zebrafish thrombosis. *Lab. Anim. Comp. Med.* **2015**, *35*, 27–31.

26. Chen, Y.S. Studies on metabolic products of *Hypochnus sasakii* Shirai: Isolation of *p*-hydroxyphenylacetic acid and its physiological activity. *Agric. Biol. Chem.* **1958**, *22*, 136–142.
27. Ohtani, K.; Fujioka, S.; Kawano, T.; Shimada, A.; Kimura, Y. Nematicidal activities of 4-hydroxyphenylacetic acid and oidiolactone D produced by the fungus *Oidiodendron* sp. *Z. Naturforsch. C. J. Biosci.* **2011**, *66*, 31–34. [CrossRef] [PubMed]
28. Flubacher, N.; Baltenweck, R.; Hugueney, P.; Fischer, J.; Thines, E.; Riemann, M.; Nick, P.; Khattab, I.M. The fungal metabolite 4-hydroxyphenylacetic acid from *Neofusicoccum parvum* modulates defence responses in grapevine. *Plant Cell Environ.* **2023**, *46*, 3575–3591. [CrossRef] [PubMed]
29. Fries, L.; Iwasaki, H. *p*-Hydroxyphenylacetic acid and other phenolic compounds as growth stimulators of the red alga *Porphyra tenera*. *Plant Sci. Lett.* **1976**, *6*, 299–307. [CrossRef]
30. An, S.; Yao, Y.; Wu, J.; Hu, H.; Wu, J.; Sun, M.; Li, J.; Zhang, Y.; Li, L.; Qiu, W.; et al. Gut-derived 4-hydroxyphenylacetic acid attenuates sepsis-induced acute kidney injury by upregulating ARC to inhibit necroptosis. *Biochim. Biophys. Acta Mol. Basis Dis.* **2024**, *1870*, 166876. [CrossRef]
31. Liu, Z.; Xi, R.; Zhang, Z.; Li, W.; Liu, Y.; Jin, F.; Wang, X. 4-Hydroxyphenylacetic acid attenuated inflammation and edema via suppressing HIF-1α in seawater aspiration-induced lung injury in rats. *Int. J. Mol. Sci.* **2014**, *15*, 12861–12884. [CrossRef] [PubMed]
32. Takahama, U.; Oniki, T.; Murata, H. The presence of 4-hydroxyphenylacetic acid in human saliva and the possibility of its nitration by salivary nitrite in the stomach. *FEBS Lett.* **2002**, *518*, 116–118. [CrossRef] [PubMed]
33. Zhao, H.; Jiang, Z.; Chang, X.; Xue, H.; Yahefu, W.; Zhang, X. 4-Hydroxyphenylacetic acid prevents acute APAP-induced liver injury by increasing phase II and antioxidant enzymes in mice. *Front. Pharmacol.* **2018**, *9*, 653. [CrossRef] [PubMed]
34. Fries, L. Growth regulating effects of phenylacetic acid and *p*-hydroxyphenylacetic acid on *Fucus spiralis* L. (Phaeophyceae, Fucales) in axenic culture. *Phycologia* **1977**, *16*, 451–455. [CrossRef]
35. Vissiennon, C.; Nieber, K.; Kelber, O.; Butterweck, V. Route of administration determines the anxiolytic activity of the flavonols kaempferol, quercetin and myricetin—are they prodrugs? *J. Nutr. Biochem.* **2012**, *23*, 733–740. [CrossRef] [PubMed]
36. Skorochod, I.; Kurdish, I. P-62—Quantum-chemical study of the antioxidant mechanisms of 4-hydroxyphenylacetic acid a metabolite of *Bacillus subtilis* IMV V-7023 in gas phase. *Free Radic. Biol. Med.* **2018**, *120*, S63. [CrossRef]
37. Liu, Y.; Shi, C.; Zhang, G.; Zhan, H.; Liu, B.; Li, C.; Wang, L.; Wang, H.; Wang, J. Antimicrobial mechanism of 4-hydroxyphenylacetic acid on *Listeria monocytogenes* membrane and virulence. *Biochem. Biophys. Res. Commun.* **2021**, *572*, 145–150.
38. Ko, H.S.; Jin, R.D.; Krishnan, H.B.; Lee, S.B.; Kim, K.Y. Biocontrol ability of *Lysobacter antibioticus* HS124 against *Phytophthora* blight is mediated by the production of 4-hydroxyphenylacetic acid and several lytic enzymes. *Curr. Microbiol.* **2009**, *59*, 608–615. [CrossRef] [PubMed]
39. Choi, J.H.; Sapkota, K.; Park, S.E.; Kim, S.; Kim, S.J. Thrombolytic, anticoagulant and antiplatelet activities of codiase, a bi-functional fibrinolytic enzyme from *Codium fragile*. *Biochimie* **2013**, *95*, 1266–1277. [CrossRef] [PubMed]
40. Mourão, P.A. Perspective on the use of sulfated polysaccharides from marine organisms as a source of new antithrombotic drugs. *Mar. Drugs* **2015**, *13*, 2770–2784. [CrossRef] [PubMed]
41. Doshi, G.; Nailwal, N. A Review on molecular mechanisms and patents of marine-derived anti-thrombotic agents. *Curr. Drug Targets* **2021**, *22*, 318–335. [CrossRef] [PubMed]
42. Haque, N.; Parveen, S.; Tang, T.; Wei, J.; Huang, Z. Marine natural products in clinical use. *Mar. Drugs* **2022**, *20*, 528. [CrossRef] [PubMed]
43. Shi, Y.P.; Zhang, Y.G.; Li, H.N.; Kong, H.T.; Zhang, S.S.; Zhang, X.M.; Li, X.B.; Liu, K.C.; Han, L.W.; Tian, Q.P. Discovery and identification of antithrombotic chemical markers in Gardenia Fructus by herbal metabolomics and zebrafish model. *J. Ethnopharmacol.* **2020**, *253*, 112679. [CrossRef] [PubMed]
44. Qi, Y.; Zhao, X.; Liu, H.; Wang, Y.; Zhao, C.; Zhao, T.; Zhao, B.; Wang, Y. Identification of a quality marker (Q-Marker) of danhong injection by the zebrafish thrombosis model. *Molecules* **2017**, *22*, 1443. [CrossRef] [PubMed]
45. Zhang, M.; Li, P.; Zhang, S.; Zhang, X.; Wang, L.; Zhang, Y.; Li, X.; Liu, K. Study on the mechanism of the danggui-chuanxiong herb pair on treating thrombus through network pharmacology and zebrafish models. *ACS Omega* **2021**, *6*, 14677–14691. [CrossRef]
46. Zhu, H.; Lan, C.; Zhao, D.; Wang, N.; Du, D.; Luo, H.; Lu, H.; Peng, Z.; Wang, Y.; Qiao, Z.; et al. Wuliangye *Baijiu* but not ethanol reduces cardiovascular disease risks in a zebrafish thrombosis model. *NPJ Sci. Food* **2022**, *6*, 55. [CrossRef] [PubMed]
47. Stark, K.; Massberg, S. Interplay between inflammation and thrombosis in cardiovascular pathology. *Nat. Rev. Cardiol.* **2021**, *18*, 666–682. [CrossRef] [PubMed]
48. Schrijvers, D.M.; De Meyer, G.R.Y.; Martinet, W. Autophagy in atherosclerosis: A potential drug target for plaque stabilization. *Arterioscler. Thromb. Vasc. Biol.* **2011**, *31*, 2787–2791. [CrossRef] [PubMed]
49. Denton, D.; Xu, T.; Kumar, S. Autophagy as a pro-death pathway. *Immunol. Cell Biol.* **2015**, *93*, 35–42. [CrossRef] [PubMed]
50. Martinet, W.; De Meyer, G.R.Y. Autophagy in atherosclerosis: A cell survival and death phenomenon with therapeutic potential. *Circ. Res.* **2009**, *104*, 304–317. [CrossRef] [PubMed]
51. Cosemans, J.M.; Angelillo-Scherrer, A.; Mattheij, N.J.; Heemskerk, J.W. The effects of arterial flow on platelet activation, thrombus growth, and stabilization. *Cardiovasc. Res.* **2013**, *99*, 342–352. [CrossRef] [PubMed]
52. Koupenova, M.; Kehrel, B.E.; Corkrey, H.A.; Freedman, J.E. Thrombosis and platelets: An update. *Eur. Heart J.* **2017**, *38*, 785–791. [CrossRef] [PubMed]

53. Ampofo, E.; Später, T.; Müller, I.; Eichler, H.; Menger, M.D.; Laschke, M.W. The marine-derived kinase inhibitor fascaplysin exerts anti-thrombotic activity. *Mar. Drugs* **2015**, *13*, 6774–6791. [CrossRef]
54. Fruman, D.A.; Chiu, H.; Hopkins, B.D.; Bagrodia, S.; Cantley, L.C.; Abraham, R.T. The PI3K pathway in human disease. *Cell* **2017**, *170*, 605–635. [CrossRef] [PubMed]
55. Shen, C.; Liu, M.; Xu, R.; Wang, G.; Li, J.; Chen, P.; Ma, W.; Mwangi, J.; Lu, Q.; Duan, Z.; et al. The 14-3-3ζ-c-Src-integrin-β3 complex is vital for platelet activation. *Blood* **2020**, *136*, 974–988. [CrossRef] [PubMed]
56. Fan, D.; Tian, Z.Z.; Ma, X.L.; Zuo, X.; Ya, F.L.; Yang, Y. Fruitflow, a water-soluble tomato concentrate, inhibits platelet activation, aggregation and thrombosis by regulating the signaling pathway of PI3K/Akt and MAPKs. *J. Sun Yat-Sen Univ. Med. Sci.* **2020**, *41*, 243–250.
57. Aslan, J.E.; Tormoen, G.W.; Loren, C.P.; Pang, J.; McCarty, O.J. S6K1 and mTOR regulate Rac1-driven platelet activation and aggregation. *Blood* **2011**, *118*, 3129–3136. [CrossRef]
58. Fang, S.; Wan, X.; Zou, X.; Sun, S.; Hao, X.; Liang, C.; Zhang, Z.; Zhang, F.; Sun, B.; Li, H.; et al. Arsenic trioxide induces macrophage autophagy and atheroprotection by regulating ROS-dependent TFEB nuclear translocation and AKT/mTOR pathway. *Cell Death Dis.* **2021**, *12*, 88. [CrossRef] [PubMed]
59. Shao, B.Z.; Han, B.Z.; Zeng, Y.X.; Su, D.F.; Liu, C. The roles of macrophage autophagy in atherosclerosis. *Acta Pharmacol. Sin.* **2016**, *37*, 150–156. [CrossRef] [PubMed]
60. Zhao, K.; Xu, X.S.; Meng, X.; Li, Y.L.; Li, J.F.; Chen, W.Q. Autophagy of monocytes attenuates the vulnerability of coronary atherosclerotic plaques. *Coron. Artery Dis.* **2013**, *24*, 651–656. [CrossRef] [PubMed]
61. Wang, X.; Fang, Y.; Huang, Q.; Xu, P.; Lenahan, C.; Lu, J.; Zheng, J.; Dong, X.; Shao, A.; Zhang, J. An updated review of autophagy in ischemic stroke: From mechanisms to therapies. *Exp. Neurol.* **2021**, *340*, 113684. [CrossRef] [PubMed]
62. Lekli, I.; Haines, D.D.; Balla, G.; Tosaki, A. Autophagy: An adaptive physiological countermeasure to cellular senescence and ischaemia/reperfusion-associated cardiac arrhythmias. *J. Cell. Mol. Med.* **2017**, *21*, 1058–1072. [CrossRef] [PubMed]
63. Yao, R.Q.; Ren, C.; Xia, Z.F.; Yao, Y.M. Organelle-specific autophagy in inflammatory diseases: A potential therapeutic target underlying the quality control of multiple organelles. *Autophagy* **2021**, *17*, 385–401. [CrossRef] [PubMed]
64. Wang, X.J.; Xie, X.; Luo, X.; Song, Y.L.; Zhao, Y.W.; Huang, W.Z.; Wang, Z.Z.; Xiao, W. Chemical constituents from *Rhodiola wallichiana* var. *cholaensis* (I). *Chin. Tradit. Herb. Drugs* **2015**, *46*, 3471–3474.
65. Parkhomchuk, D.; Borodina, T.; Amstislavskiy, V.; Banaru, M.; Hallen, L.; Krobitsch, S.; Lehrach, H.; Soldatov, A. Transcriptome analysis by strand-specific sequencing of complementary DNA. *Nucleic Acids Res.* **2009**, *37*, e123. [CrossRef]

Disclaimer/Publisher's Note: The statements, opinions and data contained in all publications are solely those of the individual author(s) and contributor(s) and not of MDPI and/or the editor(s). MDPI and/or the editor(s) disclaim responsibility for any injury to people or property resulting from any ideas, methods, instructions or products referred to in the content.

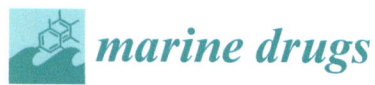 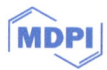

Article

Two New Sesquiterpenoids and a New Shikimic Acid Metabolite from Mangrove Sediment-Derived Fungus *Roussoella* sp. SCSIO 41427

Zimin Xiao [1,†], Jian Cai [2,†], Ting Chen [3], Yilin Wang [3], Yixin Chen [1], Yongyan Zhu [1], Chunmei Chen [2], Bin Yang [2], Xuefeng Zhou [2] and Huaming Tao [1,*]

[1] Guangdong Provincial Key Laboratory of Chinese Medicine Pharmaceutics, School of Traditional Chinese Medicine, Southern Medical University, Guangzhou 510515, China; 15917491112@163.com (Z.X.); 13676126834@163.com (Y.C.); yongyanzhu0521@163.com (Y.Z.)

[2] CAS Key Laboratory of Tropical Marine Bio-Resources and Ecology, Guangdong Key Laboratory of Marine Materia Medica, South China Sea Institute of Oceanology, Chinese Academy of Sciences, Guangzhou 510301, China; caijian19@mails.ucas.ac.cn (J.C.); chenchunmei18@mails.ucas.ac.cn (C.C.); yangbin@scsio.ac.cn (B.Y.); xfzhou@scsio.ac.cn (X.Z.)

[3] School of Stomatology, Southern Medical University, Guangzhou 510515, China; chent@smu.edu.cn (T.C.); FOURCWATER@outlook.com (Y.W.)

* Correspondence: taohm@smu.edu.cn; Tel.: +86-020-61648770

† These authors contributed equally to this work.

Abstract: Two new sesquiterpenoid derivatives, elgonenes M (**1**) and N (**2**), and a new shikimic acid metabolite, methyl 5-*O*-acetyl-5-*epi*-shikimate (**3**), were isolated from the mangrove sediment-derived fungus *Roussoella* sp. SCSIO 41427 together with fourteen known compounds (**4**–**17**). The planar structures were elucidated through nuclear magnetic resonance (NMR) and mass spectroscopic (MS) analyses. The relative configurations of **1**–**3** were ascertained by NOESY experiments, while their absolute configurations were determined by electronic circular dichroism (ECD) calculation. Elgonene M (**1**) exhibited inhibition of interleukin-1β (IL-1β) mRNA, a pro-inflammatory cytokine, at a concentration of 5 µM, with an inhibitory ratio of 31.14%. On the other hand, elgonene N (**2**) demonstrated inhibition at a concentration of 20 µM, with inhibitory ratios of 27.57%.

Keywords: mangrove sediment-derived fungi; sesquiterpenoid; IL-1β; anti-inflammatory

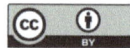

1. Introduction

As a defensive response to injury, inflammation is not always harmful; however, excessive expression of inflammatory mediators can lead to immune system dysregulation, resulting in inflammatory diseases [1]. Currently, the most widely used anti-inflammatory drugs worldwide are nonsteroidal anti-inflammatory drugs (NSAIDs), but they come with serious gastrointestinal side effects and cardiovascular risks [2]. Therefore, exploring new anti-inflammatory drugs is crucial research. Scientists are actively investigating natural sources, including marine organisms, plants, and microorganisms, in the quest for new therapeutic agents with potent anti-inflammatory properties and improved safety profiles.

The ocean is a treasure trove of resources, and the search for new natural products from the marine environment for drug development has become an international research hotspot. Statistics show that, in the year 2021 alone, researchers discovered 1425 new compounds with a wide range of biological activities from marine-derived organisms [3]. Among these, mangrove sediment-derived microorganisms (MSMs) are an important source of various natural products. As of 2021, researchers have isolated and identified 519 new natural products from MSMs, with 57% of these compounds originating from fungi and exhibiting broad and effective biological activities. These compounds from marine-derived fungi have shown promising antimicrobial properties against various pathogens, significant anticancer potential, anti-inflammatory effects, antioxidant activity, and additional biological activities, such as antiviral, antiparasitic, and immunomodulatory effects [4]. The discovery of these 519 new natural products from MSMs, particularly with a significant proportion originating from fungi, highlights the immense potential of marine ecosystems as a source of bioactive compounds. The exploration of marine-derived fungi and other MSMs continues to be a fruitful area of research, offering new avenues for drug discovery and development. By harnessing the diverse chemical structures and biological activities of these natural products, scientists aim to address various health challenges and improve the well-being of humans.

Roussoella sp. SCSIO 41427 belongs to the Ascomycota phylum, and, in previous research reports, numerous structurally novel and biologically active secondary metabolites have been discovered from strains of this kind [5] (for instance, from *Roussoella hysterioides* KT1651, tetracyclic diterpene fusicoccanes, roussoellols A and B, with unique bent structural frameworks [6]. Additionally, a novel dehydroacetic acid derivative, roussoellenic acid, isolated from *Roussoella* sp. (MFLUCC 17-2059), displayed excellent inhibitory activity against biofilm formation in *Staphylococcus aureus* [7].

In our previous research, we successfully isolated a multitude of structurally novel compounds from marine-derived fungi. These compounds encompass a variety of new polyketides, alkaloids, and other metabolites, each showcasing a diverse array of noteworthy biological activities. Notably, these compounds demonstrate promising anti-inflammatory, antifungal, and antitumor properties [8–10]. In this study, we extracted, isolated, and identified seventeen compounds (Figure 1) from the rice fermentation products of the strain *Roussoella* sp. SCSIO 41427, sourced from mangrove sediment. Among them are two new sesquiterpenoids, elgonenes M (**1**) and N (**2**), one new natural product (**3**) (previously reported synthetically [11]), along with seven known isocoumarins derivatives (**4–10**) and some other known compounds (**11–17**). Notably, elgonenes M (**1**) and N (**2**) demonstrated a reduction in the expression of endogenous inflammatory factor IL-1β mRNA at concentrations of 5 µM and 20 µM, with inhibition rates of 31.14% and 27.57%, respectively. This paper focuses on the isolation, structural elucidation, and details of the biological activities of these compounds.

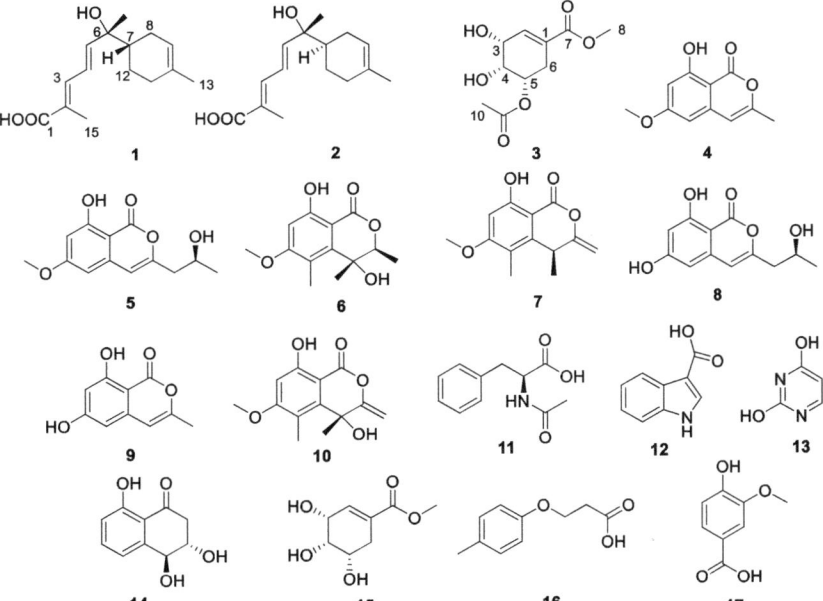

Figure 1. Structures of compounds **1–17**.

2. Results and Discussion

2.1. Structural Determination

Compound **1** was obtained as a pale yellow oil, and its molecular formula of $C_{15}H_{22}O_3$ was deduced from the negative HRESIMS ion peak at m/z 249.1499 [M-H]$^-$ (calculated for $C_{15}H_{21}O_3^-$, 249.1496), implying five degrees of hydrogen deficiency. The ^{1}H NMR data (Table 1) showed three methyls at δ_H 1.33 (s, H$_3$-14), 1.64 (s, H$_3$-13), and 1.96 (s, H$_3$-15); three methylenes at δ_H 1.81/2.03 (H$_2$-8), 1.99 (m, H$_2$-11), and 1.24/1.90 (H$_2$-12); and five olefinic protons at 7.29 (d, J = 11.4 Hz, H-3), 6.59 (dd, J = 11.4, 15.1 Hz, H-4), 6.17 (d, J = 15.1 Hz, H-5), 1.63 (m, H-7), and 5.36 (m, H-9). Analysis of the ^{13}C, DEPT135 and HSQC NMR spectra displayed 15 carbon signals, including one carbonyl carbons at δ_C 173.5 (C-1); two olefinic tertiary carbons at δ_C 126.1 (C-2), and 134.2 (C-10); four olefinic methine carbons at δ_C 140.1 (C-3), 123.5 (C-4), 148.0 (C-5), and 120.3 (C-9); three methyl carbons at δ_C 23.5 (C-13), 26.1 (C-14), and 12.6 (C-15); three methylene carbons at 26.9 (C-8,), 30.8 (C-11), and 23.6 (C-12); and two methine carbon (including one oxygenated) at 75.3 (C-6) and 44.3 (C-7). The ^{1}H-^{1}H COSY correlations (Figure 2) of H$_2$-11/H$_2$-12/H$_2$-7/H$_2$-8/H-9 and the HMBC correlations from H$_3$-13 to C-9, C-10, and C-11 revealed a six-membered ring with a methyl at C-10. A chain system with hydroxyl and carboxyl groups was confirmed by the ^{1}H-^{1}H COSY correlations of H-3/H-4/H-5 and the HMBC correlations from H-2 to C-1 and C-4, as well as from H-4 to C-6 and from H-5 to H$_3$-14. The HMBC correlation from H$_3$-14 to C-7 suggested that methine carbon C-6 at the end of the chain was located at C-7 on the ring. Furthermore, the NMR data indicated that the planar structure of **1** was similar to that of the known compound, sesquiterpene elgonene D [12]. Also, Compound **2** was obtained as a pale yellow oil, and its molecular formula of $C_{15}H_{22}O_3$ was deduced from the negative HRESIMS ion peak at m/z 249.1498 [M-H]$^-$ (calculated for $C_{15}H_{21}O_3^-$, 249.1496). The NMR spectroscopic data (Table 1) comparison between **2** and **1** revealed that they possess identical planar structures.

Table 1. The NMR data of **1–3** (600 and 150 MHz, δ in ppm, CDCl$_3$).

Pos.	1		2		3	
	δ_C, Type	δ_H, (J in Hz)	δ_C, Type	δ_H, (J in Hz)	δ_C, Type	δ_H, (J in Hz)
1	173.5, C		173.1, C		129.2, C	
2	126.1, C		126.0, C		140.5, CH	6.79, brs
3	140.1, CH	7.29, d, (11.4)	140.1, CH	7.30, d, (11.4)	69.2, CH	4.42, m
4	123.5, CH	6.59, dd, (15.1, 11.4)	123.3, CH	6.61, dd, (15.2, 11.4)	69.7, CH	4.08, m
5	148.0, CH	6.17, d, (15.1)	148.8, CH	6.17, d, (15.2)	72.4, CH	5.05, m
6	75.3, C		75.5, C		26.5, CH$_2$	2.63, m
7	44.3, CH	1.63, m	44.2, CH	1.63, m	168.1, C	
8	26.9, CH$_2$	1.81, m; 2.03, m	25.8, CH$_2$	1.81, m; 2.03, m	52.4, CH$_3$	3.76, s
9	120.3, CH	5.36, m	120.4, CH	5.36, m	172.3, C	
10	134.2, C		134.2, C		21.0, CH$_3$	2.11, s
11	30.8, CH$_2$	1.99, m	30.9, CH$_2$	1.99, m		
12	23.6, CH$_2$	1.24, m; 1.90, m	24.2, CH$_2$	1.24, m; 1.90, m		
13	23.5, CH$_3$	1.64, s	23.5, CH$_3$	1.64, s		
14	26.1, CH$_3$	1.33, s	26.3, CH$_3$	1.32, s		
15	12.6, CH$_3$	1.96, s	12.6, CH$_3$	1.97, s		

As for their configuration, $\Delta^{2,3}$ and $\Delta^{4,5}$ double bonds in **1** and **2** were both deduced as E by the NOESY correlation of H$_3$-15/H-3 (Figure 2) and the large coupling constant $J_{H-4/H-5}$ = 15.1/15.2 Hz. Due to the consistent trends observed in their experimental CD curves, the ECD calculations of **1/2** (Figure 3) indicated that the configuration was established as 6R,7S/6R,7R. Thus, compounds **1** and **2** are a pair of diastereomers, with both having an R configuration of C-6. To differentiate between the diastereomers **1** and **2**, a detailed conformational analysis was performed. The dominant conformation of the 6R,7S stereoisomer was characterized by a close spatial proximity between H$_3$-14 and H-7, indicating the presence of a NOESY effect of H$_3$-14/H-7 (Figure 2). Compared with the NMR experimental data, the NOESY correlation of H$_3$-14/H-7 in **1** suggested its absolute configuration as 6R,7S. Similarly, the absence of a NOESY correlation of H$_3$-14/H-7 in **2** suggested its absolute configuration as 6R,7R. Therefore, the gross structures, as depicted in Figure 1, were constructed and have been designated as elgonenes M (**1**) and N (**2**).

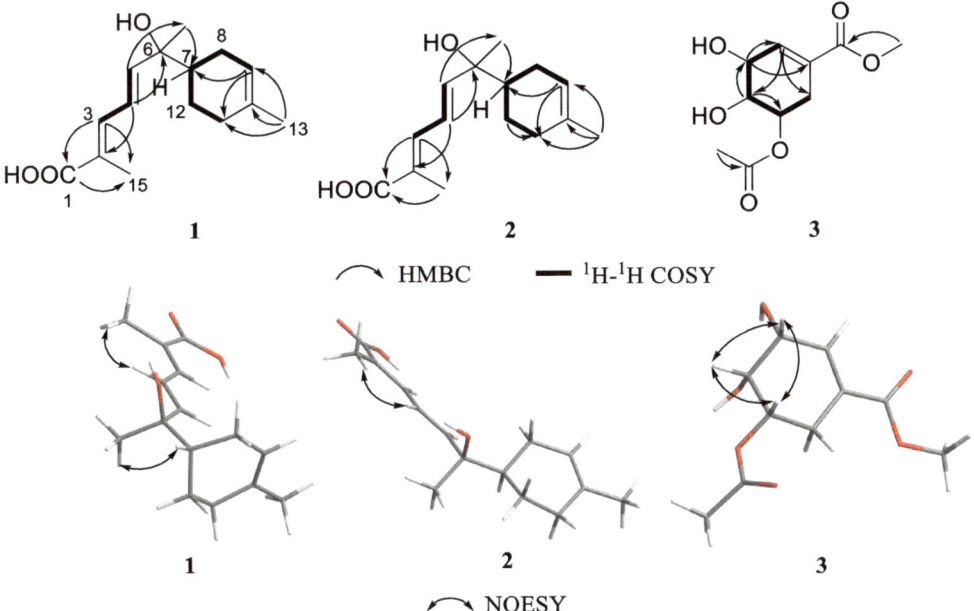

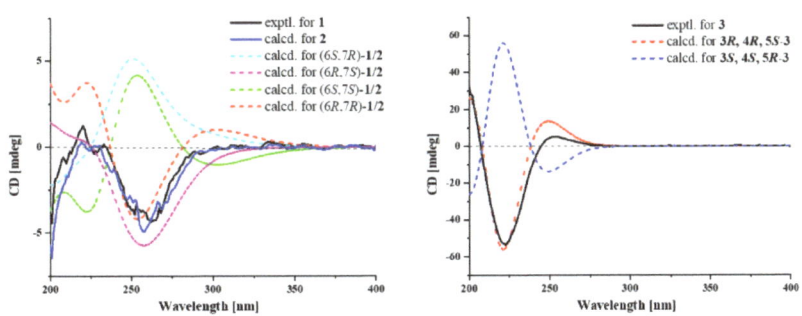

Figure 2. Key ^{1}H-^{1}H COSY, HMBC, and NOESY correlations of **1**–**3**.

Figure 3. Experimental and calculational ECD spectrum of **1**–**3**.

Compound **3** was isolated as pale yellow oil, and its molecular formula was determined as C$_{10}$H$_{14}$O$_6$ by HRESIMS ion peak at m/z 231.0870 [M+H]$^+$ (calculated for C$_{10}$H$_{15}$O$_6^+$, 231.0863), corresponding to four indices of hydrogen deficiency. The ^{1}H NMR spectrum exhibited two methyl singlets at δ_H 2.10 (H$_3$-10) and 3.76 (H$_3$-8). Analysis of the ^{13}C NMR (Table 1) and DEPT135 NMR spectra suggested the presence of three quaternary carbons, one CH$_2$ group, including two carbonyl/ester-bearing quaternary carbons at δ_C 168.1 (C-7) and 172.3 (C-9), and one double-bond-bearing quaternary carbon at δ_C 129.2 (C-1). Additionally, the ^{1}H NMR and HSQC data indicated the presence of four CH groups, including three oxygen-bearing CHs at δ_C 69.2 (C-3), 69.7 (C-4), and 72.4 (C-5), and one double-bond-bearing CH at δ_C 140.5 (C-2). The cyclohexene ring was determined through HMBC correlations from H-2 to C-4/C-6, H-3 to C-1/C-2, H-4 to C-2/C-3/C-5/C-6, and H$_2$-6 to C-1/C-2/C-4/C-5. The structural elucidation involved establishing two side chains through HMBC correlations (Figure 2) from H$_3$-8 to C-1/C-7 and H$_3$-10 to C-5/C-9. The connection between the side chain structure and the cyclohexene ring was revealed through HMBC correlations from H-2/H$_2$-6 to C-7, H-5 to C-9/C-10. Furthermore, ^{1}H-^{1}H COSY correlations between H-2/H-3/H-4/H-5/H-6 confirmed the cyclohexyl structure. The above NMR data indicated that the structural skeleton of **3** was identical to that of a synthesized compound, methyl 5-*O*-acetyl-5-*epi*-shikimate [11]. The NOESY correlations of H-3/H-5, H-3/H-4, and H-4/H-5 supposed that the relative configuration of **3** was rel-(3*R*, 4*R*, 5*S*). Finally, its absolute configuration was determined to be 3*R*, 4*R*, 5*S* through the ECD calculations and specific rotation compared with **15** (Figure 3).

By comparing their physicochemical properties and spectroscopic data with the reported literature values, other known compounds were determined. Compounds present in SCSIO 41427 were 8-hydroxy-6-methoxy-3-methyl-1*H*-isochromen-1-one (**4**) [13], (*S*)-8-hydroxy-3-(2-hydroxypropyl)-6-methoxy-1*H*-isochromen-1-one (**5**) [14], (3*S*,4*R*)-4,8-dihydroxy-6-methoxy-3,4,5-trimethylisochroman-1-one (**6**) [15], (*S*)-8-hydroxy-6-methoxy-4,5-dimethyl-3-methyleneisochroman-1-one (**7**) [16], (*S*)-6,8-dihydroxy-3-(2-hydroxypropyl)-1*H*-isochromen-1-one (**8**) [17], 6,8-dihydroxy-3-methyl-1*H*-isochromen-1-one (**9**) [18], 4,8-dihydroxy-6-methoxy-4,5-dimethyl-3-methyleneisochroman-1-one (**10**) [16], acetyl-*L*-phenylalanine (**11**) [19], 1*H*-indole-3-carboxylic acid (**12**) [20], pyrimidine-2,4-diol (**13**) [21], trans-3,4-dihydro-3,4,8-trihydroxynaphthalen-1(2*H*)-one (**14**) [22], methyl 5-*epi*-Shikimate (**15**) [11], 3-(*p*-tolyloxy)propanoic acid (**16**) [23], 4-hydroxy-3-methoxybenzoic acid (**17**) [24], related physicochemical and spectroscopic data shown in Supplementary Materials.

2.2. Bioactive Assay

Most acute and chronic non-infectious inflammatory diseases are associated with the pro-inflammatory cytokine interleukin-1β (IL-1β), and clinical studies have proven that blocking IL-1β can effectively resolve inflammation [25]. In order to investigate the anti-inflammatory effects of the compounds, an inflammation model was established using lipopolysaccharide (LPS)-stimulated C57BL/6 mouse primary bone marrow-derived macrophages. Dexamethasone, a well-known anti-inflammatory drug, was used as a positive control for comparison. The experimental results revealed that both **1** (5 μM) and **2** (10 and 20 μM) exerted noticeable effects on the expression of endogenous inflammatory factor IL-1β mRNA within the cells. Specifically, Compound **1** at 5 μM significantly reduced the expression of IL-1β mRNA, resulting in an impressive inhibition rate of 31.14%. Similarly, Compound **2** at a concentration of 20 μM exhibited a significant reduction in the level of IL-1β mRNA, with an inhibition rate of 27.57% (Figure 4). These findings suggested that both **1** and **2** possessed anti-inflammatory properties. Compound **1** showed activity only at 5 μM and was inactive at higher concentrations. The cellular toxicity of **1** on LPS-stimulated C57BL/6 mouse primary bone marrow-derived macrophages at 10 and 20 μM was speculated to be the reason behind these results. Therefore, the difference in activity between compounds **1** and **2** may be attributed to their distinct configurations at C-7. In addition, anti-inflammatory activities have also been found in sesquiterpene derivatives in the published literature [26,27], proving that these types of compounds indeed have certain research value in anti-inflammatory activity. Further studies are needed to elucidate the underlying mechanisms and explore their potential in the treatment of inflammatory diseases.

During the in vitro antitumor activity screening, compounds **1**, **3–6**, **8–10**, and **14** were evaluated at a concentration of 50 μM. The results indicated that the inhibition rate on MDA-MB-435 tumor cells (human breast cancer cells) was below 50%, indicating that their IC$_{50}$ values were greater than 50 μM.

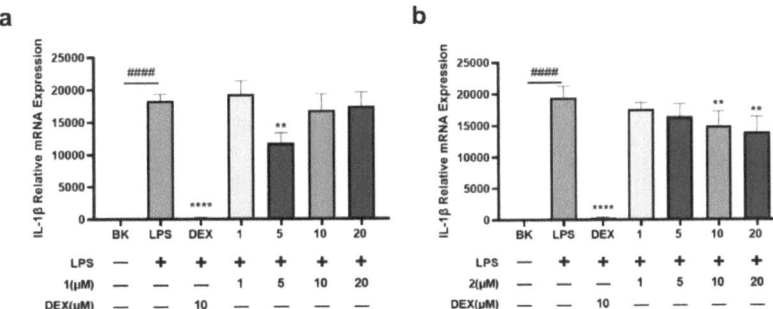

Figure 4. Inhibitory activity of **1** (**a**) and **2** (**b**) on IL-1β mRNA expression in LPS-induced macrophages. where values are expressed as mean ± standard deviation, $n \geq 3$; #### $p < 0.0001$ for LPS-stimulated model group vs. blank control group; ** $p < 0.01$, **** $p < 0.0001$ for treatment groups vs. LPS-stimulated model group.

3. Materials and Methods

3.1. General Experimental Procedures

The UV and ECD spectra was recorded on a UV-Vis spectrophotometer model 8453VU-Vis (Agilent, Beijing, China) and a chirascan circular dichroism spectrometer (Applied Photophysics, Surrey, Britain), respectively. The IR spectrum was obtained using an IR Affinity-1 spectrometer (Shimadzu, Beijing, China). HRESIMS spectra were recorded with a Bruker maXis Q-TOF mass spectrometer. The NMR spectra were recorded on a AVANCE III HD 600 MHz spectrometer (Bruker BioSpin International AG, Fällanden, Switzerland), and chemical shifts were recorded as δ-values. High-Performance Liquid Chromatograph (HPLC) was performed on the Agilent 1260 with a DAD detector using an ODS column (YMC-pack ODS-A, 10 × 250 mm, 5 μm). Thin-layer chromatography analysis (TLC) and column chromatography (CC) were carried out on plates precoated with silica gel GF254 (10–40 μm), over silica gel (200–300 mesh) (Qingdao Marine Chemical Factory, Qingdao, China) and Sephadex LH-20 (Amersham Biosciences, Uppsala, Sweden). Spots were detected on TLC (Qingdao Marine Chemical Factory) under 254 nm UV light. All solvents used, except for the liquid chromatography mobile phase, were of analytical grade (Tianjin Fuyu Chemical and Industry Factory, Tianjin, China). The mobile phase for liquid chromatography was of HPLC gradient grade (Shanghai Xingke High Purity Solvents Co., Ltd, Shanghai, China).

3.2. Fungal Source and Strain Identification

The fungal strain SCSIO 41427 was isolated from a mangrove sediment sample collected from a Gaoqiao mangrove in Lianjiang, China. The strains were stored on MB agar (malt extract 15 g, sea salt 10 g, agar 16 g, H_2O 1 L, pH 7.4–7.8) slants in liquefied petrolatum and deposited at Key Laboratory of Tropical Marine Bio-resources and Ecology, Chinese Academy of Sciences. The strain SCSIO 41427 was designated as *Roussoella* sp., due to its ITS sequence (GenBank accession No. OR574981) homology with *Roussoella* sp. LT796863.1.

3.3. Fungal Cultivation and Fermentation

The fermentation of *Roussoella* sp. SCSIO 41427 was carried out using a solid-state culture medium. The preparation of the medium involved combining 180 mL of distilled water, 3 g of sea salt, and 150 g of rice in a 1000 mL conical flask. The MB seed solution was prepared by mixing 400 mL of distilled water, 8 g of sea salt, and 6 g of malt extract in a 1000 mL conical flask, with pH adjustment set to 7.4–7.8. Both media were sterilized by autoclaving at 121 °C for 30 min and allowed to cool. The strain was activated by inoculating it into MB agar medium (or PDA medium) after being stored in paraffin oil. The activation process occurred at 26 °C for 5 days (typically 5 days), after which agar sections containing the newly cultivated *Roussoella* sp. SCSIO 41427 were transferred to MB seed liquid. This mixture was then cultured in two bottles at 27 °C with agitation at 180 rpm for 48 h to obtain the seed liquid. The seed liquid was subsequently transferred to the solid rice culture medium and allowed to ferment at 26 °C for 30 days. This process was scaled up to 60 bottles, yielding 45 bottles of fermented material (6.75 kg in dry) from *Roussoella* sp. SCSIO 41427.

3.4. Extraction and Isolation

After the fermentation product was crushed, it was subjected to ultrasonic extraction with ethyl acetate and the resulting crude extract (109.1 g) was obtained. Silica gel (200–300 mesh) column chromatography (CC) was employed using stepwise gradient elution with petroleum ether/dichloromethane (0–100%, v/v) and dichloromethane/methanol (0–100%, v/v) to obtain six fractions (Frs. A–F). Fraction C (Fr. C, 5.5 g) was separated by ODS CC using CH_3OH/H_2O (10:90–100:0) gradient elution, yielding five subfractions (C1–C5). Subfraction C5 was further purified using semi-preparative HPLC with CH_3CN/H_2O (40:60, 0.1% HCOOH) as the eluent, resulting in the isolation of **1** (3.9 mg, t_R = 34.8 min) and **2** (3.4 mg, t_R = 36.3 min). Subfraction C4, obtained from semi-preparative HPLC with CH_3OH/H_2O (58:42) as the eluent, yielded **5** (17.0 mg, t_R = 21.8 min). Subfraction C3 was isolated using semi-preparative HPLC with CH_3OH/H_2O (55:45) as the eluent, resulting in the isolation of **9** (6.9 mg, t_R = 16.7 min). Subfraction C2 was purified using semi-preparative HPLC with CH_3OH/H_2O (40:60) as the eluent, yielding **6** (2.3 mg, t_R = 34.5 min) and **16** (20.8 mg, t_R = 31.3 min). Fraction E (2.3 g) was subjected to Sephadex LH-20 CC, eluting with methanol, to obtain three subfractions (E1–E3). Subfraction E3 was further isolated using semi-preparative HPLC with CH_3CN/H_2O (18:82) as the eluent, yielding **3** (7.7 mg, t_R = 12.0 min). Fraction A (5.0 g) was separated from Fr. A by ODS CC with CH_3OH/H_2O (10:90–100:0) gradient elution and was subsequently fractionated into four subfractions (A1–A4). Subfraction A2 was further purified using semi-preparative HPLC with CH_3CN/H_2O (55:45) as the eluent, resulting in the isolation of **4** (5.0 mg, t_R = 16.8 min). Subfraction A3 was obtained using semi-preparative HPLC with CH_3OH/H_2O (68:32) as the eluent, resulting in the isolation of **7** (6.5 mg, t_R = 25.8 min). Fractions D (2.3 g), B (2.5 g), and F (2.0 g) were subjected to Sephadex LH-20 CC with methanol as the eluent, leading to the separation of four subfractions (D1–D4), five subfractions (B1–B5), and four subfractions (F1–F4), respectively. Subfraction D2 was purified using semi-preparative HPLC with CH_3OH/H_2O (25:75) as the eluent, yielding **14** (5.2 mg, t_R = 20.3 min), D3 with CH_3OH/H_2O (45:55) as the eluent, yielding **8** (7.8 mg, t_R = 21.8 min) and **17** (4.5 mg, t_R = 11.0 min), D4 with CH_3OH/H_2O (40:60, 0.1% HCOOH) as the eluent, yielding **12** (7.0 mg, t_R = 19.5 min). Subfraction B5 was isolated using semi-preparative HPLC with CH_3CN/H_2O (46:54) as the eluent, leading to the isolation of **10** (2.6 mg, t_R = 18.4 min). Subfraction F2 was purified using semi-preparative HPLC with CH_3OH/H_2O (15:85, 0.1% HCOOH) as the eluent, resulting in the isolation of **15** (22.5 mg, t_R = 13.2 min). Subfraction F3 was purified using semi-preparative HPLC with CH_3CN/H_2O (20:80, 0.1% HCOOH) as the eluent, resulting in the isolation of **11** (3.9 mg, t_R = 18.8 min). Subfraction F4 was isolated using semi-preparative HPLC with CH_3OH/H_2O (5:95) as the eluent, leading to the isolation of **13** (2.4 mg, t_R = 13.0 min).

3.5. Spectroscopic Data of **1–3**

Elgonene M (**1**): pale yellow oil; $[\alpha]_D^{25}$ −25.9 (c 0.1, CH_3OH); ECD (0.2 mg/mL, CH_3OH) λ_{max} ($\Delta\varepsilon$) 201 (−4.41), 220 (1.25), 262 (−4.35); UV (CH_3OH) λ_{max} (log ε) 261 (0.62) nm; IRυ_{max}: 3440, 2961, 2924, 2855, 1682, 1636, 1609, 1377, 978 cm^{-1}; ^{1}H and ^{13}C NMR data, as shown in Table 1; HRESIMS m/z 249.1499 [M−H]$^-$ (calculated for $C_{15}H_{21}O_3{}^-$, 249.1496).

Elgonene N (**2**): pale yellow oil; $[\alpha]_D^{25}$ −18.4 (c 0.1, CH_3OH); ECD (0.2 mg/mL, CH_3OH) λ_{max} ($\Delta\varepsilon$) 201 (−6.44), 219 (0.32), 258 (−4.91); UV (CH_3OH) λ_{max} (log ε) 260 (0.70) nm; IRυ_{max}: 3440, 2959, 2922, 2853, 1682, 1639, 1404, 1379, 1018, 980 cm^{-1}; ^{1}H and ^{13}C NMR data as shown in Table 1; HRESIMS m/z 249.1498 [M-H]$^-$ (calculated for $C_{15}H_{21}O_3^-$, 249.1496).

Methyl 5-O-acetyl-5-*epi*-shikimate (3): pale yellow oil; $[\alpha]_D^{25}$ −49.6 (c 0.1, CH$_3$OH); ECD (0.2 mg/mL, CH$_3$OH) λ_{max} ($\Delta\varepsilon$) 200 (32.65), 223 (−53.34), 254 (5.08); UV (CH$_3$OH) λ_{max} (log ε) 218 (0.65) nm; ^{1}H and ^{13}C NMR data as shown in Table 1; HRESIMS m/z 231.0870 [M+H]$^+$ (calculated for $C_{10}H_{15}O_6^+$, 231.0863) and 253.0690 [M+Na]$^+$ (calculated for $C_{10}H_{14}NaO_6^+$, 253.0683).

3.6. ECD Calculation of **1–3**

Conformational analyses of **1–3** were carried out by Spartan'14 software (v1.1.4, Wavefunction, Irvine, CA, USA) using a Molecular Merck force field. The conformers with a Boltzmann population exceeding 1% were subsequently optimized by utilizing Gaussion09 (D.01, Pittsburgh, PA, USA) at the B3LYP/6-31G (d) level in methanol using the PCM model [28]. The optimized stable conformers were chosen for further ECD calculations at the B3LYP/6-311G (d, p) level in methanol. The rotatory strengths for a total of 20 excited states were calculated. The overall ECD data were weighted by Boltzmann distribution, and the ECD curves and enantiomeric ECD curves were generated by GuassianView 6.0 software with a half-bandwidth of 0.33 eV, based on the Boltzmann-calculated contribution of each conformer after UV correction.

3.7. Anti-Inflammatory Assay

Femurs and tibias were harvested from 6–8 week old C57BL/6 mice, rinsed thrice with 2% antibiotic-containing PBS, and both ends of the bones were removed. Bone marrow cavities were flushed with PBS, and the cell suspension was passed through a 70 μm cell strainer into a centrifuge tube. The suspension was centrifuged at 500× g for 5 min at 4 °C, the supernatant was discarded, and red blood cells were lysed by adding red blood cell lysis buffer and incubating for 10 min. Following another centrifugation at 500× g for 5 min at 4 °C, the supernatant was discarded, and cells were resuspended in α-MEM containing 10% FBS. The cells were seeded in culture dishes and incubated in a 37 °C, 5% CO$_2$ incubator for 2 h. The medium was then collected in centrifuge tubes, centrifuged at 500× g for 5 min at 4 °C, and cells were resuspended in α-MEM containing 50 ng/mL M-CSF. Cells were seeded at a density of 2.5×10^6 cells/mL in a 24-well plate and cultured for 5 days for subsequent experiments. The cells were divided into a blank group, a model group, treatment groups with compounds **1** and **2** (at concentrations of 1 μM, 5 μM, 10 μM, and 20 μM), and a positive control group with dexamethasone (20 μM). Except for the blank group, all other groups were co-incubated with 100 ng/mL lipopolysaccharide (LPS) for 6 h. After 6 h, the IL-1β mRNA expression was measured. The culture medium was discarded, and the cells were washed twice with PBS. RNA was extracted using the Trizol method, and its concentration was determined with NanoDrop. RNA was reverse transcribed into cDNA using the EnzyArtisan reverse transcription kit. A 10 μL qPCR reaction was prepared according to the SYBR qPCR kit (EnzyArtisan) instructions and run on a ROCHE qPCR LightCycler96 instrument following the recommended protocol. The housekeeping gene GAPDH was used as an internal control to normalize the CT values, using the $2^{-\Delta\Delta Ct}$ formula. The results were shown as mean ± SD from three independent experiments.

3.8. Cytotoxicity Bioassay

The cytotoxicity of **1, 3–6, 8–10,** and **14** against MDA-MB-435 (human breast cancer cells) was determined by assessing cell viability through the 3-(4,5)-dimethylthiahiazo (-z-yl)-3,5-di-phenytetrazoliumromide (MTT) assay. Briefly, cells were seeded at a density of 5×10^3 cells per well in a 96-well plate and left to incubate overnight, followed by treatment with the compounds for the required duration. The optical density at 570 nm (OD$_{570}$) was measured using a Hybrid Multi-Mode Reader (Synergy H1, BioTek, Santa Clara, CA, USA). The experiment was independently repeated three times.

4. Conclusions

In summary, seventeen compounds, including two new sesquiterpenoid derivatives (**1–2**) and a new shikimic acid metabolite (**3**), were isolated from the mangrove-sediment fungus *Roussoella* sp. SCSIO 41427. The absolute configurations of the new compounds were confirmed by ECD calculations and NMR data analysis. During the screening for activity against MDA-MB-435 tumor cells, the compounds **1**, **3–6**, **8–10**, and **14** exhibited an inhibition rate below 50%, indicating a lack of significant inhibitory activity. Moreover, the newly discovered sesquiterpenoid derivatives **1** and **2** exhibited inhibitory effects on the expression of the inflammatory factor IL-1β mRNA, suggesting their potential as anti-inflammatory agents worthy of further investigation.

Supplementary Materials: The following supporting information can be downloaded at: https://www.mdpi.com/article/10.3390/md22030103/s1, Figures S1–S32: NMR, HRESIMS, UV, IR, CD and HPLC spectra of compounds **1**–**3**; Table S1 and S2: Energies of **1**–**3** at B3LYP/6–311g (d, p) level; The physicochemical and spectroscopic data of compounds **4**–**17**.

Author Contributions: Funding acquisition, C.C., X.Z. and H.T.; Investigation, Z.X., J.C., T.C., Y.W., Y.C., Y.Z. and B.Y.; Methodology, Z.X. and J.C.; Supervision, X.Z. and H.T.; Writing—original draft, Z.X. and J.C. All authors have read and agreed to the published version of the manuscript.

Funding: This research was funded by the Key-Area Research and Development Program of Guangdong Province (2023B1111050008), the Special Funds for Promoting Economic Development (Marine Economic Development) of Guangdong Province (GDNRC [2022]35), the Natural Science Foundation of Guangdong Province (2021A1515011711, 2021A1515410002 and 2020A1515110560), and the Postdoctoral Fellowship Program of CPSF (GZC20232777).

Data Availability Statement: The data presented in this study are available on request from the corresponding author.

Acknowledgments: We are grateful to Aijun Sun, Yun Zhang, and Xuan Ma in the analytical facility at SCSIO and Xin Li in the central laboratory at SMU for recording spectroscopic data.

Conflicts of Interest: The authors declare no conflicts of interest.

References

1. Sun, Y.; Chen, P.; Zhai, B.; Zhang, M.; Xiang, Y.; Fang, J.; Xu, S.; Gao, Y.; Chen, X.; Sui, X.; et al. The Emerging Role of Ferroptosis in Inflammation. *Biomed. Pharmacother.* **2020**, *127*, 110108. [CrossRef]
2. Coxib and traditional NSAID Trialists' (CNT) Collaboration; Bhala, N.; Emberson, J.; Merhi, A.; Abramson, S.; Arber, N.; Baron, J.A.; Bombardier, C.; Cannon, C.; Farkouh, M.E.; et al. Vascular and Upper Gastrointestinal Effects of Non-Steroidal Anti-Inflammatory Drugs: Meta-Analyses of Individual Participant Data from Randomised Trials. *Lancet* **2013**, *382*, 769–779. [PubMed]
3. Carroll, A.R.; Copp, B.R.; Davis, R.A.; Keyzers, R.A.; Prinsep, M.R. Marine Natural Products. *Nat. Prod. Rep.* **2023**, *40*, 275–325. [CrossRef] [PubMed]
4. Li, K.; Chen, S.; Pang, X.; Cai, J.; Zhang, X.; Liu, Y.; Zhu, Y.; Zhou, X. Natural Products from Mangrove Sediments-Derived Microbes: Structural Diversity, Bioactivities, Biosynthesis, and Total Synthesis. *Eur. J. Med. Chem.* **2022**, *230*, 114117. [CrossRef] [PubMed]
5. Muria-Gonzalez, M.J.; Chooi, Y.-H.; Breen, S.; Solomon, P.S. The Past, Present and Future of Secondary Metabolite Research in the Dothideomycetes. *Mol. Plant Pathol.* **2015**, *16*, 92–107. [CrossRef] [PubMed]
6. Takekawa, H.; Tanaka, K.; Fukushi, E.; Matsuo, K.; Nehira, T.; Hashimoto, M. Roussoellols A and B, Tetracyclic Fusicoccanes from *Roussoella Hysterioides*. *J. Nat. Prod.* **2013**, *76*, 1047–1051. [CrossRef] [PubMed]
7. Phukhamsakda, C.; Macabeo, A.P.G.; Yuyama, K.T.; Hyde, K.D.; Stadler, M. Biofilm Inhibitory Abscisic Acid Derivatives from the Plant-Associated Dothideomycete Fungus, *Roussoella* Sp. *Molecules* **2018**, *23*, 2190. [CrossRef] [PubMed]
8. Chen, C.; Ren, X.; Tao, H.; Cai, W.; Chen, Y.; Luo, X.; Guo, P.; Liu, Y. Anti-Inflammatory Polyketides from an Alga-Derived Fungus *Aspergillus ochraceopetaliformis* SCSIO 41020. *Mar. Drugs* **2022**, *20*, 295. [CrossRef] [PubMed]
9. Peng, B.; Cai, J.; Xiao, Z.; Liu, M.; Li, X.; Yang, B.; Fang, W.; Huang, Y.; Chen, C.; Zhou, X.; et al. Bioactive Polyketides and Benzene Derivatives from Two Mangrove Sediment-Derived Fungi in the Beibu Gulf. *Mar. Drugs* **2023**, *21*, 327. [CrossRef]
10. Ye, Y.; Liang, J.; She, J.; Lin, X.; Wang, J.; Liu, Y.; Yang, D.; Tan, Y.; Luo, X.; Zhou, X. Two New Alkaloids and a New Butenolide Derivative from the Beibu Gulf Sponge-Derived Fungus *Penicillium* sp. SCSIO 41413. *Mar. Drugs* **2023**, *21*, 27. [CrossRef]
11. Armesto, N.; Fernández, S.; Ferrero, M.; Gotor, V. Influence of Intramolecular Hydrogen Bonds in the Enzyme-Catalyzed Regioselective Acylation of Quinic and Shikimic Acid Derivatives. *Tetrahedron* **2006**, *62*, 5401–5410. [CrossRef]

12. Cheng, T.; Chepkirui, C.; Decock, C.; Matasyoh, J.C.; Stadler, M. Sesquiterpenes from an Eastern African Medicinal Mushroom Belonging to the Genus *Sanghuangporus*. *J. Nat. Prod.* **2019**, *82*, 1283–1291. [CrossRef] [PubMed]
13. Gremaud, G.; Tabacchi, R. Isocoumarins of the Fungus *Ceratocystis Fimbriata coffea*. *Nat. Prod. Lett.* **1994**, *5*, 95–103. [CrossRef]
14. Tang, J.; Wang, W.; Li, A.; Yan, B.; Chen, R.; Li, X.; Du, X.; Sun, H.; Pu, J. Polyketides from the Endophytic Fungus *Phomopsis* sp. Sh917 by Using the One Strain/Many Compounds Strategy. *Tetrahedron* **2017**, *73*, 3577–3584. [CrossRef]
15. Boonyaketgoson, S.; Trisuwan, K.; Bussaban, B.; Rukachaisirikul, V.; Phongpaichit, S. Isochromanone Derivatives from the Endophytic Fungus *Fusarium* sp. PDB51F5. *Tetrahedron Lett.* **2015**, *56*, 5076–5078. [CrossRef]
16. Tayone, W.C.; Kanamaru, S.; Honma, M.; Tanaka, K.; Nehira, T.; Hashimoto, M. Absolute Stereochemistry of Novel Isochromanone Derivatives from *Leptosphaeria* sp. KTC 727. *Biosci. Biotech. Bioch.* **2011**, *75*, 2390–2393. [CrossRef]
17. Zhong, J.; Chen, Y.; Chen, S.; Liu, Z.; Liu, H.; Zhang, W.; Yan, H. Study on the Secondary Metabolites from the Deep-Sea-Derived Fungus *Neoroussoella* sp. and Their Biological Activities. *Nat. Prod. Res. Dev.* **2021**, *33*, 1165.
18. Singh, B.; Parshad, R.; Khajuria, R.K.; Guru, S.K.; Pathania, A.S.; Sharma, R.; Chib, R.; Aravinda, S.; Gupta, V.K.; Khan, I.A.; et al. Saccharonol B, a New Cytotoxic Methylated Isocoumarin from *Saccharomonospora azurea*. *Tetrahedron Lett.* **2013**, *54*, 6695–6699. [CrossRef]
19. Koshti, N.; Naik, S.; Parab, B. Polymer-Bound Cationic Rh(I) Phosphine Catalyst for Homogeneous Asymmetric Hydrogenation. *Indian J. Chem. B* **2005**, *44B*, 2555–2559. [CrossRef]
20. Li, D.; Li, X.; Cui, C.; Wang, B. Chemical Constituents of Endophytic Fungus *Hypocreales* sp. Derived from the Red Alga *Symphyocladia Latiuscula*. *Haiyang Kexue*. **2008**, *32*, 51–55.
21. Lee, Y.S.; Lee, H.S.; Shin, K.H.; Kim, B.-K.; Lee, S. Constituents of the Halophyte Salicornia Herbacea. *Arch. Pharmacal Res.* **2004**, *27*, 1034–1036. [CrossRef]
22. Cui, H.; Li, X.; Li, M.; Lu, F.; Wang, Y.; Liu, D.; Kang, J. Study on Anti-HBV Secondary Metabolites from Sponge-associated Fungus *Penicillium janthinellum* LZDX-32-1. *Chin. J. Mar. Drugs* **2017**, *36*, 42–46.
23. Zou, M.; Wang, R.; Yin, Q.; Liu, L. Bioassay-Guided Isolation and Identification of Anti-Alzheimer's Active Compounds from Spiranthes Sinensis (Pers.) Ames. *Med. Chem. Res.* **2021**, *30*, 1849–1855. [CrossRef]
24. Cao, L.; Tian, H.; Wang, Y.; Zhou, X.; Jiang, R.; Liu, Y. Chemical Constituents in the Fruits of Mangrove Plant Sonneratia Apetala Buch. Ham. *J. Trop. Oceanogr.* **2015**, *34*, 77–82.
25. Dinarello, C.A. Clinical Perspective of IL-1β as the Gatekeeper of Inflammation. *Eur. J. Immunol.* **2011**, *41*, 1203–1217. [CrossRef] [PubMed]
26. Chi, M.; Dong, X.; Wei, W.; Li, X.; Li, X.; Liu, J.; Feng, T. Bisabolane and Drimane Sesquiterpenes from the Fungus *Coprinellus* sp. *Phytochem. Lett.* **2023**, *55*, 30–33. [CrossRef]
27. De Cássia Da Silveira e Sá, R.; Andrade, L.N.; De Sousa, D.P. Sesquiterpenes from Essential Oils and Anti-Inflammatory Activity. *Nat. Prod. Commun.* **2015**, *10*, 1767–1774. [CrossRef]
28. Luo, X.; Lin, X.; Tao, H.; Wang, J.; Li, J.; Yang, B.; Zhou, X.; Liu, Y. Isochromophilones A–F, Cytotoxic Chloroazaphilones from the Marine Mangrove Endophytic Fungus *Diaporthe* sp. SCSIO 41011. *J. Nat. Prod.* **2018**, *81*, 934–941. [CrossRef] [PubMed]

Disclaimer/Publisher's Note: The statements, opinions and data contained in all publications are solely those of the individual author(s) and contributor(s) and not of MDPI and/or the editor(s). MDPI and/or the editor(s) disclaim responsibility for any injury to people or property resulting from any ideas, methods, instructions or products referred to in the content.

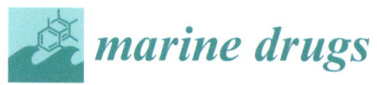

Article

The Peptide LLTRAGL Derived from *Rapana venosa* Exerts Protective Effect against Inflammatory Bowel Disease in Zebrafish Model by Regulating Multi-Pathways

Yongna Cao [1,2], Fenghua Xu [1,2], Qing Xia [1,2], Kechun Liu [1,2], Houwen Lin [1,2,3], Shanshan Zhang [1,2,*] and Yun Zhang [1,2,*]

[1] Biology Institute, Qilu University of Technology (Shandong Academy of Sciences), Jinan 250103, China; caoyn123987@163.com (Y.C.); xfh20171215@163.com (F.X.); xiaq@sdas.org (Q.X.); hliukch@sdas.org (K.L.); franklin67@126.com (H.L.)
[2] Engineering Research Center of Zebrafish Models for Human Diseases and Drug Screening of Shandong Province, Jinan 250103, China
[3] Research Center for Marine Drugs, State Key Laboratory of Oncogenes and Related Genes, Department of Pharmacy, School of Medicine, Shanghai Jiao Tong University, Shanghai 200127, China
* Correspondence: qingshuibaikai@126.com (S.Z.); xiaohan_0818@163.com (Y.Z.); Tel.: +86-531-8260-5322 (Y.Z.)

Abstract: Inflammatory bowel disease (IBD) is a chronic inflammatory bowel disease with unknown pathogenesis which has been gradually considered a public health challenge worldwide. Peptides derived from *Rapana venosa* have been shown to have an anti-inflammatory effect. In this study, peptide LLTRAGL derived from *Rapana venosa* was prepared by a solid phase synthesis technique. The protective effects of LLTRAGL were studied in a 2,4,6-trinitrobenzene sulfonic acid (TNBS)-induced zebrafish colitis model. The underlying mechanisms of LLTRAGL were predicted and validated by transcriptome, real-time quantitative PCR assays and molecular docking. The results showed that LLTRAGL reduced the number of macrophages migrating to the intestine, enhanced the frequency and rate of intestinal peristalsis and improved intestinal inflammatory damage. Furthermore, transcriptome analysis indicated the key pathways (NOD-like receptor signal pathway and necroptosis pathway) that link the underlying protective effects of LLTRAGL's molecular mechanisms. In addition, the related genes in these pathways exhibited different expressions after TNBS treatment. Finally, molecular docking techniques further verified the RNA-sequencing results. In summary, LLTRAGL exerted protective effects in the model of TNBS-induced colitis zebrafish. Our findings provide valuable information for the future application of LLTRAGL in IBD.

Keywords: *Rapana venosa*; LLTRAGL; inflammatory bowel disease; 2,4,6 trinitrobenzene sulfonic acid; zebrafish; transcriptome analysis; NOD-like receptor; necroptosis

Citation: Cao, Y.; Xu, F.; Xia, Q.; Liu, K.; Lin, H.; Zhang, S.; Zhang, Y. The Peptide LLTRAGL Derived from *Rapana venosa* Exerts Protective Effect against Inflammatory Bowel Disease in Zebrafish Model by Regulating Multi-Pathways. *Mar. Drugs* **2024**, *22*, 100. https://doi.org/10.3390/md22030100

Academic Editors: Hong Wang, Huawei Zhang and Bin Wei

Received: 29 December 2023
Revised: 19 February 2024
Accepted: 20 February 2024
Published: 22 February 2024

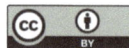

Copyright: © 2024 by the authors. Licensee MDPI, Basel, Switzerland. This article is an open access article distributed under the terms and conditions of the Creative Commons Attribution (CC BY) license (https://creativecommons.org/licenses/by/4.0/).

1. Introduction

Inflammatory bowel disease (IBD) is a chronic inflammation in the gastrointestinal tract which has been categorized into ulcerative colitis (UC) and Crohn's disease (CD) [1,2]. According to statistics, about 6.8 million cases of IBD were documented worldwide [3]. Due to unpredictable and highly variable symptoms, IBD presents a major healthcare burden of global morbidity, with the highest prevalence in Europe and North America, and rising incidence in Asia [4]. The treatment protocols for IBD mainly rely on medication therapy or surgery [4,5]. In addition to the preferred choice of anti-inflammatory drugs (antibiotics), biological agents (primarily anti-TNF-α) and immunosuppressants are also used for the treatment of IBD [4,6]. However, long-term use of these medications is often not safe for the body due to their potential side effects. In this regard, the search for new sources of drugs to improve the clinical safety and efficacy of IBD treatment remains essential.

Natural products derived from marine organisms often exhibit novel chemical structures and unique physiological effects because the living environment is different from terrestrial organisms. Marine peptides which can be isolated from algae, molluscs, fish and marine by-products [7–9] show multi-bioactivities, such as anti-inflammatory, antihypertensive, antioxidant, antimicrobial and neuroprotective activities, etc. [8,10–14]. Therefore, peptides have become important resources for new drugs, health foods, special biological functional materials and cosmetics in recent years [15]. *Rapana venosa* (*Rv*) is an important marine snail which exhibits an increasing nutritional and economic importance [16]. Some studies have demonstrated that hemocyanin and peptides from *Rv* exhibited antimicrobial and antitumor activities [14,17,18]. Additionally, a previous study in our lab indicated that peptides from *Rv* could significantly improve inflammation damage in zebrafish induced by metronidazole. Among six peptides which are disclosed in the China patent (Patent NO: 202010313278X), LLTRAGL showed positive anti-inflammatory activities without obvious side effects on zebrafish. Furthermore, in a recent study, it was proved that the anti-inflammatory peptides derived from food-resource phycocyanin had better anti-IBD activity [19]. This study provides a possibility for the study of the same food-derived anti-inflammatory peptides in anti-IBD with safety and effectiveness. However, the anti-IBD activity and fundamental mechanism of action of LLTRAGL is still unclear.

Zebrafish is an ideal model system for human disease and drug development with the advantages of high reproducibility, rapid development, small size, high throughput, low cost and high genetic and morphological similarity with the human counterpart [20,21]. Many studies have reported that zebrafish (*Danio rerio*) larvae have emerged as a useful tool for the screening and exploration of potential drugs in the treatment of IBD and gastrointestinal diseases [22,23].

Studies have proved that inflammatory reactions are a crucial factor in the development of IBD. Hence, peptides from *Rv* may be promising therapeutics for IBD. Nonetheless, there is little information about peptides from *Rv* on the application in IBD. In this study, the peptide LLTRAGL, which was purified and characterized from the enzymatic *Rv* tissue, was evaluated for its potential to alleviate IBD symptoms in 2,4,6 trinitrobenzene sulfonic acid (TNBS)-induced zebrafish for the first time; the potential molecular mechanisms of LLTRAGL were investigated.

2. Results

2.1. Effect of Peptide LLTRAGL on the Migration of Macrophages in Zebrafish Juvenile Treated with TNBS

To assess the effects of the peptide LLTRAGL on the development of colitis, a colitis model in zebrafish was established by inducing TNBS. The safe concentrations of the peptide were screened from 10 to 640 μg/mL by using a zebrafish model (Supplementary Figure S1). LLTRAGL could inhibit the migration of macrophages to the intestine at 20 μg/mL, while the effect of inhibiting the migration of macrophages to the intestine at 80–320 μg/mL was similar. Furthermore, after treating zebrafish with LLTRAGL at 640 μg/mL, they were all dead. Therefore, the dosages of LLTRAGL were chosen at 20, 40 and 80 μg/mL. Later, the colitis zebrafish larvae were treated with LLTRAGL (20, 40, 80 μg/mL) and 5-ASA (1 μg/mL) for 24 h, respectively. According to the results in Figure 1, TNBS significantly induced colitis in zebrafish with increasing numbers of neutrophils cells in the intestines and enlarging the damaged intestinal area, which was compared to the control group. However, compared with the TNBS group, the positive drug and LLTRAGL significantly improved the intestinal inflammation of zebrafish ($p \leq 0.01$ and $p \leq 0.05$). LLTRAGL can reduce the number of macrophages in the intestine with dose dependency. In particular, at the high dose group (80 μg/mL) the peptide could significantly reduce the number of macrophages migrating to the intestine ($p \leq 0.01$). The data suggest that LLTRAG is effective in ameliorating colitis and reducing inflammatory responses.

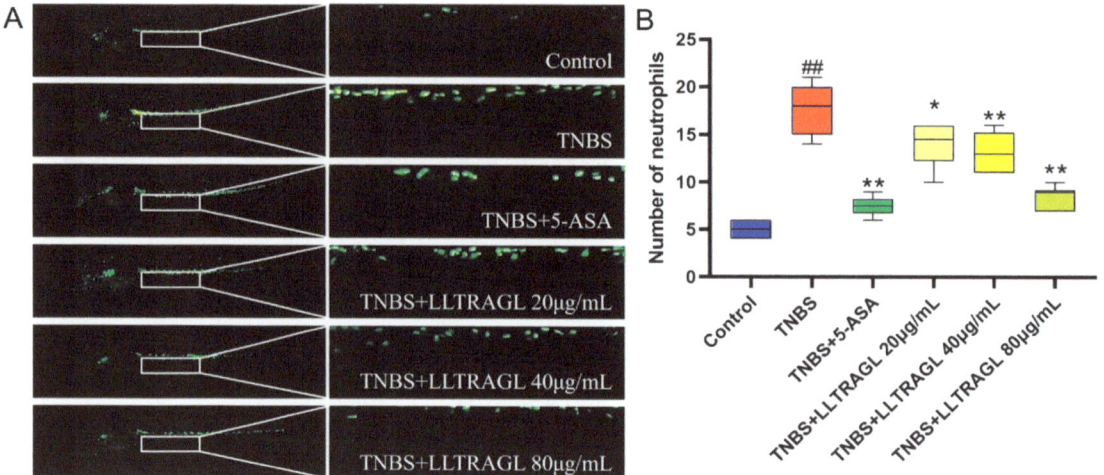

Figure 1. Effect of peptide LLTRAGL on TNBS-induced migration of zebrafish to intestinal macrophages. (**A**) Typical fluorescence images of Tg (*zlyz: EGFP*) macrophage migration in transgenic zebrafish juveniles. (**B**) Box chart showing the number of macrophages migrating from zebrafish larvae to the intestine. (**A**) the image on the right is an enlarged image of the white box on the left. Compared with the blank group, ## $p \leq 0.01$; compared with the TNBS group, * $p \leq 0.05$ and ** $p \leq 0.01$.

2.2. Effect of Peptide LLTRAGL Promote Gastrointestinal Motility in Zebrafish

It is well known that colitis causes gastrointestinal dysfunction and influences the intestinal peristalsis capacity. To further investigate the potential anti-inflammatory effect of peptide in IBD-induced zebrafish colitis, the promoted gastrointestinal motility was evaluated by using a fluorescent dye solution. TNBS-treated zebrafish showed strong fluorescence density in the intestine (Figure 2A). This result indicated that TNBS significantly depressed the intestinal efflux efficiency (IEE) and the intestinal peristalsis frequency of the control group ($p \leq 0.01$, Figure 2B,C). However, the inhibitory effect could be significantly ameliorated by 5-ASA ($p \leq 0.01$, Figure 2). Furthermore, LLTRAGL treatment could also alleviate the depressed IEE and promote the gastrointestinal peristalsis frequency of zebrafish compared with the TNBS-treated zebrafish, especially at the concentration of 80 μg/mL, demonstrating the therapeutical effects of the peptide on TNBS-induced IBD ($p \leq 0.01$, Figure 2).

2.3. Effect of Peptide LLTRAGL on TNBS-Induced Pathological Changes and Ultrastructure of Intestinal

The zebrafish intestinal histopathological changes are shown in Figure 3. The hematoxylin and eosin (H&E) images in Figure 3A clearly showed that the intestinal epithelial cells of larvae in the control group showed clear structures of mucosa, muscularis propria, and serosa, and columnar epithelial cells were neatly arranged. TNBS treatment caused a decrease in intestine folding, goblet cells, columnar epithelial cells, and an increase in inflammatory cell infiltration, cilia defects and mucus volumes. In contrast, the LLTRAGL treatment group can significantly improve the damage caused by TNBS, and the number of goblet cells and columnar epithelial cells were increased. Furthermore, the gut tissue morphology was closely similar to that of normal zebrafish. The Alcian blue (AB) staining was performed to determine the mucus levels in the intestinal goblet cells. According to the results shown in Figure 3B, compared with the control group, the mucous in the intestines of zebrafish was significantly reduced after TNBS treatment. However, an obvious recovery of mucin was observed after peptide treatment. Subsequently, the ultrastructure of the intestinal tissue of zebrafish was shown in Figure 3C. The intestinal microvilli of zebrafish in the control group were arranged neatly and were uniform in thickness. However, disrupted and shortened microvilli, defective, tight and adherent junctions of intestinal epithelial cells, and decreased goblet cell numbers were observed in TNBS-treated zebrafish. LLTRAGL treatment could recover the injured intestinal microvilli and reverse them to a state similar to that of normal zebrafish.

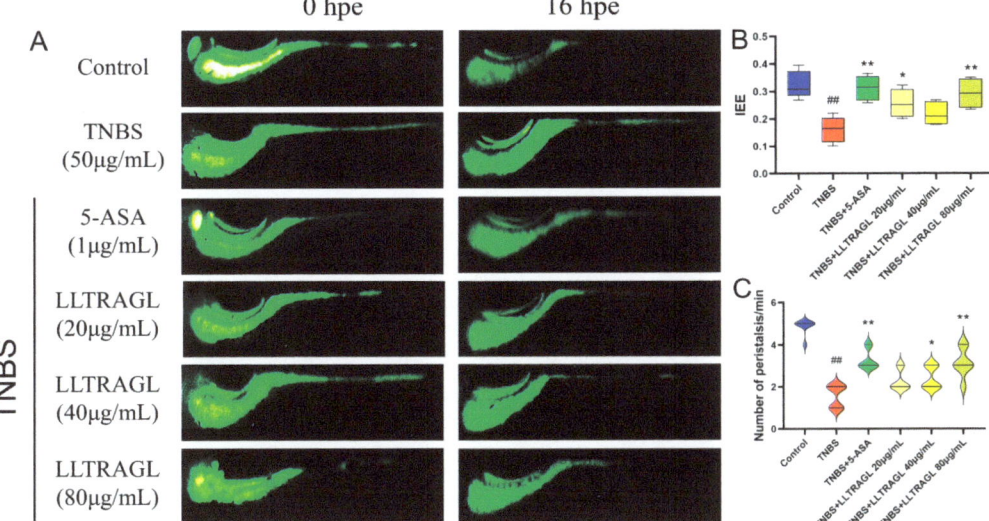

Figure 2. LLTRAGL improves TNBS-induced intestinal peristalsis damage. (**A**) Typical fluorescence images of intestinal efflux rate (IEE) of wild zebrafish juveniles. The blue box shows that after staining with calcein for 1.5 h, the drug was administered for 16 h. (**B**) Box chart showing the intestinal efflux rate of zebrafish juveniles. (**C**) Violin chart showing the number of intestinal peristalses in zebrafish juveniles. Compared with the blank group, ## $p \leq 0.01$; compared with the TNBS group, * $p \leq 0.05$ and ** $p \leq 0.01$.

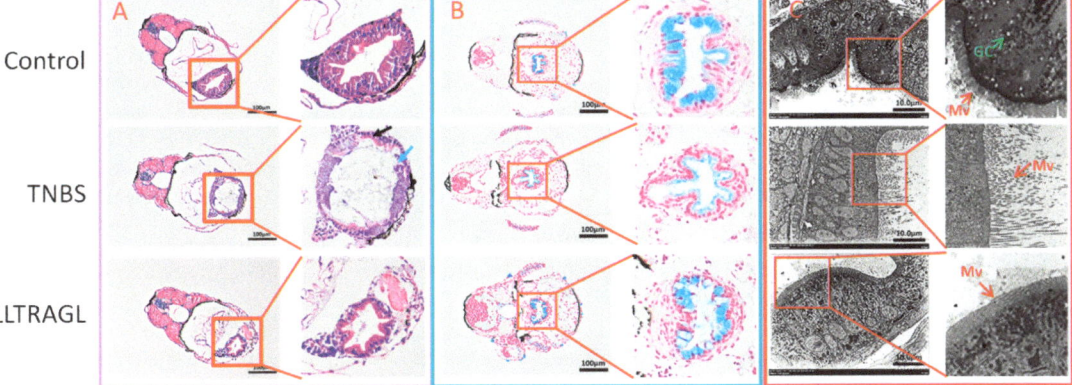

Figure 3. Effects of the peptide on TNBS-induced intestinal tissue pathology and ultrastructure of zebrafish. (**A**) H&E staining of intestinal tissues. Black arrow: sparse arrangement of cells; Blue arrow: Mucosal layer necrosis, cell lysis, enhanced cytoplasmic basophilia, disappearance of intestinal folds. Scale bar is 100 μm. (**B**) Alcian blue (AB) staining of intestinal tissues. Scale bar is 100 μm. (**C**) Electron microscopy of intestinal ultrastructure. Red arrow: intestinal microvilli status; Mv represents microvilli; Green arrow: goblet cell state; GC stands for goblet cell. Scale bar is 10.0 μm.

2.4. Transcriptome Analysis of Peptide LLTRAGL in Improving TNBS-Induced Inflammatory Bowel Disease Damage

2.4.1. Differentially Expressed Genes (DEGs) by Transcriptome Analysis

In order to further analyze the effects of LLTRAGL on the transcription level, the mRNAs from the control group, TNBS treatment group and peptide treatment group were sequenced. A total of 386 DEGs (the absolute value of log2FoldChange ≥ 1; p-value < 0.05) were identified between the TNBS group and control group. Among these genes, 231 were up-regulated and 155 were down-regulated genes. In the peptide-treated group, there were 215 DEGs compared to the TNBS group, with 141 DEGs up-regulated and 74 DEGs down-regulated (Figure 4A). The top 10 up- and down-regulated DEGs for each comparison are displayed in Figure 4B,C (Supplementary Table S1). Venn analysis showed that the two comparison groups had 35 DEGs in common (Figure 4D, Supplementary Table S2).

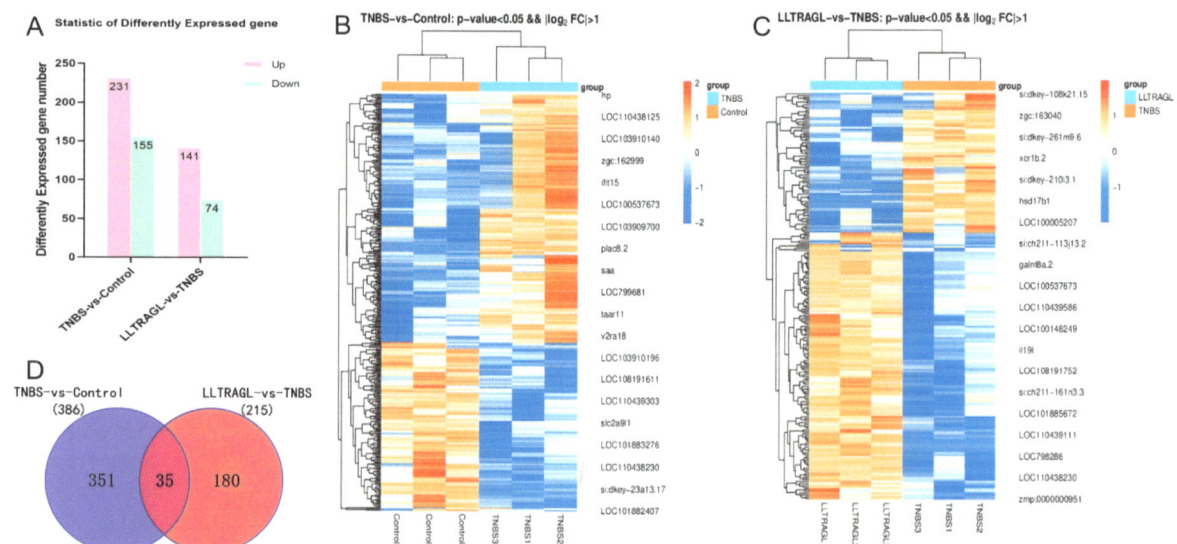

Figure 4. The differentially expressed genes among the control group, TNBS group and peptide treatment group in RNA-Seq. (**A**) Statistical histogram of differentially expressed genes in TNBS vs. Control and LLTRAGL vs. TNBS. (**B**) TNBS vs. Control differential gene grouping cluster diagram. (**C**) LLTRAGL vs. TNBS differential gene grouping cluster diagram. (**D**) Venn diagram of common and unique differentially expressed genes between the TNBS vs. Control and LLTRAGL vs. TNBS comparative groups. The red color in the figure represents genes encoding relatively high expression proteins, while the blue color represents genes encoding relatively low expression proteins.

2.4.2. GO Term Enrichment Analysis

Based on the above DEGs, the GO function of differentially expressed genes between TNBS-treated zebrafish and LLTRAGL treatment zebrafish was analyzed by Gene Set Enrichment Analysis (GSEA) to study the function of DEGs. In the GO functional concentration analysis (Figure 5A), the biological process of zebrafish enrichment in the LLTRAGL-treated group was mainly related to the inflammatory response compare with the TNBS group (Supplementary Table S3). According to GSEA and cluster mapping, the expression of inflammatory response-related genes in LLTRAGL-treated zebrafish was significantly reversed, compared with that of the TNBS-treated group (Figure 5B,C, Supplementary Table S4).

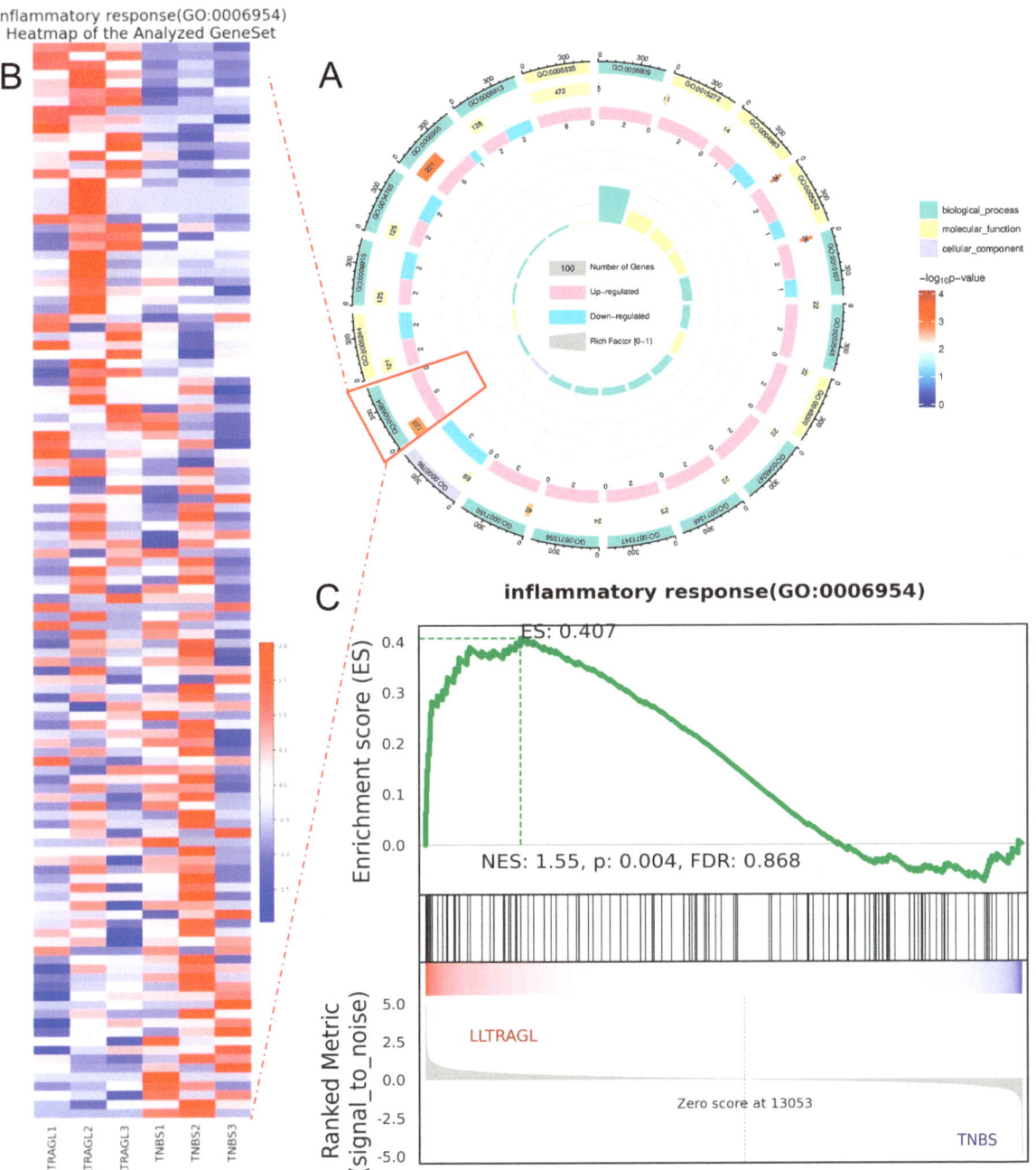

Figure 5. GO enrichment analysis of DEGs and GSEA of all tested genes. (**A**) Circle plots of the distribution of DEGs in different GO categories. The circle chart shows the distribution of DEGs in the molecular function (MF), biological process (BP), and cellular composition (CC) categories. (**B**) Grouping clustering diagram of inflammatory response in the GSEA analysis. (**C**) Analysis Results of the Inflammatory Response Gene Set, mainly including the distribution map of enrichment score (ES), gene distribution map of gene set, and distribution map of the measurement and control bar sorting matrix.

2.4.3. KEGG Pathway Enrichment Analysis

KEGG pathway analysis showed that the up-regulated genes between the TNBS and control group involve the top 10 pathways, including the NOD-like receptor signaling pathway, necroptosis, C-type lectin receptor signaling pathway and cytokine–cytokine receptor interaction. The down-regulated genes involve the top 10 pathways, including Neuroactive ligand–receptor interaction, Phenylalanine, tyrosine and tryptophan biosynthesis, Hedgehog signaling pathway and FoxO signaling pathway (Figure 6A, Supplementary Table S5). For the KEGG pathway analysis between the LLTRAGL and TNBS group, the up-regulated genes involved in the top 10 pathways are the NOD-like receptor signaling pathway, necroptosis, cytokine–cytokine receptor interaction and the MAPK signaling pathway, etc. The down-regulated genes involve the key pathways, including necroptosis and cytokine–cytokine receptor interaction signaling pathway (Figure 6B, Supplementary Table S5). KEGG pathway analysis showed that the differentially expressed genes involved inflammation-related pathways, of which NOD-like receptor signaling pathway and necroptosis pathway were the most significant pathways. Subsequently, we further validated the accuracy of the RNA-sequencing analysis by a quantitative RT-PCR of seven gene expression levels, which were related to the inflammation. Results showed that the transcription levels of *mmp9*, *il8*, *il1β*, *il12*, *il10*, *ripk3* and *bax* genes were consistent with the results of the transcriptome sequencing (Figure 7). These results indicated that the LLTRAGL peptide might alleviate zebrafish IBD via regulating multiple inflammation-related pathways.

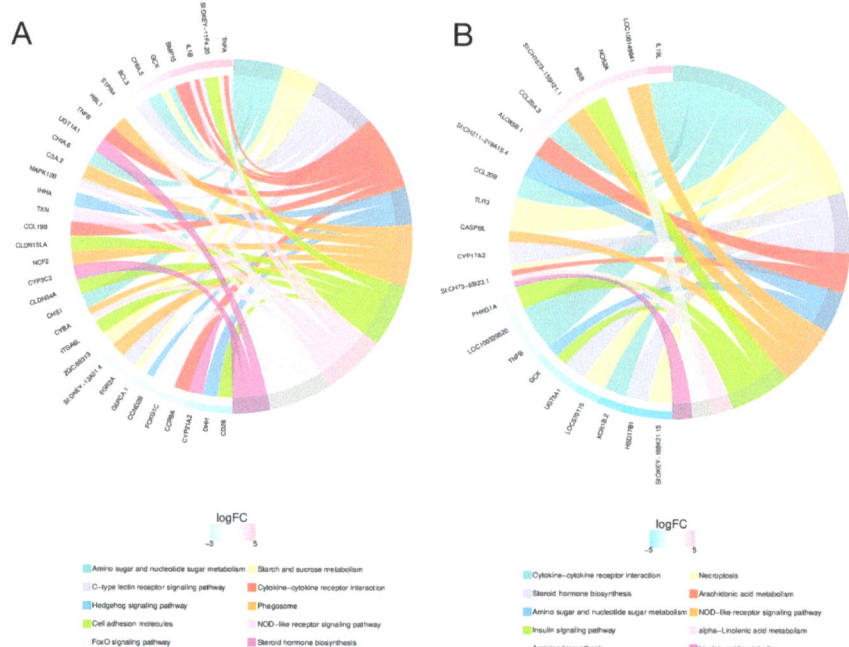

Figure 6. KEGG pathway enrichment analysis of DEGs. (**A**) KEGG-enriched top 10 chord diagram of TNBS vs. Control. (**B**) KEGG-enriched top 10 chord diagram of LLTRAGL-vs-TNBS. KEGG, Kyoto Encyclopedia of Genes and Genomes.

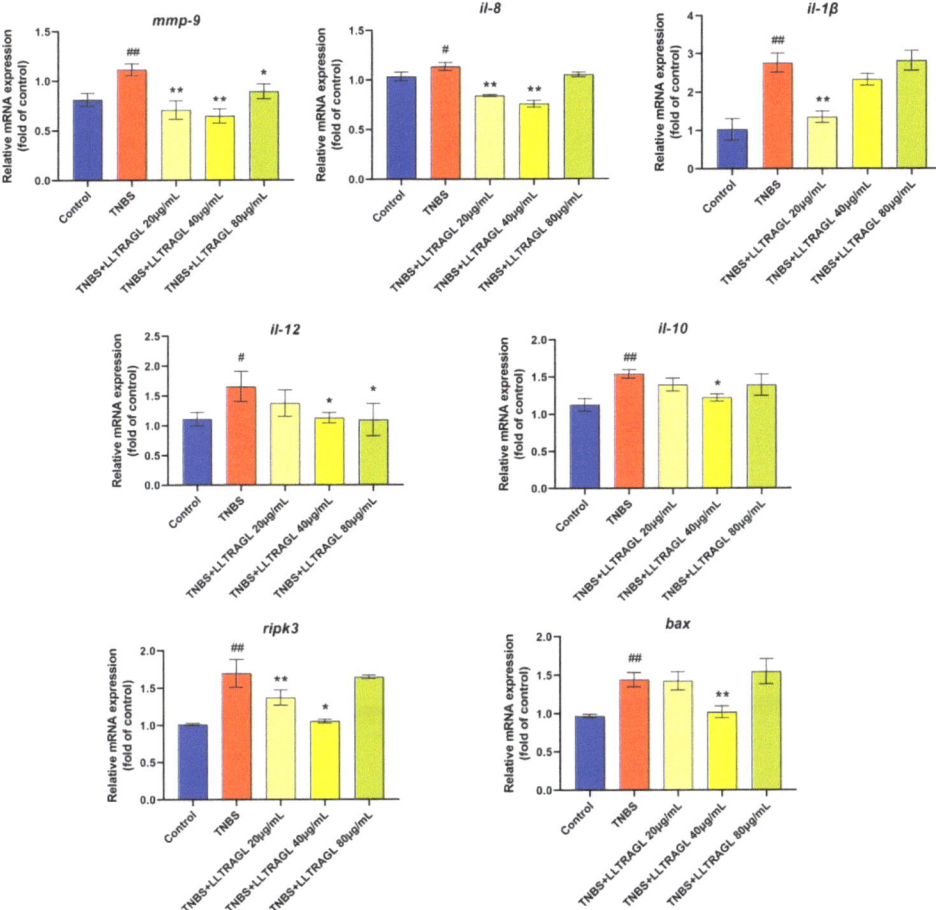

Figure 7. Effect of LLTRAG on the inflammation-related gene expression in zebrafish, determined by RT-PCR. Compared with the blank group, # $p \leq 0.05$ and ## $p \leq 0.01$; compared with the TNBS group, * $p \leq 0.05$ and ** $p \leq 0.01$.

2.5. LLTRAGL Alleviates Inflammatory Bowel Disease Damage through the NOD-Like Receptor Signaling Pathway and Necroptosis Signaling Pathway

NOD-like receptor and necroptosis signaling pathways exist in the KEGG concentration of mRNA-seq in colitis zebrafish treated with LLTRAGL. We think these two signaling pathways may be necessary for LLTRAGL to improve inflammatory bowel disease. To test our hypothesis, we quantitatively detected the expression of the NOD-like receptor and necroptosis signaling pathway-related proteins in the untreated zebrafish blank group, peptide treatment group and TNBS group. Compared with the control blank group, the TNBS group showed a significant increase in the expression of *nod2*, *myd88*, *nlrp1*, *nlrp3*, *pycard*, *nfkb*, *tnfa*, *cox-2*, *tgfβ* and *il-10* genes; moreover, *caspase-9*, *ripk1*, *caspase-1* and *tlr4* genes, which are related to necroptosis, are also up-regulated. After LLTRAGL treatment, the up-regulated gene expression by TNBS could significantly reverse (Figure 8). Combined with the mRNA-seq analysis results, we found that LLTRAGL down-regulated the expression of genes in the NOD-like receptor signal pathway and necroptosis signal pathway, thus playing a role in treating IBD in zebrafish.

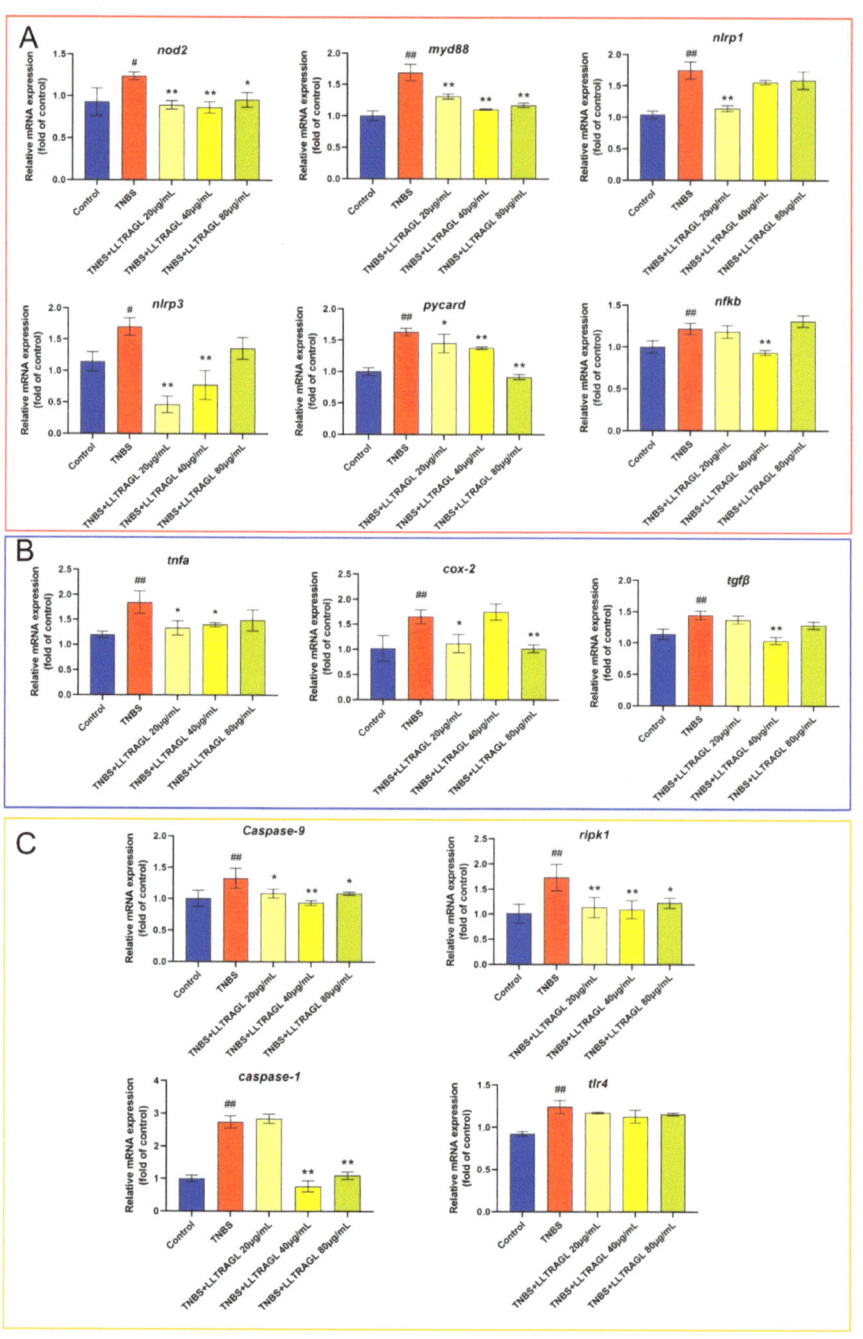

Figure 8. Effect of LLTRAG on gene expression in TNBS-induced colitis in zebrafish. (**A**) NOD-like receptor signal pathway-related genes. (**B**) Inflammatory factors-related genes. (**C**) necroptosis signal pathway-related gene. Compared with the blank group, # $p \leq 0.05$ and ## $p \leq 0.01$; compared with the TNBS group, * $p \leq 0.05$ and ** $p \leq 0.01$.

2.6. Insight into Molecular Docking Simulation

To predict the binding affinity of LLTRAGL to the target, molecular docking was performed by selecting target genes related to the NOD-like receptor signaling pathway and necroptosis signaling pathway as receptors while using 5-ASA as a positive control to assist in validating the pharmacological effects. Molecular docking was performed using LLTRAGL and 5-ASA as ligands, and the key targets of the NOD-like receptor signaling pathway and necroptosis signaling pathway genes PYCARD (6KI0), IL-8 (6WZL), IL-1β (7Z3W), Caspase-9 (5WVC) and RIPK1 (7YDX) as receptors and the docking results are shown in Table 1.

Table 1. LLTRAGL and 5-ASA, respectively, use CDOCKER to dock the CDocker energy and CDocker interaction energy of five proteins.

Protein Name (PDB ID)	−CDocker Energy (KJ/mol)		−CDocker Interaction Energy (KJ/mol)	
	LLTRAGL	5-ASA	LLTRAGL	5-ASA
PYCARD (6KI0)	122.0260	14.2595	82.2045	15.3231
IL-8 (6WZL)	89.7209	29.0584	59.6621	29.9727
IL-1β (7Z3W)	106.3360	18.3206	69.2347	19.1699
Caspase-9 (5WVC)	112.6820	14.8370	98.2614	15.6957
RIPK1 (7YDX)	138.7620	30.1659	146.1860	31.0330

Compared with the positive control 5-ASA, the binding energy of LLTRAGL to PYCARD, IL-8, IL-1β, Caspase-9 and RIPK1 proteins all had lower CDOCKER INTERACTION ENERGY, with the highest binding energy of −89.7209 and the lowest binding energy of 138.7620 KJ/mol, indicating that LLTRAGL had a good affinity with all target genes. The LLTRAGL peptide combined with receptors through the interaction forces of hydrogen bonds, as well as the electrostatic and hydrophobic forces. LLTRAGL formed more stable hydrogen bonds and hydrophobic forces with the surrounding residues in the active site of the target proteins than 5-ASA. (Figures S2 and S3)

3. Discussion

IBD is a chronic and recurrent inflammatory disease of the gastrointestinal tract [20]. As a typical inflammatory disease, research indicates that immune cell types are involved in the pathogenesis of IBD [24]. However, the mechanism of IBD pathogenesis is extremely complex and unclear, which has limited the development of effective treatments. Therefore, new therapeutic strategies for IBD are urgently needed. A growing interest has been focused on compounds obtained from natural resources.

The effects of peptide LLTRAGL derived from *Rapana venosa* on TNBS-induced colitis in zebrafish were investigated. Studies had indicated that LLTRAGL could reduce the inflammatory responses in the TNBS-induced zebrafish model of colitis by suppressing the number of neutrophil cells in the intestine, alleviating the damage in the intestinal area and promoting gastrointestinal motility. Furthermore, the ameliorative effect of the peptide on TNBS-induced colitis may be associated with the modulation of a NOD-like receptor signal pathway and necroptosis pathway-associated genes. Molecular docking further proved the efficacy of the interaction between LLTRAGL and key proteins in the inflammation-related signaling pathways.

TNBS administration can induce the IBD model with the hallmark aspects of human IBD, including the induction of pro-inflammatory pathways, the occurrence of neutrophils and macrophages in the intestine, and reduce the intestinal peristalsis [25,26]. An increase in the intestinal neutrophil numbers and gastrointestinal motility disorders in zebrafish were found in TNBS-treated zebrafish, which validated the applicability of TNBS for generating the colitis models [26]. After LLTRAGL treatment, the colitis symptoms of TNBS-induced zebrafish were significantly ameliorated.

The complete intestinal epithelium [27] and intestinal barrier [28] are crucial for maintaining normal intestinal physiological function. In this study, LLTRAGL and TNBS co-treatment zebrafish can improve the infiltration of inflammatory cells, decreasing goblet cells, and crypt damage. Furthermore, the similar intestinal morphology improvement effects of drugs with anti-IBD activities can be observed in the mouse model [28–30]. These suggested that the peptide LLTRAGL may reduce inflammatory bowel disease by improving the integrity of the intestinal epithelial tissue and intestinal barrier.

The transcriptome analysis is used to study gene expression at the RNA level. The annotation results of GO showed that the differential genes between LLTRAGL- and TNBS-induced colitis zebrafish were mainly enriched in biological processes, such as inflammatory response and cell apoptosis. As shown in the KEGG pathway analysis results, there were significant changes in NOD-like receptor signaling and necroptosis pathway in LLTRAGL treatment zebrafish and TNBS treatment zebrafish.

Numerous experiments in vitro and in vivo have indicated the production of anti-IBD functions by regulating NOD-like receptor signaling [31,32]. NOD1 and NOD2, as sensors of peptidoglycan and cellular stress and activators of multiple signaling pathways involved in immune response, are critical players in the resistance to inflammatory diseases [33]. NOD2 is involved in the recognition of infectious bacteria, induction of immune responses, and protection of the intestinal mucosal barrier from bacterial erosion through the activation of nuclear factor kappa B (NF-κB) [34]. NLRP1 is the first pattern recognition receptor (PRR) discovered to form an inflammasome, and genome-wide association studies have identified NLRP1 mutations linked with IBD [35]. The NLRP3 can produce IL-1β and IL-18 and initiate inflammatory processes [31]. In addition, IL-1β promotes the production of IL-22 and IL-10 to maintain epithelial integrity [36,37]. In the previous study, the genes related to the NOD-like receptor signaling pathway, include *myd88*, *nod2*, *nlrp1*, *nlrp3* and *pycard* were significantly up-regulated in TNBS treatment zebrafish. However, LLTRAGL could effectively reverse the up-regulation of the key genes in zebrafish.

Necroptosis is a cell death pathway that is supposed to be of importance in the pathogenesis of many diseases such as cancer, IBD and other intestinal diseases [38,39]. The transcriptome analysis of the colon tissue of DSS-induced colitis mice indicates that the necroptosis pathway plays an anti-inflammatory role in IBD [40]. In addition, the necrotic apoptotic pathway was also enriched in KEGG analysis according to the transcriptome analysis of TNBS zebrafish. The key genes involved in the necroptosis signaling pathway, *caspase-9*, *ripk1*, *ripk3*, *caspase-1*, *tlr4* and *bax*, were significantly up-regulated in TNBS treatment zebrafish. Significant reversals of gene expression levels were found in the peptide-treated zebrafish.

A combination of the transcription analysis and RT-PCR results demonstrates that the level gene expression of *pycard*, *il-8*, *il-1β*, *caspase-9* and *ripk1* is critical to the efficacy of IBD inhibition. Thus, the proteins PYCARD, IL-8, IL-1β, Caspase-9 and RIPK1 involved in the NOD-like receptor and necroptosis signaling pathway were selected as receptors [41–43]. Molecular docking was used to further verify the mRNA-sequencing results. The docking results showed that LLTRAGL had a lower binding energy compared to 5-ASA, indicating that LLTRAGL had a higher affinity for all five proteins, which further confirmed that the mechanism of LLTRAGL treatment for zebrafish colitis might be related to the activation of the NOD-like receptor signaling pathway and necroptosis signaling pathway.

In a comprehensive analysis of the phenotypic and mechanistic results, there were some differences in the trend of LLTRAGL. According to the phenotypic results in the zebrafish model, the group with the optimal concentration of 80 μg/mL was selected for transcriptome analysis. This phenomenon may be because LLTRAGL regulates the influence of changes in gene level first, then affects protein level, regulates various reactions in the body, and finally shows the reduction in macrophages. The 80 μg/mL concentration may be due to the body's own regulation of gene overexpression.

4. Materials and Methods

4.1. Chemicals and Reagents

2,4,6-trinitrobenzenesulfonic acid (TNBS), 5-aminosalicylic acid (5-ASA), and calcein were purchased from Sigma-Aldrich (Shanghai, China). All other chemicals and reagents were of analytical grade from local commercial sources.

4.2. LLTRAGL Peptide Preparation

LLTRAGL peptide was isolated and purified from Rv enzymolysis protein by an activity-directed separation technique, then the amino acid sequence was identified by LC-MS omics. The LLTRAGL peptide consisted of Leu-Leu-Thr-Arg-Ala-Gly-Leu and had a molecular weight 742 Da. Its anti-inflammation activity was proved by the zebrafish model. According to the patent records and previous research studies, it was found that the observed inflammatory activity of the peptide is attributed to its low molecular weight, high proportion of hydrophobic and positively charged amino acids [44,45]. The synthetic peptide of LLTRAGL was used in the study (CelLmano Biotech Co., Ltd., Hefei, China) with a purity of 95%.

4.3. Zebrafish Maintenance

The wild-type AB strain and transgenic zebrafish (zlyz: EGFP) strain were used for animal experiments which were obtained from the Engineering Research Center of Zebrafish Models for Human Diseases and Drug Screening of Shandong Province (Jinan, China). The zebrafish embryos were kept under a constant temperature (28 ± 0.5 °C) and 14 h-light/10 h-dark cycles. The healthy zebrafish were paired with a sex ratio at 2:2 (female:male) overnight and embryos were collected the next morning. Then, zebrafish embryos were transferred into clean culture water (5 mM NaCl, 0.17 mM KCl, 0.33 mM $CaCl_2$, and 0.33 mM $MgSO_4$) containing 2 mg/L methylene blue solution after three washes [46].

4.4. TNBS-Induced Colitis Experiment

Colitis in zebrafish was induced by TNBS to evaluate the effects of LLTRAGL on mitigating the colitis according to the published literature [26]. The 3 dpf (days post-fertilization) zebrafish larvae of the Tg: zlyz-EGFP strain were randomly placed into 24-well plates (10 per well), and then randomly divided into six groups. Four parallel holes per group were set in the experiment. Except for the blank group, which was incubated in fish water without TNBS, the zebrafish in the other groups were incubated in water with TNBS (60 µM) under the same conditions. After 48 h of incubation, the positive control group and peptide treatment groups were added into 5-ASA and three different concentrations of peptide (20, 40, 80 µg/mL). Then, the zebrafish larvae were anesthetized with tricaine (0.2%, w/v) after 24 h of incubation. The number of neutrophil cells in the zebrafish intestines was used as an evaluation index which was observed and photographed via a microscope (Olympus, SZX2-ILLTQ, Tokyo, Japan).

4.5. Intestinal Efflux Efficiency Experiment

AB zebrafish embryos at 3 dpf were randomly divided into six groups; namely, the blank control group; the 5-ASA positive control group; the TNBS model group; and the low-, medium-, and high-dosage peptide groups, with 4 repeat holes per group (10 per well). Next, the zebrafish colitis model was constructed by exposing larvae to TNBS. After 48 h, each group was stained with 0.2% calcein solution for 1.5 h. Then the dye was removed by washing the zebrafish three times with phosphate-buffered saline (PBS). The intestinal fluorescence of zebrafish was determined by using an Olympus SZX16 fluorescence microscope (Tokyo, Japan) equipped with a digital color camera (DP2-BSW, cellSens Standard software 2.2). The integrated option density (IOD) of each zebrafish was analyzed using Image Pro-Plus 5.1. The average IOD of the control group was defined as IOD0, and the average IOD of the TNBS group was defined as IOD1. Then, the positive drug and different concentrations of peptide LLTRAGL (20, 40, 80 µg/mL) were added into positive control group and peptide treatment groups. All the zebrafish were cultured in a dark environment for 16 h. After that, the fluorescence intensities of the zebrafish guts were captured using the fluorescent microscope, and the IOD was determined (IOD2). The intestinal efflux efficiency (IEE) was calculated according to Equation (1) [47].

$$IEE = (IOD0/IOD1 - IOD2)/(IOD0/IOD1) \tag{1}$$

4.6. Peristalsis-Promoting Effect

In this experiment, AB zebrafish embryos at 3 dpf were randomly divided into six groups and colitis zebrafish was induced as described in Section 4.4, for a total of 6 groups with 4 repeat holes per group (10 per well). Then, each group was stained with 0.2% calcein for 1.5 h. After that, the zebrafish were rinsed three times in PBS. The peristalsis-promoting effect was evaluated according to intestinal peristalsis frequency of each zebrafish in 1 min, which was recorded by an Olympus SZX16 fluorescence microscope (Tokyo, Japan).

4.7. Pathological Observation and Ultrastructure of the Intestinal Tissue of Zebrafish

The pathological observation of the intestinal tissue of zebrafish was examined by using the hematoxylin and eosin (H&E) [48] and Alcian blue (AB) [49] methods. In this experiment, AB zebrafish embryos at 3 dpf were randomly divided into six groups and colitis zebrafish was induced as described in Section 4.4. Following drug treatment, ten zebrafish larvae were randomly collected from each group and fixed in 4% paraformaldehyde for 24 h. Then, the fixed larvae were dehydrated in gradient ethanol, immersed in xylene, and embedded in paraffin. The tissue sections were observed and photographed under the Olympus SZX16 fluorescence microscope (Tokyo, Japan).

The ultrastructure of the intestinal tissue of zebrafish was observed by using the scanning electron microscopy method [49]. After drug treatment, ten zebrafish larvae were randomly collected from each group and fixed in an electron microscope fixation liquid containing 5% glutaraldehyde. Then, the fixed larvae were dehydrated in propanol, embedded in epoxy resin, and double stained with uranium acetate and lead citrate. Finally, ultra-thin intestinal tissue sections were observed by using the HT7800/HT7700 projection electron microscope (HITACHI, Chiyoda, Japan).

4.8. Differential Expression and Enrichment Analysis of RNA-Seq

The wild-type AB strain was used in this experiment. Zebrafish were randomly divided into blank group, modeling group and 80 µg/mL drug administration group, with three repeat holes in each group (30 zebrafish per hole). RNA-sequencing analysis was performed on zebrafish larvae samples with the assistance of OE Biotech Co., Ltd. (Shanghai, China). The differential expression analysis of two conditions/groups (two biological replicates per condition) was performed using the DESeq2 R package (1.20.0). Genes with an adjusted p-adjust ≤ 0.05 and absolute fold change ≥ 2 found by DESeq2 were assigned as differentially expressed. The Gene Ontology (GO) enrichment analysis of differentially expressed genes (DEGs) and test the statistical enrichment of differential expression genes in the Kyoto Encyclopedia of Genes and Genomes (KEGG) pathways [50,51] were performed on an online OECloud tools (https://cloud.oebiotech.cn, accessed on 13 February 2023).

4.9. Qualification of Gene Expression

The transcripts of several genes involved in the key signaling pathways—*mmp9*, *il8*, *il1β*, *il12*, *il10*, *ripk3* and *bax*—were selected and identified by qRT-PCR. Moreover, the expression levels of key genes in inflammatory-related signaling pathways were also determined. Total RNA was extracted from drug-treated zebrafish samples using the SPARKeasy RNA isolation kit (Sparkjade, Qingdao, China) according to the manufacturer's instructions. cDNAs were generated using the SPAPKscript II RT Plus Kit (Sparkjade,

Qingdao, China) with a random primer, and quantitative RT-PCR reactions were carried out using the ChamQ Universal SYBR qPCR Master Mix. In this study, *β-actin* was chosen as a standard control gene. The sequences of primers in RT-qPCR were listed in Table S6. The RT-qPCR amplification reaction conditions were as follows: 95 °C for 1 min followed by 40 cycles of 95 °C for 20 s and 72 °C for 30 s. The relative mRNA expression changes relative to *β-actin* were calculated using the $2^{-\Delta\Delta CT}$ method. Relevant primers were designed against zebrafish genes.

4.10. Molecular Docking

In the docking study, the key target proteins in the NOD-like receptor signal pathway and necroptosis pathway were chosen as the receptors, and the active peptide and positive control were selected as ligands. The three-dimensional (3D) crystal structure of PYCARD (6KI0), IL-8 (6WZL), IL-1β (7Z3W), Caspase-9 (5WVC) and RIPK1 (7YDX) were obtained from the Protein Data Bank (https://www.rcsb.org/structure/1O8A). The 3D structure of LLTRAGL and 5-ASA were constructed and the energy minimized by using the MM2 molecular mechanics method with Chem3D Pro 14.0 (CambridgeSoft Co., Waltham, MA, USA). Before docking, water molecules and other irrelevant ions were removed from the structure of protein receptors. Subsequently, the receptors and two ligands were energetically minimized by the CHARMm force field. The automated molecular docking studies at the receptor binding sites were performed using the CDOCKER module [12]. The binding site sphere of the PYCARD was set as x: −37.5115, y: 7.0317 and z: 40.2425. The binding site sphere of IL-8 was set as x: −11.1982, y: 25.1655 and z: 46.2784. The binding site sphere of the IL-1β was set as x: 13.6831, y: 44.2132 and z: 60.4207. The binding site sphere of the Caspase-9 was set to x: 67,3437, y: −68.4981 and z: −12.8687. The binding site sphere of the RIPK1 was set to x: −16.7095, y: −5.2390 and z: 37.9227; the radius was set to 20 Å during the simulation. The values of -CDOCKER ENERGY and -CDCKER INTERACTION ENERGY were considered as an evaluation. The best conformation of the ligand and receptor showed the highest values of -CDOCKER ENERGY and -CDCKER INTERACTION ENERGY.

4.11. Statistical Analysis

All the results were expressed as the mean ± SEM, and a one-way analysis of variance (ANOVA) was used to identify each group's significant differences. The statistical significance was set as # $p < 0.05$, ## $p < 0.01$ vs. the blank control group; and * $p < 0.05$, ** $p < 0.01$ vs. the TNBS group.

5. Conclusions

In summary, this study showed that the peptide LLTRAGL, derived from *Rapana venosa*, had significant ameliorative effects on TNBS-induced colitis in zebrafish. The underlying alleviative effect of LLTRAGL might plausibly be due to its regulating effect in the NOD-like receptor signal pathway and necroptosis pathway associated genes. Hence, the peptide might be a promising therapeutic candidate against colitis, which provides valuable information for future application of LLTRAGL in IBD.

Supplementary Materials: The following supporting information can be downloaded at: https://www.mdpi.com/article/10.3390/md22030100/s1, Table S1: Up-regulation and down-regulation of TOP10 genes in TNBS vs. Control and LLTGRAGL vs. TNBS; Table S2: Common differential genes between TNBS vs. Control and LLTGRAGL vs. TNBS; Table S3: Differentially expressed genes in GO enrichment analysis circle; Table S4: Gene names included in inflammatory reactions in GO enrichment analysis circle (order from top to bottom); Table S5: Corresponding Paths in the Chord Graph of TNBS vs. Control and LLTGRAGL vs. TNBS KEGG Analysis; Table S6: Sequence of Primers Used in qPCR; Figure S1: The safe doses screening of LLTRAGL at 10, 20, 40, 80, 160, 320 and 640 µg/mL; Figure S2: 3D diagrams of LLTRAGL and 5-ASA docked with 6KI0, 6WZL, 7Z3W, 5WVC and 7YDX molecules; Figure S3: 2D diagrams of LLTRAGL and 5-ASA docked with 6KI0, 6WZL, 7Z3W, 5WVC and 7YDX molecules.

Author Contributions: Conceptualization, S.Z. and Y.Z.; methodology, Y.C. and S.Z.; validation, Y.Z.; formal analysis, Y.C., F.X. and Q.X.; data curation, Y.C., S.Z. and Y.Z; writing—original draft preparation, Y.C. and S.Z.; writing—review and editing, K.L. and Y.Z.; supervision, K.L., H.L. and Y.Z.; project administration, K.L. and Y.Z.; funding acquisition, S.Z., H.L. and Y.Z. All authors have read and agreed to the published version of the manuscript.

Funding: This research was funded by National Key R&D Program of China (2022YFC2804600), National Natural Science Foundation of China (22137006, 42006090), Taishan Scholars Program (tsqn202211204), Jinan Talent Project for University (2021GXRC047) and Industry Integration Innovation Pilot Project-Basic Research Project of Qilu University of Technology (Shandong Academy of Sciences) (2023PY042).

Institutional Review Board Statement: The animal study was reviewed and approved by Animal Care and Ethics Committee of Biology Institute, Qilu University of Technology (Shandong Academy of Sciences).

Data Availability Statement: The data presented in the current study are available on request from the corresponding author.

Conflicts of Interest: The authors declare no conflicts of interest.

References

1. Hodson, R. Inflammatory bowel disease. *Nature* **2016**, *540*, S97. [CrossRef] [PubMed]
2. Liu, D.; Saikam, V.; Skrada, K.A.; Merlin, D.; Iyer, S.S. Inflammatory bowel disease biomarkers. *Med. Res. Rev.* **2022**, *42*, 1856–1887. [CrossRef] [PubMed]
3. Kudelka, M.R.; Stowell, S.R.; Cummings, R.D.; Neish, A.S. Intestinal epithelial glycosylation in homeostasis and gut microbiota interactions in IBD. *Nat. Rev. Gastroenterol. Hepatol.* **2020**, *17*, 597–617. [CrossRef] [PubMed]
4. Bilal, M.; Nunes, L.V.; Duarte, M.T.S.; Ferreira, L.F.R.; Soriano, R.N.; Iqbal, H.M.N. Exploitation of Marine-Derived Robust Biological Molecules to Manage Inflammatory Bowel Disease. *Mar. Drugs* **2021**, *19*, 196. [CrossRef] [PubMed]
5. Jimenez, K.M.; Gasche, C. Management of Iron Deficiency Anaemia in Inflammatory Bowel Disease. *Acta Haematol.* **2019**, *142*, 30–36. [CrossRef] [PubMed]
6. Besednova, N.N.; Zaporozhets, T.S.; Kuznetsova, T.A.; Makarenkova, I.D.; Kryzhanovsky, S.P.; Fedyanina, L.N.; Ermakova, S.P. Extracts and Marine Algae Polysaccharides in Therapy and Prevention of Inflammatory Diseases of the Intestine. *Mar. Drugs* **2020**, *18*, 289. [CrossRef] [PubMed]
7. Cunha, S.A.; Pintado, M.E. Bioactive peptides derived from marine sources: Biological and functional properties. *Trends Food Sci. Technol.* **2022**, *119*, 348–370. [CrossRef]
8. Sila, A.; Bougatef, A. Antioxidant peptides from marine by-products: Isolation, identification and application in food systems. A review. *J. Funct. Foods* **2016**, *21*, 10–26. [CrossRef]
9. Xu, F.H.; Qiu, Y.Z.; Zhang, Y.; Yang, F.H.; Ji, M.M.; Liu, K.C.; Jin, M.; Zhang, S.S.; Li, B. The molecular mechanism of three novel peptides from C-phycocyanin alleviates MPTP-induced Parkinson's disease-like pathology in zebrafish. *Food Funct.* **2023**, *14*, 6157–6171. [CrossRef]
10. Zhang, X.; Li, H.; Wang, L.; Zhang, S.; Wang, F.; Lin, H.; Gao, S.; Li, X.; Liu, K. Anti-inflammatory peptides and metabolomics-driven biomarkers discovery from sea cucumber protein hydrolysates. *J. Food Sci.* **2021**, *86*, 3540–3549. [CrossRef]
11. Zhang, X.; Cao, D.; Sun, X.; Sun, S.; Xu, N. Preparation and identification of antioxidant peptides from protein hydrolysate of marine alga Gracilariopsis lemaneiformis. *J. Appl. Phycol.* **2019**, *31*, 2585–2596. [CrossRef]
12. Zhang, S.S.; Han, L.W.; Shi, Y.P.; Li, X.B.; Zhang, X.M.; Hou, H.R.; Lin, H.W.; Liu, K.C. Two Novel Multi-Functional Peptides from Meat and Visceral Mass of Marine Snail Neptunea arthritica cumingii and Their Activities In Vitro and In Vivo. *Mar. Drugs* **2018**, *16*, 473. [CrossRef] [PubMed]
13. Ren, Q.; Jiang, X.; Zhang, S.; Gao, X.; Paudel, Y.N.; Zhang, P.; Wang, R.; Liu, K.; Jin, M. Neuroprotective effect of YIAEDAER peptide against Parkinson's disease like pathology in zebrafish. *Biomed. Pharmacother.* **2022**, *147*, 112629. [CrossRef] [PubMed]
14. Dolashka, P.; Moshtanska, V.; Borisova, V.; Dolashki, A.; Stevanovic, S.; Dimanov, T.; Voelter, W. Antimicrobial proline-rich peptides from the hemolymph of marine snail Rapana venosa. *Peptides* **2011**, *32*, 1477–1483. [CrossRef]
15. Gogineni, V.; Hamann, M.T. Marine natural product peptides with therapeutic potential: Chemistry, biosynthesis, and pharmacology. *Biochim. Biophys. Acta Gen. Subj.* **2018**, *1862*, 81–196. [CrossRef]
16. Luo, F.; Xing, R.; Wang, X.; Peng, Q.; Li, P. Proximate composition, amino acid and fatty acid profiles of marine snail Rapana venosa meat, visceral mass and operculum. *J. Sci. Food Agric.* **2017**, *97*, 5361–5368. [CrossRef]
17. Arnulf, S.; Alexander, D.; Stefan, S.; Wolfgang, V.; Wilhelm, A.; Pavlina, D. Cytotoxic Effects of Rapana venosa Hemocyanin on Bladder Cancer Permanent Cell Lines. *J. US-China Med. Sci.* **2016**, *13*, 179–188. [CrossRef]
18. Dolashka, P.; Dolashki, A.; Velkova, L.; Stevanovic, S.; Molin, L.; Traldi, P.; Velikova, R.; Voelter, W. Bioactive compounds isolated from garden snails. *J. BioSci. Biotechnol.* **2015**, special edition/online. 147–155.

19. Xu, F.H.; Yang, F.; Qiu, Y.Z.; Wang, C.S.; Zou, Q.l.; Wang, L.Z.; Li, X.B.; Jin, M.; Liu, K.C.; Zhang, S.S.; et al. The alleviative effect of C-phycocyanin peptides against TNBS-induced inflammatory bowel disease in zebrafish via the MAPK/Nrf2 signaling pathways. *Fish. Shellfish. Immun.* **2024**, *145*, 109351. [CrossRef]
20. Ni, Y.; Zhang, Y.; Zheng, L.; Rong, N.; Yang, Y.; Gong, P.; Yang, Y.; Siwu, X.; Zhang, C.; Zhu, L.; et al. Bifidobacterium and Lactobacillus improve inflammatory bowel disease in zebrafish of different ages by regulating the intestinal mucosal barrier and microbiota. *Life Sci.* **2023**, *324*, 121699. [CrossRef]
21. Wheeler, M.A.; Jaronen, M.; Covacu, R.; Zandee, S.E.J.; Scalisi, G.; Rothhammer, V.; Tjon, E.C.; Chao, C.C.; Kenison, J.E.; Blain, M.; et al. Environmental Control of Astrocyte Pathogenic Activities in CNS Inflammation. *Cell* **2019**, *176*, 581–596.e18. [CrossRef] [PubMed]
22. Mousavi, T.; Hassani, S.; Baeeri, M.; Rahimifard, M.; Vakhshiteh, F.; Gholami, M.; Ghafour-Broujerdi, E.; Abdollahi, M. Comparison of the safety and efficacy of fingolimod and tofacitinib in the zebrafish model of colitis. *Food Chem. Toxicol.* **2022**, *170*, 113509. [CrossRef] [PubMed]
23. Marjoram, L.; Bagnat, M. Infection, Inflammation and Healing in Zebrafish: Intestinal Inflammation. *Curr. Pathobiol. Rep.* **2015**, *3*, 147–153. [CrossRef]
24. Huang, X.; Ai, F.; Ji, C.; Tu, P.; Gao, Y.; Wu, Y.; Yan, F.; Yu, T. A Rapid Screening Method of Candidate Probiotics for Inflammatory Bowel Diseases and the Anti-inflammatory Effect of the Selected Strain Bacillus smithii XY1. *Front. Microbiol.* **2021**, *12*, 760385. [CrossRef]
25. Oehlers, S.H.; Flores, M.V.; Okuda, K.S.; Hall, C.J.; Crosier, K.E.; Crosier, P.S. A chemical enterocolitis model in zebrafish larvae that is dependent on microbiota and responsive to pharmacological agents. *Dev. Dyn.* **2011**, *240*, 288–298. [CrossRef] [PubMed]
26. Sheng, Y.; Li, H.; Liu, X.; Xie, B.; Wei, W.; Wu, J.; Meng, F.; Wang, H.Y.; Chen, S. A Manganese-Superoxide Dismutase From Thermus thermophilus HB27 Suppresses Inflammatory Responses and Alleviates Experimentally Induced Colitis. *Inflamm. Bowel Dis.* **2019**, *25*, 1644–1655. [CrossRef]
27. Zhu, X.; Tian, X.; Yang, M.; Yu, Y.; Zhou, Y.; Gao, Y.; Zhang, L.; Li, Z.; Xiao, Y.; Moses, R.E.; et al. Procyanidin B2 Promotes Intestinal Injury Repair and Attenuates Colitis-Associated Tumorigenesis via Suppression of Oxidative Stress in Mice. *Antioxid. Redox Signal* **2021**, *35*, 75–92. [CrossRef]
28. Yin, S.; Yang, H.; Tao, Y.; Wei, S.; Li, L.; Liu, M.; Li, J. Artesunate ameliorates DSS-induced ulcerative colitis by protecting intestinal barrier and inhibiting inflammatory response. *Inflammation* **2020**, *43*, 765–776. [CrossRef]
29. Yu, J. Gut microbiome and metabolome: The crucial players in inflammatory bowel disease. *J. Gastroenterol. Hepatol.* **2023**, *38*, 5–6. [CrossRef]
30. Wang, X.; Huang, S.; Zhang, M.; Su, Y.; Pan, Z.; Liang, J.; Xie, X.; Wang, Q.; Chen, J.; Zhou, L.; et al. Gegen Qinlian decoction activates AhR/IL-22 to repair intestinal barrier by modulating gut microbiota-related tryptophan metabolism in ulcerative colitis mice. *J. Ethnopharmacol.* **2023**, *302 Pt B*, 115919. [CrossRef]
31. Rubino, S.J.; Selvanantham, T.; Girardin, S.E.; Philpott, D.J. Nod-like receptors in the control of intestinal inflammation. *Curr. Opin. Immunol.* **2012**, *24*, 398–404. [CrossRef]
32. Chuphal, B.; Rai, U.; Roy, B. Teleost NOD-like receptors and their downstream signaling pathways: A brief review. *Fish. Shellfish. Immunol. Rep.* **2022**, *3*, 100056. [CrossRef]
33. Trindade, B.C.; Chen, G.Y. NOD1 and NOD2 in inflammatory and infectious diseases. *Immunol. Rev.* **2020**, *297*, 139–161. [CrossRef] [PubMed]
34. Kufer, T.A.; Kremmer, E.; Banks, D.J.; Philpott, D.J. Role for erbin in bacterial activation of Nod2. *Infect. Immun.* **2006**, *74*, 3115–3124. [CrossRef]
35. Cummings, J.R.; Cooney, R.M.; Clarke, G.; Beckly, J.; Geremia, A.; Pathan, S.; Hancock, L.; Guo, C.; Cardon, L.R.; Jewell, D.P. The genetics of NOD-like receptors in Crohn's disease. *Tissue Antigens* **2010**, *76*, 48–56. [CrossRef] [PubMed]
36. Sugimoto, K.; Ogawa, A.; Mizoguchi, E.; Shimomura, Y.; Andoh, A.; Bhan, A.K.; Blumberg, R.S.; Xavier, R.J.; Mizoguchi, A. IL-22 ameliorates intestinal inflammation in a mouse model of ulcerative colitis. *J. Clin. Investig.* **2008**, *118*, 534–544. [CrossRef]
37. Bishop, J.L.; Roberts, M.E.; Beer, J.L.; Huang, M.; Chehal, M.K.; Fan, X.; Fouser, L.A.; Ma, H.L.; Bacani, J.T.; Harder, K.W. Lyn activity protects mice from DSS colitis and regulates the production of IL-22 from innate lymphoid cells. *Mucosal Immunol.* **2014**, *7*, 405–416. [CrossRef]
38. Li, S.; Ning, L.G.; Lou, X.H.; Xu, G.Q. Necroptosis in inflammatory bowel disease and other intestinal diseases. *World J. Clin. Cases* **2018**, *6*, 745–752. [CrossRef]
39. Qi, J.; Wang, J.; Zhang, Y.; Long, H.; Dong, L.; Wan, P.; Zuo, Z.; Chen, W.; Song, Z. High-Salt-Diet (HSD) aggravates the progression of Inflammatory Bowel Disease (IBD) via regulating epithelial necroptosis. *Mol. Biomed.* **2023**, *4*, 28. [CrossRef] [PubMed]
40. Yang, W.; Tao, K.; Wang, Y.; Huang, Y.; Duan, C.; Wang, T.; Li, C.; Zhang, P.; Yin, Y.; Gao, J.; et al. Necrosulfonamide ameliorates intestinal inflammation via inhibiting GSDMD-medicated pyroptosis and MLKL-mediated necroptosis. *Biochem. Pharmacol.* **2022**, *206*, 115338. [CrossRef]
41. Bryant, A.H.; Bevan, R.J.; Spencer-Harty, S.; Scott, L.M.; Jones, R.H.; Thornton, C.A. Expression and function of NOD-like receptors by human term gestation-associated tissues. *Placenta* **2017**, *58*, 25–32. [CrossRef] [PubMed]

42. Coelho, M.M.; Bezerra, E.M.; da Costa, R.F.; de Alvarenga, E.C.; Freire, V.N.; Carvalho, C.R.; Pessoa, C.; Albuquerque, E.L.; Costa, R.A. In silico description of the adsorption of cell signaling pathway proteins ovalbumin, glutathione, LC3, TLR4, ASC PYCARD, PI3K and NF-Kbeta on 7.0 nm gold nanoparticles: Obtaining their Lennard-Jones-like potentials through docking and molecular mechanics. *RSC Adv.* **2023**, *13*, 35493–35499. [CrossRef] [PubMed]
43. Molnar, T.; Pallagi, P.; Tel, B.; Kiraly, R.; Csoma, E.; Jenei, V.; Varga, Z.; Gogolak, P.; Odile Hueber, A.; Mate, Z.; et al. Caspase-9 acts as a regulator of necroptotic cell death. *FEBS J.* **2021**, *288*, 6476–6491. [CrossRef] [PubMed]
44. Guha, S.; Majumder, K. Structural-features of food-derived bioactive peptides with anti-inflammatory activity: A brief review. *J. Food Biochem.* **2019**, *43*, e12531. [CrossRef]
45. Rakesh, K.P.; Suhas, R.; Gowda, D.C. Anti-inflammatory and Antioxidant Peptide-Conjugates: Modulation of Activity by Charged and Hydrophobic Residues. *Int. J. Pept. Res. Ther.* **2017**, *25*, 227–234. [CrossRef]
46. Xu, F.; Zhang, Y.; Qiu, Y.; Yang, F.; Liu, G.; Dong, X.; Chen, G.; Cao, C.; Zhang, Q.; Zhang, S.; et al. Three novel antioxidant peptides isolated from C-phycocyanin against H2O2-induced oxidative stress in zebrafish via Nrf2 signaling pathway. *Front. Mar. Sci.* **2022**, *9*, 1098091. [CrossRef]
47. Wang, X.X.; Zou, H.Y.; Cao, Y.N.; Zhang, X.M.; Sun, M.; Tu, P.F.; Liu, K.C.; Zhang, Y. Radix Panacis quinquefolii Extract Ameliorates Inflammatory Bowel Disease through Inhibiting Inflammation. *Chin. J. Integr. Med.* **2023**, *29*, 825–831. [CrossRef]
48. Faal, M.; Manouchehri, H.; Changizi, R.; Bootorabi, F.; Khorramizadeh, M.R. Assessment of resveratrol on diabetes of zebrafish (*Danio rerio*). *J. Diabetes Metab. Disord.* **2022**, *21*, 823–833. [CrossRef]
49. Mhalhel, K.; Briglia, M.; Aragona, M.; Porcino, C.; Abbate, F.; Guerrera, M.C.; Laura, R.; Krichen, Y.; Guerbej, H.; Germana, A.; et al. Nothobranchius as a model for anorexia of aging research: An evolutionary, anatomical, histological, immunohistochemical, and molecular study. *Ann. Anat.* **2023**, *250*, 152116. [CrossRef]
50. Lu, W.; Yang, F.; Meng, Y.; An, J.; Hu, B.; Jian, S.; Yang, G.; Lu, H.; Wen, C. Immunotoxicity and transcriptome analysis of zebrafish embryos exposure to Nitazoxanide. *Fish. Shellfish. Immunol.* **2023**, *141*, 108977. [CrossRef]
51. Ma, J.; Chen, J.; Louro, B.; Martins, R.S.T.; Canario, A.V.M. Somatostatin 3 loss of function impairs the innate immune response to intestinal inflammation. *Aquac. Fish.* **2021**, *6*, 548–557. [CrossRef]

Disclaimer/Publisher's Note: The statements, opinions and data contained in all publications are solely those of the individual author(s) and contributor(s) and not of MDPI and/or the editor(s). MDPI and/or the editor(s) disclaim responsibility for any injury to people or property resulting from any ideas, methods, instructions or products referred to in the content.

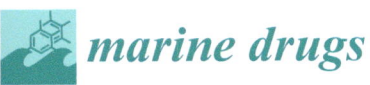 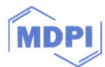

Article

Development of Integrated Vectors with Strong Constitutive Promoters for High-Yield Antibiotic Production in Mangrove-Derived *Streptomyces*

Mingxia Zhao †, Zhiqiang Yang †, Xinyue Li, Yaqi Liu, Yingying Zhang, Mengqian Zhang, Yangli Li, Xincheng Wang, Zixin Deng, Kui Hong * and Dongqing Zhu *

Key Laboratory of Combinatorial Biosynthesis and Drug Discovery, Ministry of Education, School of Pharmaceutical Sciences, Wuhan University, Wuhan 430071, China; zmingxia2021@163.com (M.Z.); nilealexed@gmail.com (Z.Y.); lixinyue0880@163.com (X.L.); liuyaqi2019@163.com (Y.L.); yingying199603@163.com (Y.Z.); zhangmengqian0331@163.com (M.Z.); 13512775882@163.com (Y.L.); ww709693222@163.com (X.W.); zxdeng@sjtu.edu.cn (Z.D.)
* Correspondence: kuihong31@whu.edu.cn (K.H.); dzhu2011@whu.edu.cn (D.Z.)
† These authors contributed equally to this work.

Abstract: It is important to improve the production of bioactive secondary products for drug development. The *Escherichia coli*—*Streptomyces* shuttle vector pSET152 and its derived vector pIB139 containing a strong constitutive promoter *ermE*p* are commonly used as integrative vectors in actinomycetes. Four new integrative vectors carrying the strong constitutive promoter *kasO*p*, *hrdB*p, *SCO5768*p, and SP44, respectively, were constructed and proven to be functional in different mangrove-derived *Streptomyces* host strains by using kanamycin resistance gene *neo* as a reporter. Some biosynthetic genes of elaiophylins, azalomycin Fs, and armeniaspirols were selected and inserted into these vectors to overexpress in their producers including *Streptomyces* sp. 219807, *Streptomyces* sp. 211726, and *S. armeniacus* DSM 43125, resulting in an approximately 1.1–1.4-fold enhancement of the antibiotic yields.

Keywords: marine *Streptomyces*; integrative vector; constitutive promoter; elaiophylin; azalomycin F; armeniaspirol

1. Introduction

Natural products are critical sources of drug resources. *Streptomyces* strains, harboring complex secondary metabolic gene clusters, are the most important producers of antibiotics and other bioactive secondary metabolites. The *Escherichia coli*—*Streptomyces* shuttle vector pSET152 [1] and its derived vector pIB139 [2,3] containing strong constitutive promoter *ermE*p* are commonly employed in high-yield strain breeding. They are non-replicative in streptomycetes but integrate into the chromosome to yield stable recombinant strains, thus avoiding the possible problems associated with autonomously replicating plasmids. pSET152 and pIB139 were widely used in gene function analysis, secondary metabolite biosynthetic gene cluster mining, and silent gene cluster activation [4–6]. They also introduced some homologous or heterologous genes into *Streptomyces* to increase antibiotic production [7–10].

*ermE*p* is a mutated promoter of the erythromycin resistance gene of *Saccharopolyspora erythrea* [2]. During our research, we found that the *ermE*p* did not express a high level in some *Streptomyces* spp. It is necessary to enrich molecular tools for gene manipulation by constructing new pSET152-derived vectors with other strong constitutive promoters. *kasO*p* and *hrdB*p, an engineered promoter of the SARP family regulator gene and a native promoter of the principal sigma factor gene in *S. coelicolor*, constitutively transcribe gene expression more strongly than the *ermE*p* [11,12]. *SCO5768*p is also a strong constitutive

promoter scanned from the *Streptomyces* species, which was twice as strong as *ermEp** in *S. venezuelae* [13]. SP44 is a synthesized constitutive promoter, which was twice as strong as *kasOp** in *S. avermitilis* [14]. As we all know, the promoter strength comparisons were performed using particular genes in special strains under specific conditions, so these findings should not be extrapolated to draw general conclusions.

In this work, we constructed four pSET152-derived vectors with the strong constitutive promoters reported [15], such as *kasOp**, *hrdBp*, *SCO5768p*, and SP44. Kanamycin resistance gene *neo* was used as a reporter to test their transcriptional levels in *Streptomyces* strains. These vectors were applied in gene overexpression to increase the antibiotic production of the mangrove-derived *Streptomyces* strains, including elaiophylin producer *Streptomyces* sp. 219807 [16], azalomycin F producer *Streptomyces* sp. 211726 [17–19], and armeniaspirol producer *S. armeniacus* DSM 43125 [4,20].

2. Results

2.1. Construction of Recombinant Plasmids Harboring Strong Constitutive Promoters and the Corresponding Reporter Plasmids

The native promoters *hrdBp*, *SCO5768p*, and *kasOp** were amplified by PCR, and the synthetic promoter SP44 was synthetized to develop four new integrating vectors pWHU1288-pWHU1291 (Figure 1). The construction of the following plasmids is listed in Table S1. Agarose gel electrophoresis analysis of PCR products or recombinant plasmids digested with restriction enzymes is shown in Figures S1 and S2.

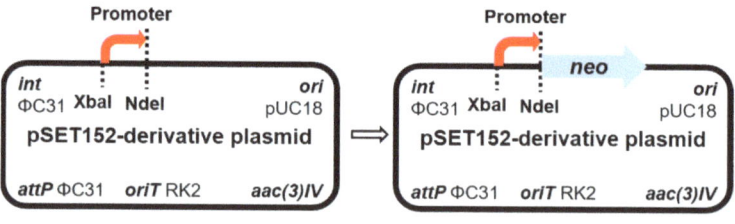

Promoter	+pSET152 ⟹	Plasmid	+ neo ⟹	Plasmid
None		pSET152		pWHU1292
ermEp*		pIB139		pLXY37
hrdBp		pWHU1288		pLXY39
SCO5768p		pWHU1289		pLXY40
kasOp*		pWHU1290		pLXY41
SP44		pWHU1291		pWXC4

Figure 1. Genetic map of the base vectors.

Next, we need a reporter gene to test whether the four promoters express normally in *Streptomyces* strains. The kanamycin resistance gene *neo* was amplified from plasmid pHZ1358 [21] and inserted into pIB139 to generate plasmid pLXY37; the *neo* gene is controlled by the promoter *ermEp**. pLXY37 was conjugated into *Streptomyces* strains, including *S. coelicolor* M145, *S. lividans* TK24, *S. albus* J1074, and *S. venezuelae* ISP5230. The recombinant strains and their corresponding wild-type strains were inoculated in TSBY liquid medium containing 0–50 µg/mL kanamycin and cultured at 30 °C for 48 h. The recombinant strains harboring pLXY37 showed obvious kanamycin resistance, as compared to the wild-type strains (Figure S3). The results proved the *neo* gene is functional, and can be used to reveal the strength of promoters.

The gene *neo* was also inserted into pSET152 to generate a promoter-less reporter plasmid pWHU1292 as the negative control. pWHU1292 was conjugated into *S. ceolicolor* M145 and the recombinant strain *S. ceolicolor* M145::pWHU1292 was inoculated in TSBY liquid medium containing 0–25 µg/mL kanamycin and cultured at 30 °C for 48 h. Compared with *S. ceolicolor* M145::pLXY37 as the positive control and the wild-type strain *S. ceolicolor* M145 as the negative control, *S. ceolicolor* M145::pWHU1292 was inhibited completely at the concentration of 18–25 µg/mL kanamycin (Figure S4). The results revealed that the *neo* gene can be used to test the promoter when the concentration of kanamycin is above 20 µg/mL. Then the *neo* gene was inserted into pWHU1288-pWHU1291, respectively, to generate the corresponding reporter plasmids pLXY39-pLXY41 and pWXC4 to test the strength of promoters in host strains (Figure 1).

2.2. Comparison of Promoter Strength in Different Streptomyces Strains

The reporter plasmids were conjugated into six different *Streptomyces* strains, including *S. coelicolor* M145, *S. lividans* TK24, *S. olivaceus* CGMCC 4.1369, *Streptomyces* sp. 219807, *Streptomyces* sp. 211726, and *S. armeniacus* DSM 43125, respectively. The kanamycin resistance level of the recombinant strains (Table 1 and Figures S5–S10) is a direct reflection of promoter activity.

Table 1. Kanamycin resistance levels conferred by different promoters in different *Streptomyces* strains.

Strain	Medium	Kanamycin Resistance Levels (µg/mL)					
		None	ermEp*	hrdBp	SCO5768p	kasOp*	SP44
S. coelicolor M145	SFM [1]	0	200	400	0	200	800–1000
S. lividans TK24	SFM	0	200	200	1000	400–800	1500–2000
S. olivaceus CGMCC 4.1369	SFM	0–50	400	400	400	400	1000
Streptomyces sp. 219807	FM [2]	0	200	800–1000	0	800–1000	1000–1200
Streptomyces sp. 211726	FM	0	100–200	300–400	100–200	200	600
S. armeniacus DSM 43125	FM	0	900	900	2200	2200	1800

[1] SFM, Soy Flour Mannitol medium; [2] FM, fermentation medium.

In *S. coelicolor* M145, the strength of promoters is placed in the order of SP44 > *hrdB*p > *kasO*p*, *ermE*p* > *SCO5768*p. *S. lividans* and *S. coelicolor* are closely related species belonging to the *S. violaceouruber* sub-clade, but the promoter strengths in *S. lividans* TK24 and *S. coelicolor* M145 are different. The strength of promoters in *S. lividans* TK24 is placed in the order of SP44 > *SCO5768*p > *kasO*p* > *hrdB*p, *ermE*p*. Firstly, *SCO5768*p, the weakest promoter in *S. ceolicolor* M145, exhibited higher activity than the other natural promoters and ranked second only to the artificial promoter SP44 in *S. lividans* TK24. Secondly, contrary to the result in *S. ceolicolor* M145, the activity of *kasO*p* was higher than *ermE*p* and the expression level of *hrdB*p was similar to *ermE*p* in *S. lividans* TK24.

S. olivaceus is a member of glucose isomerase producers as food enzymes approved by the National Health Commission of the P. R. China (GB 2760-2014). The artificial promoter SP44 is also the most potent in *S. olivaceus* CGMCC 4.1369. The other promoters have similar expression levels.

In elaiophylin producer *Streptomyces* sp. 219807, the strength of promoters is placed in the order of SP44 > *hrdB*p, *kasO*p* > *ermE*p* > *SCO5768*p. The strength of promoters in azalomycin F producer *Streptomyces* sp. 211726 is placed in the order of SP44 > *hrdB*p > *kasO*p*, *ermE*p*, *SCO5768*p.

S. armeniacus DSM 43125 has been found to biosynthesize armeniaspirols, which are potent antibiotics against Gram-positive bacteria [4,22,23]. In *S. armeniacus* DSM 43125, *SCO5768*p and *kasO*p* show the best performances with kanamycin resistance up to 2200 µg/mL. The activities of SP44 (1800 µg/mL) are also superior to those of *ermE*p*. The strength of *hrdB*p is similar to *ermE*p*. The strength of promoters in *S. armeniacus* DSM 43125 is placed in the order of *kasO*p*, *SCO5768*p > SP44 > *hrdB*p, *ermE*p*.

In summary, the promoters SP44, *kasO*p*, and *hrdB*p showed better or similar activities compared with *ermE*p* in the *Streptomyces* strains tested. The strength of *SCO5768*p varies significantly among diverse strains. Next, we selected pWHU1288 containing *hrdB*p or pWHU1290 containing *kasO*p* to construct plasmids for overexpressing genes in *Streptomyces* sp. 219807, *Streptomyces* sp. 211726, and *S. armeniacus* DSM 43125.

2.3. Enhancement of Elaiophylin Production

Elaiophylin (ELA) is a glycosylated macrodiolide antibiotic with various biological activities (Figure 2a). *Streptomyces* sp. 219807 is an elaiophylin producer from mangrove soil collected in Sanya of China [16] (Figure 2b). In order to obtain the biosynthetic gene cluster of elaiophylin, the whole genome of *Streptomyces* sp. 219807 was sequenced. A DNA region about 64-kb carrying 28 ORFs (Figure 2c, Table S3, accession no. PP236859) was believed to be involved in elaiophylin biosynthesis based on the proposed functions of the genes. Based on the reported elaiophylin biosynthetic gene cluster and biosynthetic pathway in other *Streptomyces* strains, the roles of biosynthetic genes in the cluster can be suggested (Figure S11).

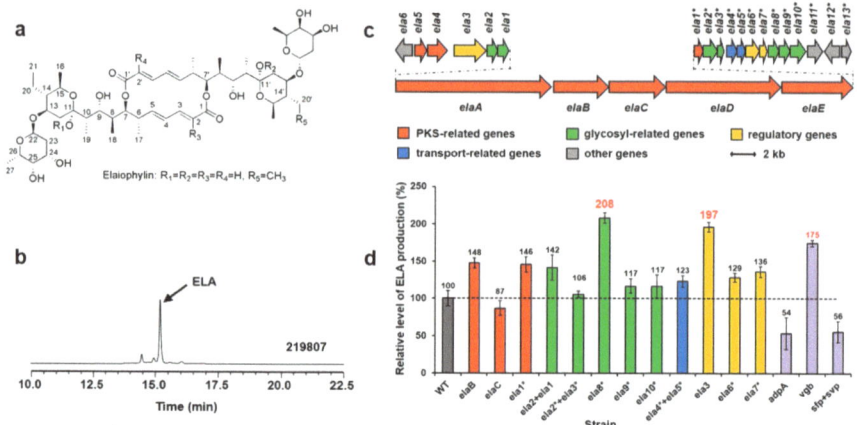

Figure 2. Structures of elaiophylins (**a**). HPLC analysis (252 nm) of extracts from *Streptomyces* sp. 219807 culture (**b**). ELA, elaiophylin. The elaiophylin biosynthetic gene cluster in *Streptomyces* sp. 219807 (**c**). Relative levels of elaiophylin production by *Streptomyces* sp. 219807 derivative strains detected and quantified by HPLC (**d**): WT, 219807::pWHU1288; *elaB*, 219807::pNN1; *elaC*, 219807::pDQ139; *ela1**, 219807::pDQ137; *ela2* + *ela1*, 219807::pLXY45; *ela2** + *ela3**, 219807::pLXY44; *ela8**, 219807::pLXY48; *ela9**, 219807::pLXY50; *ela10**, 219807::pLXY49; *ela4** + *ela5**, 219807::pLXY47; *ela3*, 219807::pLXY51; *ela6**, 219807::pLXY52; *ela7**, 219807::pLXY46; *adpA*, 219807::pLXY55; *vgb*, 219807::pLXY56; *sfp* + *svp*, 219807::pWHU2449. Error bars indicate the standard deviation ($n = 3$).

Three polyketide synthases (PKS) genes (Figure 2c,d, red), seven sugar biosynthesis-related genes (green), two transfer-related genes (blue), and three regulator genes (yellow) in the cluster were amplified from the chromosome of *Streptomyces* sp. 219807 by PCR, inserted into pWHU1288 (the vector carrying *hrdB*p) to generate recombinant plasmids, which were conjugated in *Streptomyces* sp. 219807, respectively. The resulting recombinant strains were confirmed by PCR. The cultures of the derivative strains were extracted and tested by using HPLC and LC-MS. The results showed that the elaiophylin production of the *Streptomyces* sp. 219807 wild-type strain was about 0.98 g/L in this work and that the best two genes at increasing elaiophylin production were the NAD(P)-dependent oxidoreductase gene *ela8** (about 2.04 g/L, increase of 108%) and the LuxR family transcriptional regulator gene *ela3* (about 1.93 g/L, increase of 97%). Then *ela8** and *ela3* were selected and inserted into pWHU1291 (the vector carrying the promoter SP44) to generate recombinant plasmids, which were conjugated in *Streptomyces* sp. 219807 to increase the elaiophylin production further, respectively. However, the results showed that the production decreased about 30% unexpectedly (Figure S12a).

Three heterologous genes were also conjugated in strain *Streptomyces* sp. 219807, respectively, including AraC family transcriptional global regulator gene *adpA* from *S. coelicolor*, synthetic Vitreoscilla hemoglobin gene *vgb*, phosphopantetheinyl transferase (PPtase) gene *sfp* from *Bacillus subtilis*, and *svp* from *S. verticillus*. These genes have been proven to increase antibiotic production or activate silent gene clusters [7,8]. HPLC analysis showed that the overexpression of *vgb* increased the elaiophylin production about 75% (Figure 2d purple). The overexpression of *adpA* or *sfp* + *svp* decreased the elaiophylin production about 50%.

2.4. Enhancement of Azalomycin F production

Azalomycin F (Azl F) is a complex of ployhydroxy macrocyclic lactones with broad-spectrum antimicrobial activities (Figure 3a). *Streptomyces* sp. 211726 isolated from mangrove soil is a remarkable producer of azalomycin F (Figure 3b) [17,18]. A circa 130-kb DNA region carrying 23 ORFs (Figure 3c) was proved to be involved in azalomycin F biosynthesis [18,19]. Several genes, as shown in Figure 3c and d: four precursor biosynthesis-related genes (green), two transfer-related genes (blue), and three regulator genes (yellow) in the cluster, were amplified from the chromosome of *Streptomyces* sp. 211726 by PCR, and inserted into pWHU1288 to generate recombinant plasmids, which were conjugated in the strain *Streptomyces* sp. 211726 for overexpression, respectively. The derivative strains were fermented and the cultures were extracted and tested by using HPLC and LC-MS. Compared to the wild-type strain *Streptomyces* sp. 211726 as control (about 2.80 g/L), the best two genes increasing azalomycin F production were the 4-guanidinobutyryl-CoA ligase gene *azl4* (about 6.61 g/L, increase of 136%) and the TetR family transcriptional regulator gene *azl6* (about 5.43 g/L, increase of 94%), as shown in Figure 3d. pWHU1291 was also used to overexpress *azl4* and *azl6* in *Streptomyces* sp. 211726, respectively, in order to further improve the azalomycin F production. The analysis showed a decrease in production, similar to the results observed in *Streptomyces* sp. 219807 (Figure S12b).

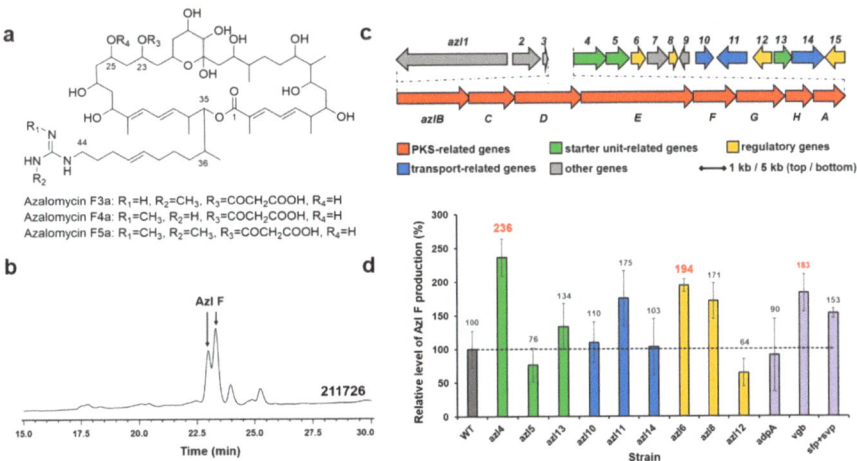

Figure 3. Structures of azalomycin Fs (**a**). HPLC analysis (241 nm) of extracts from *Streptomyces* sp. 211726 culture (**b**). Azl F, azalomycin F mixtures. The azalomycin biosynthetic gene cluster in *Streptomyces* sp. 211726 (**c**). Relative levels of azalomycin F production by *Streptomyces* sp. 211726 derivative strains detected and quantified by HPLC (**d**): WT, 211726::pWHU1288; *azl4*, 211726::pMX301; *azl5*, 211726::pMX302; *azl13*, 211726::pMX308; *azl10*, 211726::pMX305; *azl11*, 211726::pMX306; *azl14*, 211726::pMZ309; *azl6*, 211726::pMX303; *azl8*, 211726::pMX304; *azl12*, 211726::pMX307; *adpA*, 211726::pLXY55; *vgb*, 211726::pLXY56; *sfp* + *svp*, 211726::pWHU2449. Error bars indicate the standard deviation (n = 3).

The genes *adpA*, *vgb*, *sfp*, and *svp* were also conjugated in *Streptomyces* sp. 211726, respectively. HPLC analysis showed that the best gene increasing azalomycin F production was *vgb* (increase of 83%), as shown in Figure 3d (purple).

2.5. Enhancement of Armeniaspirol Production

Armeniaspirols (Arm A, B, and C as shown in Figure 4a,b), with a unique chlorinated spiro[4.4]non-8-ene scaffold, are potent antibiotics against *Helicobacter pylori* and Gram-positive pathogens [20,22]. We cloned the armeniaspirol biosynthetic gene cluster from *S. armeniacus* DSM 43125 in previous work (Figure 4c) [4]. Two PKS genes (*arm6* and *arm7*) and three regulator genes (*arm1*, *arm24* and *arm25*) in the cluster were amplified from the chromosome of *S. armeniacus* DSM 43125 by PCR, and inserted into pWHU1290 (the vector carrying *kasO*p*) to generate recombinant plasmids, which were conjugated in the strain *S. armeniacus* DSM 43125 for overexpression, respectively. The cultures of *S. armeniacus* DSM 43125 and its derivative strains were extracted and tested by using HPLC and LC-MS. The results are shown in Figure 4d. The armeniaspirol production of the wild-type strain *S. armeniacus* DSM 43125 was 0.95 mg/L. The best two genes increasing armeniaspirol production were the PKS gene *arm6* (about 2.03 mg/L, increase of 114%) and the regulator gene *arm24* (about 1.69 mg/L, increase of 78%).

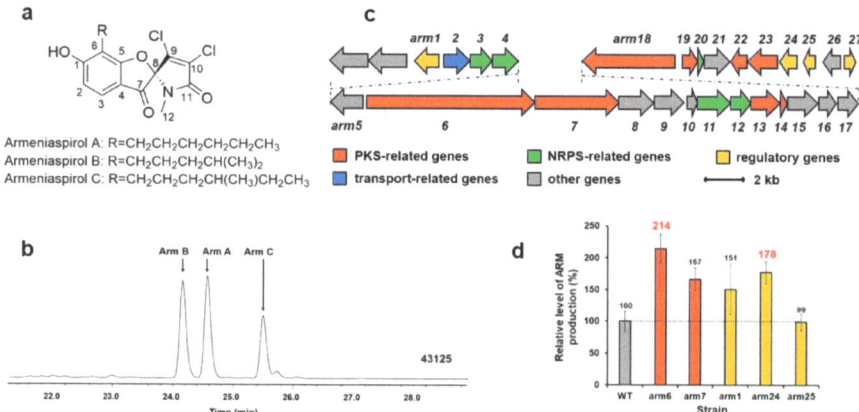

Figure 4. Structures of armeniaspirol (**a**). HPLC analysis (300 nm) of extracts from *S. armeniacus* DSM 43125 culture (**b**). Arm, armeniaspirol. The armeniaspirol biosynthetic gene cluster in *S. armeniacus* DSM 43125 (**c**). Relative levels of armeniaspirol production by *S. armeniacus* DSM 43125 derivative strains detected and quantified by HPLC (**d**): WT, 43125::pWHU1290; *arm6*, 43125::pZQ11; *arm7*, 43125::pZQ12; *arm1*, 43125::pYQ1; *arm24*, 43125::pYQ2; *arm25*, 43125::pYQ3. Error bars indicate the standard deviation (*n* = 3).

3. Discussion

Based on the comparison of promoter strength using kanamycin resistance gene *neo* as a reporter, SP44 is the strongest promoter in most of the tested strains with *S. armeniacus* being an exception. However, for unknown reasons, SP44 was ineffective in enhancing the yield of elaiophylin and azalomycin F. *kasO*p* and *hrdB*p showed similar or higher activity than the *ermE*p* in all the tested strains and they also had good performance in the improvement of antibiotic production. The activity of *SCO5768*p was not detected in some strains and the reason remains unexplained. In summary, pWHU1288 harboring *hrdB*p and pWHU1290 harboring *kasO*p* are favorable choices for the genetic manipulation of *Streptomyces* species.

pWHU1288 and pWHU1290 were used in gene overexpression to increase the antibiotic production of three *Streptomyces* strains, and we obtained high-yielding strains compared with the wild-type strains. Gene *ela8**, *azl4*, and *arm6* overexpression doubled elaiophylin, azalomycin F, and armeniaspirol production, respectively. They are all biosynthetic genes of their corresponding gene clusters, which suggests that the products of these genes may be rate-limiting enzymes in the biosynthetic pathway. The gene cluster for a secondary metabolite harbors variable amounts of biosynthetic genes. Identifying the gene responsible for the rate-limiting step is challenging, especially when dealing with a gene cluster containing numerous biosynthetic genes. Trying each one individually becomes unrealistic. Therefore, pathway-specific activator genes of a one-component regulatory system are viable choices. Gene *ela3* is the only one-component regulatory system gene of the elaiophylin biosynthetic gene cluster, and overexpression of *ela3* increased elaiophylin production about 97%. The same goes for azalomycin F biosynthesis and armeniaspirol biosynthesis. Overexpression of the histidine kinase gene or the response regulator gene of a two-component regulatory system individually did not explicitly improve antibiotic production in the elaiophylin producer and armeniaspirol producer. We also tried co-overexpression of two genes of a two-component regulatory system, but no apparent effects were observed in this work (not shown).

Vitreoscilla hemoglobin is an oxygen-binding protein that promotes oxygen delivery under low oxygen conditions to increase the efficiency of cell metabolism. Normally, oxygen supply is insufficient during the shake flask fermentation, so overexpression of *vgb* increased antibiotic production in *Streptomyces* sp. 219807 and *Streptomyces* sp. 211726, as expected. Gene *adpA* did not improve the biosynthesis of azalomycin Fs in *Streptomyces* sp. 211726 and even repressed the biosynthesis of elaiophylins in *Streptomyces* sp. 219807. AdpA is a global transcriptional activator triggering morphological differentiation and secondary metabolism in *Streptomyces*. However, genes repressed by AdpA were also reported [24]. It is reasonable that the expressions of secondary biosynthetic gene clusters are either unaffected or repressed by AdpA. Phosphopantetheinyl transferase catalyzes the conversion of the carrier proteins of polyketide synthases and nonribosomal peptide synthases from the *apo* form to the active form (*holo* form). Overexpression of the corresponding genes into actinomycete strains achieved a significantly high activation ratio at which strains produced new metabolites [8,25,26]. At the same time, the metabolites produced in some wild-type strains were either eliminated or diminished in their PPtase-overexpressing strains [8]. Thus, it was not inevitable that azalomycin F production went up and elaiophylin production went down when PPtase genes were overexpressed in the producers. In summary, gene *vgb* is a promising candidate for enhancing antibiotic production.

4. Materials and Methods

4.1. General Materials and Experimental Procedures

The bacterial strains and plasmids used in this work are listed in Table S1. Primer sequences are listed in Table S2. Reagents and solvents purchased from Sigma-Aldrich were of the highest quality available and were used without further purification. Restriction enzymes, T4 DNA ligase, and DNA polymerase were purchased from New England Biolabs and used according to the manufacturer's specifications. DNA primers were synthesized by TsingKe Co. Ltd. (Wuhan, China). Growth media and conditions used for *E. coli* and *Streptomyces* strains and standard methods for handling *E. coli* and *Streptomyces* in vivo and in vitro were as described previously, unless otherwise noted. All DNA manipulations were performed following standard procedures. DNA sequencing was carried out at TsingKe Co. Ltd. (Wuhan, China). Genome sequencing of *Streptomyces* sp. 219807 was performed by BGI Co. Ltd. (Wuhan, China) using the Illumina HiSeq 2000 System. ORFs of the secondary metabolite biosynthetic gene clusters were identified using antiSMASH (http://antismash.secondarymetabolites.org, accessed on 22 July 2018) [27], FramePlot (http://nocardia.nih.go.jp/fp4/, accessed on 22 August 2018) [28], and secondFind (http://biosyn.nih.go.jp/2ndfind/, accessed on 22 August 2018). The NRPS-PKS online tools (http://www.nii.ac.in/~pksdb/sbspks/master.html, accessed on 11 September 2018) and (http://nrps.igs.umaryland.edu/, accessed on 11 September 2018) were used to analyze PKSs [29].

The construction of plasmids is listed in Table S1. The plasmids were transferred into *E. coli* ET12567/pUZ8002, and the unmethylated plasmid was conjugated into *Streptomyces* strains, using apramycin to select the respective exconjugants. The exconjugants were confirmed by PCR.

4.2. Determination of Promoter Strength in Streptomyces Strains

Spores of the *Streptomyces* strains were harvested and resuspended in sterile water, and optical density at 450 nm was measured and normalized to the same level. Kanamycin-resistant analyses were carried out using either method 1: the spore suspension was inoculated in the liquid TSBY medium (0.5% yeast extract, 3% tryptone soya broth, 10.3% sucrose, pH 7.2) with different concentrations of kanamycin and cultured at 28 °C and 200 rpm for 3 days before the photograph was taken; or method 2: the spore suspension was series diluted, spotted on SFM medium (2% soy flour, 2% mannitol, 2% agar) or fermentation medium (FM medium, formula as shown below) with 2% agar supplemented with different concentrations of kanamycin, and the plates were incubated at 30 °C for 6 days before the photograph was taken.

4.3. Fermentation, Extraction, and Quantitative Analysis of Elaiophylins

The cultivation of *Streptomyces* sp. 219807-derived strains and the analysis of the resulting products were as previously described [16]. The strains were cultured in liquid TSBY medium at 28 °C and 200 rpm for 3 days, respectively. Then 10% (v/v) of the culture was transferred in 50 mL of fresh fermentation medium (0.2% yeast extract, 1% glucose, 2.5% dextrin, 2% oatmeal, 1% cotton seed flour, 0.5% Fish meal, 0.3% $CaCO_3$, pH 7.2) and fermented at 30 °C and 200 rpm for 8 days.

The mycelium and the culture supernatant were separated by centrifugation. The clarified supernatant after centrifugation was extracted with an equal volume of ethyl acetate three times. The ethyl acetate extracts were dried with anhydrous Na_2SO_4, filtered, and evaporated to dryness under reduced pressure. The mycelium was extracted with 30 mL of 80% (v/v) acetone water solution, which was combined with the culture supernatant extracts. The products were filtered through a 0.22 μm Nylon membrane before subjection to HPLC or LC-ESI-HRMS.

HPLC (Shimadzu, SPD-M20A/LC-20AT, Kyoto, Japan) and LC-ESI-HRMS (Thermo Scientific LTQ Orbitrap XL, positive ion mode, Waltham, MA, USA) were used to analyze samples. The HPLC conditions (Thermo Scientific C18 reversed-phase HPLC column, 250 × 4.6 mm, 5 μm; mobile phase A: water; mobile phase B: acetonitrile; UV detection λ: 252 nm) were as follows: elution gradient I (for HPLC): 10% B for 2 min, 10–100% B for 13 min, 100% B for 10 min, 100–10% B for 10 min, 10% B for 10 min at a flow rate of 1 mL/min; elution gradient II (for LC-ESI- HRMS): 10–100% B for 40 min, 100% B for 20 min, 100–10% B for 10 min, 10% B for 5 min at a flow rate of 0.5 mL/min.

The identity of resultant elaiophylin metabolites was confirmed by direct comparison of retention time and mass spectra with pure authentic standards. The production of elaiophylins was measured with the external standard law. The identities of azalomycin Fs and armeniaspirols were the same unless otherwise noted.

4.4. Fermentation, Extraction, and Quantitative Analysis of Azalomycin Fs

Streptomyces sp. 211726 and all derived strains were cultured in liquid TSBY medium at 30 °C with shaking at 200 rpm for 2 days, respectively. Then 10% (v/v) of the culture was transferred in 25 mL of fresh fermentation medium (0.2% yeast extract, 1% glucose, 3.5% soluble starch, 0.4% casein, pH 7.2–7.4) and fermented at 30 °C and 200 rpm for 10 days.

The mycelium and the culture supernatant were separated by centrifugation. The mycelium was extracted with 25 mL of methanol, which was combined with the clarified culture supernatant after centrifugation. The products were filtered through a microporous membrane (0.22 μm, nylon) before HPLC analysis.

Each sample was analyzed by HPLC (Shimadzu, SPD-M20A/LC 20AT, Kyoto, Japan) with a SHIMADZU Shim-pack VP-ODS C18 column (250 × 4.6 mm, 5 μm) at a flow rate of 1 mL/min using a mobile phase of (A) water and (B) methanol. The separation gradient was as follows: 70% B for 2 min, 70–90% B for 23 min, 90–70% B for 3 min, 70% B for 2 min. Azalomycin F was analyzed by LC-ESI-HRMS (Thermo Electron LTQ-ESI-HRMS, positive ion mode, Waltham, MA, USA) with a SHIMADZU Shim-pack VP-ODS C18 column (250 × 4.6 mm, 5 μm) at a flow rate of 0.2 mL/min using a mobile phase of (A) H_2O with 0.1% formic acid and (B) methanol. The separation gradient was as follows: 0–2 min, 80% B; 2–25 min, 80–100% B; 25–28 min, 100–80% B; 28–43 min, 80% B. The mass spectrometer was set to full scan (from 200 to 2000 m/z).

4.5. Fermentation, Extraction, and Quantitative Analysis of Armeniaspirols

The cultivation of *S. armeniacus* strains and the analysis of the resulting products were as previously described [4]. The *S. armeniacus* strains were cultured in liquid ISP-2 medium (0.4% yeast extract, 1% malt extract, 0.4% glucose, pH 7.0) containing 2 g/L $CaCO_3$ at 30 °C and 200 rpm for 3 days, respectively. Then 10% (*v/v*) of the culture was transferred in 50 mL of fresh ISP-2 medium and fermented at 30 °C and 200 rpm for 6 days.

The culture was separated from the biomass fraction and the supernatant fraction by centrifugation. The supernatant fraction was extracted with an equal volume of ethyl acetate twice. The biomass fraction was extracted with methanol, disrupted by sonication, and centrifuged to remove the cell debris. The retained supernatant was evaporated under reduced pressure, resuspended in water, and twice extracted with an equal volume of ethyl acetate. The combined organic extracts were dried over anhydrous Na_2SO_4, filtered, and concentrated on a rotovap. The residue was re-dissolved in methanol and filtered with a microporous membrane (0.22 μm, nylon).

HPLC (Shimadzu, SPD-M20A/LC-20AT, Kyoto, Japan) and LC-ESI-HRMS (Thermo Scientific LTQ Orbitrap XL, negative ion mode, Waltham, MA, USA) were used to analyze each sample. The HPLC conditions (mobile phase A: water; mobile phase B: acetonitrile; UV detection λ: 300 nm) were as follows: elution gradient I (for Thermo Scientific C18 reversed-phase HPLC column, 250 × 4.6 mm, 5 μm, used in HPLC and LC-ESI-HRMS): 5–95% B for 25 min, 95% B for 10 min, 95–5% B for 5 min, 5% B for 5 min at a flow rate of 1 mL/min.

5. Conclusions

Four strong constitutive promoters, *kasO*p*, *hrdB*p, *SCO5768*p, and SP44, were inserted in the integrative vector pSET152 to generate four new vectors, and three of them, pWHU1288 with *hrdB*p, pWHU1290 with *kasO*p*, and pWHU1291 with SP44, were proven to be functional in different host strains of six *Streptomyces* species, namely *S. coelicolor* M145, *S. lividans* TK24, *S. olivaceus* CGMCC 4.1369, *Streptomyces* sp. 219807, *Streptomyces* sp. 211726, and *S. armeniacus* DSM 43125. Furthermore, pWHU1288 was selected to overexpress NAD(P)-dependent oxidoreductase gene *ela8** in marine *Streptomyces* sp. 219807 and the elaiophylin production increased about 108%. Similarly, pWHU1288 harboring the 4-guanidinobutyryl-CoA ligase gene *azl4* enhanced the elaiophylin production of marine *Streptomyces* sp. 211726 about 136%. In addition, pWHU1290 was used to overexpress the PKS gene *arm6* in *S. armeniacus* DSM 43125 and armeniaspirol production improved about 114%. In brief, pWHU1288 and pWHU1290 exhibit efficient gene activation and expression, and flexible host compatibility, which are useful in synthetic biology.

Supplementary Materials: The following supporting information can be downloaded at: https://www.mdpi.com/article/10.3390/md22020094/s1, Table S1: Bacterial strains and plasmids used in this study; Table S2: Primers used in this study; Figures S1–S2: Agarose gel electrophoresis analysis of PCR products or recombinant plasmids digested with restriction enzymes; Figures S3–S10: Determination of promoter activity by using kanamycin resistance gene *neo* as a reporter gene; Table S3: Deduced functions and sequence comparison of elaiophylin biosynthetic genes; Figure S11: Proposed biosynthetic pathway of elaiophylin; Figure S12: Relative levels of elaiophylin (and azalomycin F) production by *Streptomyces* sp. 219807 (and 211726) derivative strains detected and quantified by HPLC.

Author Contributions: D.Z., K.H., and Z.D. conceived and designed the research. M.Z. (Mingxia Zhao), Z.Y., X.L., Y.L. (Yaqi Liu), Y.Z., M.Z. (Mengqian Zhang), Y.L. (Yangli Li), and X.W. performed the experiments. M.Z. (Mingxia Zhao), Z.Y., X.L., and Y.L. (Yaqi Liu) analyzed data. D.Z., K.H., M.Z. (Mingxia Zhao), and Z.Y. wrote the paper. All authors have read and agreed to the published version of the manuscript.

Funding: This research was funded by the National Science and Technology Fundamental Resources Investigation Program of China (2021FY100900) and the National Key R&D Program of China (2018YFC0311004).

Institutional Review Board Statement: Not applicable.

Data Availability Statement: The authors declare that all data of this study are available within the article and its Supplementary Materials file or from the corresponding authors upon request.

Acknowledgments: We thank Xudong Qu (Shanghai Jiao Tong University, Shanghai, China) for providing the template DNA carrying *kasO*p* and the plasmid carrying *sfp* and *svp*. We thank Delin You (Shanghai Jiao Tong University, Shanghai, China) for providing the plasmid carrying *adpA* and *vgb*. We thank Huarong Tan's Group (State Key Laboratory of Microbial Resources, Institute of Microbiology, Chinese Academy of Sciences, Beijing, China) for providing the template DNA carrying *hrdB*p. We also thank Yuhui Sun (Wuhan University, Wuhan, China) for the template DNA carrying *neo*.

Conflicts of Interest: The authors declare no conflicts of interest.

References

1. Bierman, M.; Logan, R.; O'Brien, K.; Seno, E.T.; Rao, R.N.; Schoner, B.E. Plasmid cloning vectors for the conjugal transfer of DNA from *Escherichia coli* to *Streptomyces* spp. *Gene* **1992**, *116*, 43–49. [CrossRef]
2. Bibb, M.J.; Janssen, G.R.; Ward, J.M. Cloning and analysis of the promoter region of the erythromycin resistance gene (ermE) of *Streptomyces erythraeus*. *Gene* **1985**, *38*, 215–226. [CrossRef] [PubMed]
3. Wilkinson, C.J.; Hughes-Thomas, Z.A.; Martin, C.J.; Bohm, I.; Mironenko, T.; Deacon, M.; Wheatcroft, M.; Wirtz, G.; Staunton, J.; Leadlay, P.F. Increasing the efficiency of heterologous promoters in actinomycetes. *J. Mol. Microbiol. Biotechnol.* **2002**, *4*, 417–426. [PubMed]
4. Qiao, Y.; Yan, J.; Jia, J.; Xue, J.; Qu, X.; Hu, Y.; Deng, Z.; Bi, H.; Zhu, D. Characterization of the Biosynthetic Gene Cluster for the Antibiotic Armeniaspirols in *Streptomyces armeniacus*. *J. Nat. Prod.* **2019**, *82*, 318–323. [CrossRef] [PubMed]
5. Chen, K.; Wu, S.; Zhu, L.; Zhang, C.; Xiang, W.; Deng, Z.; Ikeda, H.; Cane, D.E.; Zhu, D. Substitution of a Single Amino Acid Reverses the Regiospecificity of the Baeyer-Villiger Monooxygenase PntE in the Biosynthesis of the Antibiotic Pentalenolactone. *Biochemistry* **2016**, *55*, 6696–6704. [CrossRef] [PubMed]
6. Martinez-Burgo, Y.; Santos-Aberturas, J.; Rodriguez-Garcia, A.; Barreales, E.G.; Tormo, J.R.; Truman, A.W.; Reyes, F.; Aparicio, J.F.; Liras, P. Activation of Secondary Metabolite Gene Clusters in *Streptomyces clavuligerus* by the PimM Regulator of *Streptomyces natalensis*. *Front. Microbiol.* **2019**, *10*, 580. [CrossRef] [PubMed]
7. Wang, T.; Bai, L.; Zhu, D.; Lei, X.; Liu, G.; Deng, Z.; You, D. Enhancing macrolide production in *Streptomyces* by coexpressing three heterologous genes. *Enzym. Microb. Technol.* **2012**, *50*, 5–9. [CrossRef] [PubMed]
8. Zhang, B.; Tian, W.; Wang, S.; Yan, X.; Jia, X.; Pierens, G.K.; Chen, W.; Ma, H.; Deng, Z.; Qu, X. Activation of Natural Products Biosynthetic Pathways via a Protein Modification Level Regulation. *ACS Chem. Biol.* **2017**, *12*, 1732–1736. [CrossRef]
9. Liu, K.; Hu, X.R.; Zhao, L.X.; Wang, Y.; Deng, Z.; Tao, M. Enhancing Ristomycin A Production by Overexpression of ParB-Like StrR Family Regulators Controlling the Biosynthesis Genes. *Appl. Environ. Microbiol.* **2021**, *87*, e0106621. [CrossRef]
10. Yun, K.; Zhang, Y.; Li, S.; Wang, Y.; Tu, R.; Liu, H.; Wang, M. Droplet-Microfluidic-Based Promoter Engineering and Expression Fine-Tuning for Improved Erythromycin Production in *Saccharopolyspora erythraea* NRRL 23338. *Front. Bioeng. Biotechnol.* **2022**, *10*, 864977. [CrossRef]
11. Wang, W.; Li, X.; Wang, J.; Xiang, S.; Feng, X.; Yang, K. An engineered strong promoter for streptomycetes. *Appl. Environ. Microbiol.* **2013**, *79*, 4484–4492. [CrossRef]
12. Du, D.; Zhu, Y.; Wei, J.; Tian, Y.; Niu, G.; Tan, H. Improvement of gougerotin and nikkomycin production by engineering their biosynthetic gene clusters. *Appl. Microbiol. Biotechnol.* **2013**, *97*, 6383–6396. [CrossRef]
13. Li, S.; Wang, J.; Li, X.; Yin, S.; Wang, W.; Yang, K. Genome-wide identification and evaluation of constitutive promoters in streptomycetes. *Microb. Cell Factories* **2015**, *14*, 172. [CrossRef]
14. Bai, C.; Zhang, Y.; Zhao, X.; Hu, Y.; Xiang, S.; Miao, J.; Lou, C.; Zhang, L. Exploiting a precise design of universal synthetic modular regulatory elements to unlock the microbial natural products in *Streptomyces*. *Proc. Natl. Acad. Sci. USA* **2015**, *112*, 12181–12186. [CrossRef] [PubMed]
15. Lee, N.; Hwang, S.; Lee, Y.; Cho, S.; Palsson, B.; Cho, B.K. Synthetic Biology Tools for Novel Secondary Metabolite Discovery in *Streptomyces*. *J. Microbiol. Biotechnol.* **2019**, *29*, 667–686. [CrossRef] [PubMed]

16. Han, Y.; Tian, E.; Xu, D.; Ma, M.; Deng, Z.; Hong, K. Halichoblelide D a New Elaiophylin Derivative with Potent Cytotoxic Activity from Mangrove-Derived *Streptomyces* sp. 219807. *Molecules* **2016**, *21*, 970. [CrossRef]
17. Yuan, G.; Lin, H.; Wang, C.; Hong, K.; Liu, Y.; Li, J. 1H and 13C assignments of two new macrocyclic lactones isolated from *Streptomyces* sp. 211726 and revised assignments of azalomycins F3a, F4a and F5a. *Magn. Reson. Chem. MRC* **2011**, *49*, 30–37. [CrossRef]
18. Yuan, G.; Hong, K.; Lin, H.; She, Z.; Li, J. New azalomycin F analogs from mangrove *Streptomyces* sp. 211726 with activity against microbes and cancer cells. *Mar. Drugs* **2013**, *11*, 817–829. [CrossRef] [PubMed]
19. Xu, W.; Zhai, G.; Liu, Y.; Li, Y.; Shi, Y.; Hong, K.; Hong, H.; Leadlay, P.F.; Deng, Z.; Sun, Y. An Iterative Module in the Azalomycin F Polyketide Synthase Contains a Switchable Enoylreductase Domain. *Angew. Chem.* **2017**, *56*, 5503–5506. [CrossRef]
20. Jia, J.; Zhang, C.; Liu, Y.; Huang, Y.; Bai, Y.; Hang, X.; Zeng, L.; Zhu, D.; Bi, H. Armeniaspirol A: A novel anti-Helicobacter pylori agent. *Microb. Biotechnol.* **2022**, *15*, 442–454. [CrossRef]
21. Sun, Y.; Zhou, X.; Liu, J.; Bao, K.; Zhang, G.; Tu, G.; Kieser, T.; Deng, Z. '*Streptomyces nanchangensis*', a producer of the insecticidal polyether antibiotic nanchangmycin and the antiparasitic macrolide meilingmycin, contains multiple polyketide gene clusters. *Microbiology* **2002**, *148 (Pt 2)*, 361–371. [CrossRef]
22. Dufour, C.; Wink, J.; Kurz, M.; Kogler, H.; Olivan, H.; Sable, S.; Heyse, W.; Gerlitz, M.; Toti, L.; Nusser, A.; et al. Isolation and structural elucidation of armeniaspirols A–C: Potent antibiotics against gram-positive pathogens. *Chemistry* **2012**, *18*, 16123–16128. [CrossRef] [PubMed]
23. Fu, C.; Xie, F.; Hoffmann, J.; Wang, Q.; Bauer, A.; Bronstrup, M.; Mahmud, T.; Muller, R. Armeniaspirol Antibiotic Biosynthesis: Chlorination and Oxidative Dechlorination Steps Affording Spiro[4.4]non-8-ene. *Chembiochem A Eur. J. Chem. Biol.* **2019**, *20*, 764–769. [CrossRef] [PubMed]
24. Higo, A.; Hara, H.; Horinouchi, S.; Ohnishi, Y. Genome-wide distribution of AdpA, a global regulator for secondary metabolism and morphological differentiation in Streptomyces, revealed the extent and complexity of the AdpA regulatory network. *DNA Res. Int. J. Rapid Publ. Rep. Genes Genomes* **2012**, *19*, 259–273. [CrossRef] [PubMed]
25. Fang, C.; Zhang, Q.; Zhu, Y.; Zhang, L.; Zhang, W.; Ma, L.; Zhang, H.; Zhang, C. Proximicins F and G and Diproximicin A: Aminofurans from the Marine-Derived *Verrucosispora* sp. SCSIO 40062 by Overexpression of PPtase Genes. *J. Nat. Prod.* **2020**, *83*, 1152–1156. [CrossRef] [PubMed]
26. Jiang, K.; Yan, X.; Deng, Z.; Lei, C.; Qu, X. Expanding the Chemical Diversity of Fasamycin Via Genome Mining and Biocatalysis. *J. Nat. Prod.* **2022**, *85*, 943–950. [CrossRef] [PubMed]
27. Blin, K.; Shaw, S.; Kloosterman, A.M.; Charlop-Powers, Z.; van Wezel, G.P.; Medema, M.H.; Weber, T. antiSMASH 6.0: Improving cluster detection and comparison capabilities. *Nucleic Acids Res.* **2021**, *49*, W29–W35. [CrossRef]
28. Ishikawa, J.; Hotta, K. FramePlot: A new implementation of the frame analysis for predicting protein-coding regions in bacterial DNA with a high G + C content. *FEMS Microbiol. Lett.* **1999**, *174*, 251–253. [CrossRef]
29. Anand, S.; Prasad, M.V.; Yadav, G.; Kumar, N.; Shehara, J.; Ansari, M.Z.; Mohanty, D. SBSPKS: Structure based sequence analysis of polyketide synthases. *Nucleic Acids Res.* **2010**, *38*, W487–W496. [CrossRef]

Disclaimer/Publisher's Note: The statements, opinions and data contained in all publications are solely those of the individual author(s) and contributor(s) and not of MDPI and/or the editor(s). MDPI and/or the editor(s) disclaim responsibility for any injury to people or property resulting from any ideas, methods, instructions or products referred to in the content.

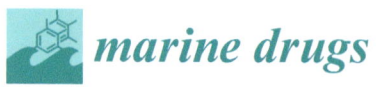 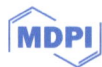

Article

Purification and Properties of a Plasmin-like Marine Protease from Clamworm (*Perinereis aibuhitensis*)

Tingting Jiang [1,†], Bing Zhang [1,2,†], Haixing Zhang [1], Mingjun Wei [1], Yue Su [1], Tuo Song [1], Shijia Ye [1], Yuping Zhu [3,*] and Wenhui Wu [1,4,*]

[1] Department of Marine Biopharmacology, College of Food Science and Technology, Shanghai Ocean University, Shanghai 201306, China; j15037793607@163.com (T.J.); bling9803@163.com (B.Z.); starfishhx@163.com (H.Z.); weimj98@163.com (M.W.); suyue0616@163.com (Y.S.); 15026952710@163.com (T.S.); yyyesj@163.com (S.Y.)
[2] Marine Biomedical Science and Technology Innovation Platform of Lin-gang Special Area, Lane 218, Haiji Sixth Road, Shanghai 201306, China
[3] Basic Medical Experimental Teaching Center, Basic Medical College, Naval Medical University, Shanghai 200433, China
[4] East China Sea Marine Biological Resources Engineering Technology Center, Zhongke Road, Putuo District, Zhoushan 316104, China
* Correspondence: ypz@smmu.edu.cn (Y.Z.); whwu@shou.edu.cn (W.W.)
† These authors contributed equally to this work.

Abstract: Marine organisms are a rich source of enzymes that exhibit excellent biological activity and a wide range of applications. However, there has been limited research on the proteases found in marine mudflat organisms. Based on this background, the marine fibrinolytic enzyme FELP, which was isolated and purified from clamworm (*Perinereis aibuhitensis*), has exhibited excellent fibrinolytic activity. We demonstrated the FELP with a purification of 10.61-fold by precipitation with ammonium sulfate, ion-exchange chromatography, and gel-filtration chromatography. SDS-PAGE, fibrin plate method, and LC–MS/MS indicated that the molecular weight of FELP is 28.9 kDa and identified FELP as a fibrinolytic enzyme-like protease. FELP displayed the maximum fibrinolytic activity at pH 9 (407 ± 16 mm^2) and 50 °C (724 ± 27 mm^2) and had excellent stability at pH 7–11 (50%) or 30–60 °C (60%), respectively. The three-dimensional structure of some amino acid residues of FELP was predicted with the SWISS-MODEL. The fibrinolytic and fibrinogenolytic assays showed that the enzyme possessed direct fibrinolytic activity and indirect fibrinolysis via the activation of plasminogen; it could preferentially degrade Aα-chains of fibrinogen, followed by Bβ- and γ-chains. Overall, the fibrinolytic enzyme was successfully purified from *Perinereis aibuhitensis*, a marine Annelida (phylum), with favorable stability that has strong fibrinolysis activity in vitro. Therefore, FELP appears to be a potent fibrinolytic enzyme with an application that deserves further investigation.

Keywords: *Perinereis aibuhitensis*; plasmin-like protease; amino acid residue sequences; fibrinolysis in vitro

Citation: Jiang, T.; Zhang, B.; Zhang, H.; Wei, M.; Su, Y.; Song, T.; Ye, S.; Zhu, Y.; Wu, W. Purification and Properties of a Plasmin-like Marine Protease from Clamworm (*Perinereis aibuhitensis*). *Mar. Drugs* 2024, 22, 68. https://doi.org/10.3390/md22020068

Academic Editors: Hong Wang, Huawei Zhang and Bin Wei

Received: 14 December 2023
Revised: 22 January 2024
Accepted: 23 January 2024
Published: 27 January 2024

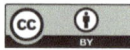

Copyright: © 2024 by the authors. Licensee MDPI, Basel, Switzerland. This article is an open access article distributed under the terms and conditions of the Creative Commons Attribution (CC BY) license (https://creativecommons.org/licenses/by/4.0/).

1. Introduction

The ocean is a large potential source of bioactives [1,2]. Due to the particular living environment, marine organisms have generated bioactive substances with significant specialization [3], especially enzymes, which have properties related to their living environment, such as thermal stability, salt tolerance, cold adaptation, etc., and offer good prospects for industrial applications [4] and biomedicine [5]. Marine organisms are important resources for the production of enzymes, and through isolation and purification from marine microorganisms, a variety of enzymes have been obtained, which exhibit antimicrobial activity [3,6–8], hydrolytic activity against blood proteins [9], collagen solubilizing activity [10] and hydrolysis of alginate for efficient production of alginate oligosaccharides [11], and others. In addition to microorganisms, there are also a wide variety of enzymes, such as cellulases [12] and digestive enzymes [13], in marine animals and plants.

It is noteworthy that enzymes with fibrinolytic activity are found in marine animals as well as in microorganisms. Marine microorganisms of the genus *Bacillus* and *Aspergillus* are considered an important source of fibrinolytic enzyme production [4,14–16]. The fibrinolytic enzymes derived from the fungus demonstrate promising thrombolytic and anticoagulant activities [17]. The purified protease production by the strain *Aspergillus brasiliensis* BCW2 has de-clotting and blood stain removal properties [18]. Che et al. (2020) successfully employed, for the high production of fibrinolytic enzymes, fibase from marine *Bacillus subtilis*, which was expressed in *Komagataella phaffii* GS115 [19]. Members of Annelida (phylum) and Echinodermata in marine organisms contain proteases with fibrinolytic and anticoagulant effects; e.g., Qingqing Bi et al. (2013) purified a fibrinolytically active UFEII from marine echiuroid worms that exhibits fibrin-direct solubilizing and fibrinogen-activating activities [20]. Yahui Ge et al. (2018) purified a novel antithrombotic enzyme from *Sipunculus nudus*, which could improve the coagulation system and inhibit thrombus formation [21]. Marine proteases have shown a good potential for application due to their high safety profile, a wide range of biological activities, and natural origin in the past decades. However, little attention has been paid to the marine mudflat organisms known as *Perinereis aibuhitensis (P. aibuhitensis)*, which also belong to Annelida (phylum). They are often present as bait in aquaculture [22]. They have been explored as research subjects to investigate the potential impacts of marine pollutants [23]. The *P. aibuhitensis* extract obtained in one study exhibited antithrombotic activity, but the specific substances responsible for fibrinolytic effects were not identified [24]. Therefore, it is necessary to investigate the fibrinolytically active components in the *P. aibuhitensis* extract.

In this study, FELP (a protease with plasmin-like activity) was isolated and purified from Annelida (phylum), *P. aibuhitensis*, in a marine mudflat. The amino acid residues were analyzed, and it was confirmed to possess fibrinolytic activity in vitro. FELP shows promise in treating and preventing thrombosis due to its exceptional stability and fibrinolytic activity. Collectively, these results provide the direction and theoretical basis for the development of marine fibrinolytic enzymes.

2. Results

2.1. Isolation and Purification of FELP with Activity Monitoring

FELP from *P. aibuhitensis* was isolated and purified using the purification process mentioned later. The activity of the fractions obtained from each isolation and purification step was monitored using fibrinolysis as an evaluation index. The relationship between the activity of the samples obtained at each ammonium sulphate saturation gradient and ammonium sulfate saturation is shown in Figure 1A. Obviously, the highest enzyme activity was found at 70% ammonium sulphate saturation, so 70% was chosen as the optimum ammonium sulphate saturation for the extraction of FELP.

The crude enzyme was re-dissolved in Tris-HCl (0.02 M), filtered through a 0.45 μm membrane, and then applied to the DEAE-sepharose FF column. The crude sample was eluted with 0–0.5 M NaCl, and the mixtures of protease samples were collected at 280 nm to obtain six fractions (I, II, III, IV, V, and VI) with the DEAE-sepharose FF column (Figure 1B). Surprisingly, fraction III was found to have better fibrinolytic activity according to the fibrin plate than the other fractions (Figure 1D). Fraction III was then dialyzed, freeze-dried, and carried with the Sephadex G-50 column. The first peak (fraction i) in Figure 1B showed excellent fibrinolytic activity. Throughout the purification process, FELP from *P. aibuhitensis* was purified 10.61-fold. The active fractions of the purification process were assayed for fibrinolytic activity and corresponding protein amount (Table 1).

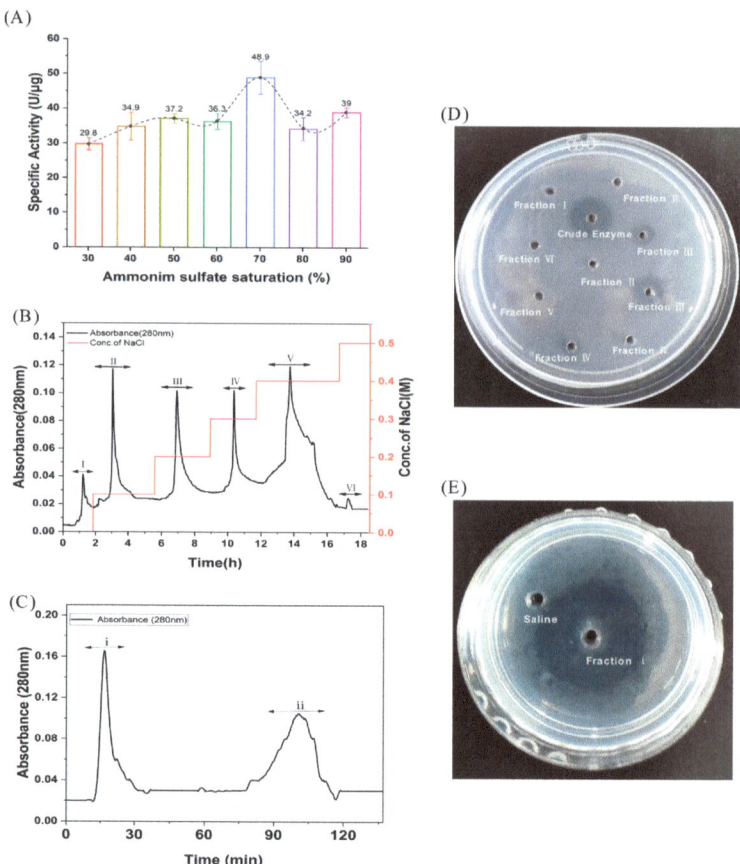

Figure 1. Isolation and purification of FELP from *P. aibuhitensis*. (**A**) The isolation of fibrinolytic enzyme from supernatant through ammonium sulfate precipitation; (**B**) An ion-exchange chromatography of crude enzyme (200 mg) with DEAE-sepharose FF column; (**C**) Gel-filtration chromatography of fraction III (1 g) with Superdex G-50. (**D**) The fibrinolytic activity of fraction I–VI. (**E**) The fibrinolytic activity of fraction i.

Table 1. Purification table of FELP from *P. aibuhitensis*.

Purification Steps	Purification Media	Activity (U) [1]	Protein (μg) [2]	Specific Activity (U/μg)	Purification Folds
Crude isolation	Ammonium sulphate precipitation	7894.06	170.21	46.38	1.00
Ion-exchange chromatography	DEAE-Sepharose FF	677.42	4.52	150.00	3.23
Gel-filtration chromatography	Sephadex G-50	1398.14	2.84	492.30	10.61

[1] Activity was measured in 1 mg of the sample at each purification step; [2] Protein was measured in 1 mg of the sample at each purification step.

2.2. SDS-PAGE

The five main bands in the crude extract were purified into a single band (Figure 2). The molecular weight analysis of FELP showed 28.9 kDa by comparing the relative mobility of the enzyme to a marker. According to the previous reports, the molecular weight of proteases with fibrinolytic activity ranges from 14 to 97 kDa with an average of 27–29 kDa [25]. The molecular weight of FELP was within this interval. Furthermore, the first peak of Superdex G-50 was protein-free in all tubes except tube 4.

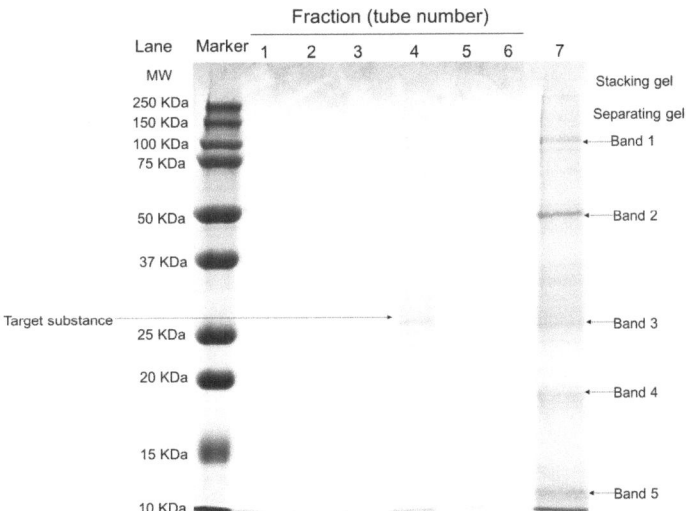

Figure 2. SDS-PAGE analysis of the purified enzyme. The crude extract and the fractions were separated by 12.5% SDS-PAGE; the bands were stained with Coomassie brilliant blue R-250 and then were transferred to the decolorizing fluid ($V_{Ethanol}:V_{Acetic\ acid}:V_{H2O}$ = 2:1:7). Lanes: Marker, protein marker (10–250 kDa); 1–6, Different tubes of elution collected in fraction i (50 mg/mL); 7, The crude exact of *P. aibuhitensis* (5 mg/mL).

2.3. Biochemical Properties of the Purified Fibrinolytic Enzyme

2.3.1. Effect of Inhibitors

The enzyme activity of FELP was affected by different protease inhibitors: soybean trypsin inhibitor (SBTI), phenylmethanesulfonyl fluoride (PMSF) at 5 mM concentration (Figure 3), ethylene diamine tetraacetic acid (EDTA) slightly inhibited the enzyme activity at 5 mM, and epsilon amino caproic acid (EACA) still weakly inhibited protease activity at 10 mM. The enzyme activity was significantly inhibited by SBTI and serine protease inhibitor-like PMSF.

2.3.2. Effect of Temperature and Thermal Stability of FELP

From Figure 4A, it is clear that the transparent circle of fibrinolysis in the fibrin plates displayed a trend of increasing and then decreasing as the temperature increased. As shown in Figure 4B, the enzyme activity was highest when the temperature reached 50 °C; as the holding time increased, the protease activity decreased. The higher the temperature, the worse was the protease stability. FELP has better temperature stability at 30 to 60 °C; even if incubated for 2 h, it still maintained more than 60% of the protease viability (Figure 4C). Furthermore, following incubation for 2 h at each temperature, the residual activity of FELP was significantly reduced at 70 °C and 80 °C compared to the other temperatures.

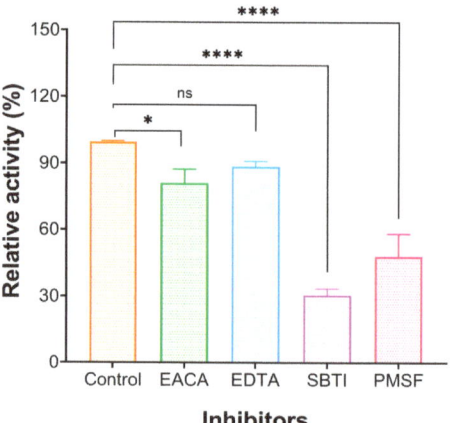

Figure 3. Effect of protease inhibitors on the activity of FELP. FELP (50 mg/mL) was mixed with EACA (10 mM), EDTA (5 mM), SBTI (5 mM), and PMSF (5 mM) at 37 °C, pH 7.4 for 18 h. The data represent mean ± SD, $n = 3$. *, and ns: not significant, * $p < 0.05$, and **** $p < 0.0001$ compared with control, respectively.

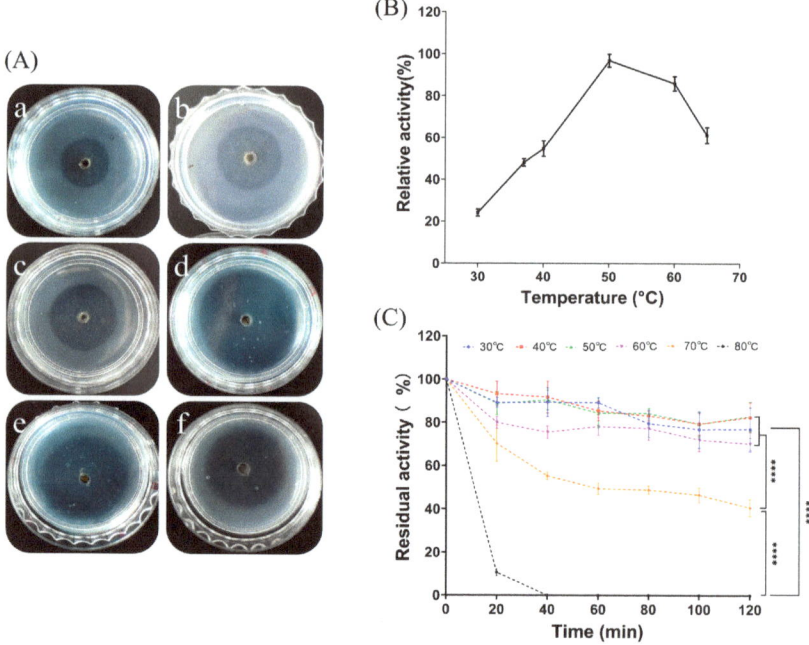

Figure 4. Optimum temperature and thermal stability were determined by evaluating the enzyme activity at different temperatures. Formation of transparent circles (**A**) and relative enzyme activity (**B**) of FELP (50 mg/mL) at 30–65 °C ((**a–f**) in (**A**) correspond to 30 °C, 37 °C, 40 °C, 50 °C, 60 °C, and 65 °C, respectively). (**C**) Determination of changes in fibrinolytic activity with incubation at different temperatures for 0, 20, 40, 60, 80, 100, and 120 min. The data represent mean ± SD, $n = 3$. **** indicate $p < 0.0001$ compared with each other in any groups.

2.3.3. Effect of pH and Stability of FELP

The influence of pH on enzyme activity was measured by treating with a pH of 3, 4, 5, 6, 7, 8, 9, 10, and 11 using different buffers (Figure 5A). The optimal enzyme activity for FELP was pH 9; either peracid or peralkaline environments inactivated the fibrinolytic enzymes (Figure 5B). At pH 7–11, the activity of FELP slowly decreased and remained above 50% for 10 h. At pH 3, the activity of the protease fell below 50% after 4 h. After incubating at each pH for 10 h, the residual activity of FELP was significantly lower at pH 3 compared to the other pH levels.

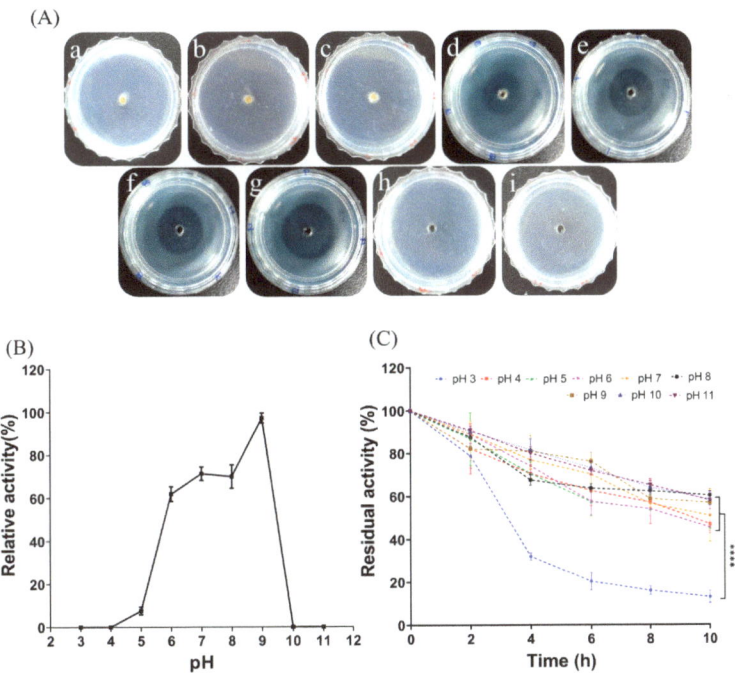

Figure 5. Influence of pH on the fibrinolytic activity of FELP (50 mg/mL) with different buffers (**B**) and the transparent circles in the fibrin plate (**A**) ((**a–i**) in (**A**) correspond to pH 3–11, respectively). (**C**) Determination of changes in fibrinolytic activity with incubation in different buffers for 0, 2, 4, 6, 8, and 10 h. The data represent mean ± SD, $n = 3$. **** indicate $p < 0.0001$ compared with each other in any groups.

2.4. Analysis of Amino Acid Residue Sequences of FELP

FELP was obtained from a clearly visible SDS-PAGE protein band; then, the gels with the target protein bands were reduced and alkylated for enzymatic digestion. The peptide mixture was sorted according to the polarity with a liquid chromatography column. The peptide segments were made with dots through an ESI ion source and then entered into the mass spectrometer to collect a primary mass spectrum; the ions with the highest ionic strengths from the primary mass spectrum were selected and typed into their secondary mass spectra. The secondary mass spectra obtained from the experiment were compared with the secondary mass spectra of fragment ions obtained through simulated hydrolysis and simulated fragmentation in the uniprotkb_Perinereis_245_2023_08_20 database to obtain the peptide identified results (Table 2). With the exception of VSTYMNWIGL, all peptide fragments had high scores, and we believed the identification results were genuine. Three peptides were created by joining the six peptide fragments in Table 2.

Table 2. Peptide fragments were obtained by comparison with the database.

Sequence	Proteins	Missed Cleavages	Ions Score
[R].NWIMTAAHCTAGDSASDLYLMVGEHDR.[S]	1	0	58
[R].IVGGQESRPNEFPWQVSMQSSFGSHYCGAIIINR.[N]	1	0	51
[R].LSTDACQGDSGGPLVVK.[D]	1	0	94
[R].VSTYMNWIGL.[-]	1	0	9
[R].SGGPCCPQILQYVQVPVISNNECNTIDYPGDITDGMICAGNR.[L]	1	0	49
[R].TAVVSGWGTLR.[S]	1	0	58

Peptide 1:
IVGGQESRPNEFPWQVSMQSSFGSHYCGAIIINRNWIMTAAHCTAGDSASDLYLMVGEHDR

Peptide 2:
TAVVSGWGTLRSGGPCCPQILQYVQVPVISNNECNTIDYPGDITDGMICAGNRLSTDACQGDSGGPLVVK

Peptide 3:
VSTYMNWIGL

The identified peptides were then used to match the proteins in the database. Notably, the above peptides were matched with a protease B8Y626 from *P. aibuhitensis* (Korean lugworm), which was not reviewed. Homology modeling of the spliced peptides was performed using the SWISS-MODEL to obtain the 3D structure (Figure 6E,F). The secondary structure of the peptides had an alpha helix, beta-sheet, and coil (Figure 6A).

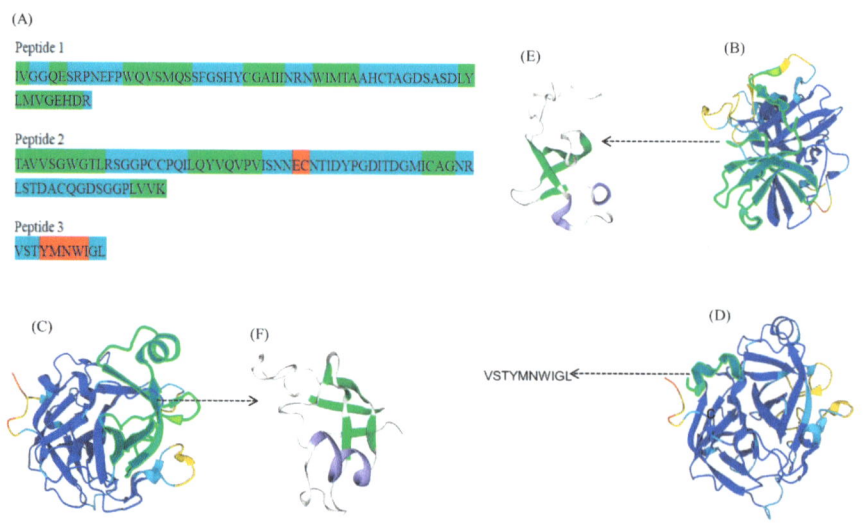

Figure 6. Predicted structures of peptides and B8Y626. (**A**): The predicted secondary structure of the three peptide chains (red indicates alpha helix, green indicates beta-sheet, and blue indicates coil). (**B–D**): The 3D structure of B8Y626 (the green fluorescently labeled fragments in (**B–D**) are the parts of FELP that match with mass spectrometry). (**E,F**): The 3D structure of peptides (green indicates beta-sheet, blue indicates alpha helix, and white indicates coil).

2.5. Fibrinolytic Activity

The fibrinolytic activity of FELP was investigated with fibrin-plate assays. Compared to saline, FELP had a distinctive transparent circle, which indicated that FELP had fibrinolytic activity. As illustrated in Figure 7A, in plasminogen-rich fibrin plates, urokinase (1000 U) and FELP both showed distinct transparent circles. On the plate that had been extinguished with fibrinogen (Figure 7B), the transparent circle of FELP was significantly smaller than that of the plate that had not been extinguished, and the edges appeared blurry. The fibrinolytic activity of FELP (348.67 ± 28.59 mm^2) was 7.86 times that of UK (44.33 ± 7.23 mm^2) in plasminogen-rich fibrin plates, and the fibrinolytic activity of FELP in plasminogen-rich fibrin plates was 2.63 times that of FELP (132.33 ± 11.5 mm^2) in plasminogen-free fibrin plates.

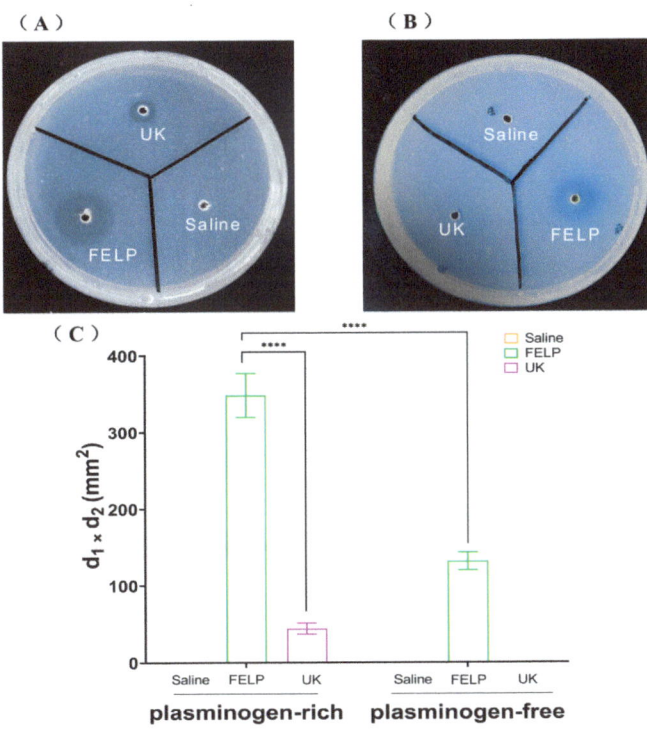

Figure 7. Fibrinolytic activity of FELP. The samples were applied to the wells in the plasminogen-rich fibrin plate (**A**) and plasminogen-free fibrin plate. (**B**) Saline, UK (1000 U), and FELP (50 mg/mL) were incubated at 37 °C for 18 h. (**C**) The fibrinolytic activity of saline, urokinase (1000 U), and FELP (The fibrinolytic activity was indicated by the two perpendicular diameters of the transparent circles). The data represent mean ± SD, $n = 3$. **** indicate $p < 0.0001$ between any concentration and FELP in the plasminogen-rich fibrin plate.

2.6. Degradation of Fibrinogen In Vitro

To elucidate the degradation mechanism of fibrinogen by FELP, it was analyzed with 12.5% SDS-PAGE. FELP could hydrolyze the three chains of fibrinogen and showed dose and time dependency. As shown in Figure 8A, at low enzyme concentrations, the Aα-chain was completely degraded, and as the enzyme concentration increased, the Bβ-chain was gradually and completely degraded, while the γ-chain was the most difficult to hydrolyze and could not be completely degraded at the sample concentration of 50 mg/mL. As the reaction time increased (Figure 8B), the Aα-chain of fibrinogen was degraded first, followed by the Bβ-chain, which began to disappear, and after 24 h, the γ-chain was eventually hydrolyzed as well.

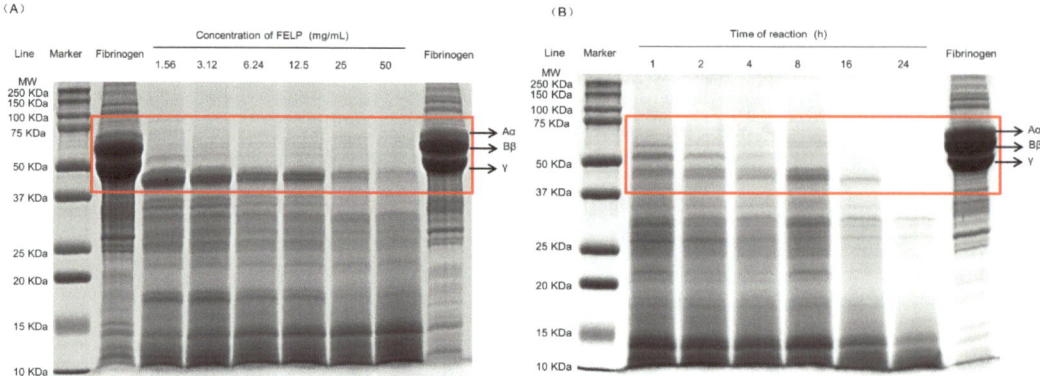

Figure 8. Fibrinogenolytic activity of FELP. (**A**) Degradation pattern of fibrinogen by FELP in a dose-dependent manner. Lanes: Fibrinogen on the left was unincubated. Fibrinogen on the right (10 mg/mL) incubated at 37 °C for 24 h. (**B**) Cleavage pattern of human fibrinogen by FELP (50 mg/mL) in a time-dependent manner. The Aα-, Bβ-, and γ- chains of fibrinogen were shown in the red rectangular frame.

3. Discussion

Streptokinase, urokinase, pro-urokinase, reteplase, and alteplase are examples of fibrinolytic enzymes and thrombolytic drugs currently used in clinical settings. These drugs have significant unintended physiological side effects, including excessive bleeding, a short plasma half-life, limited fibrin specificity, and high therapeutic doses. As a vicarious therapy, traditional medicinal animals, such as earthworms, snakes, and leeches, have attracted more attention in the past few decades [26]. A novel fibrinolytic protein DPf3, which was purified from *Pheretima vulgaris*, possesses the potential to be developed into a promising antithrombotic agent [27]. The antithrombotic protein named EPf3, purified from *Pheretima guillelmi*, was found to confer excellent anticoagulant and thrombolytic activity and could be developed into a promising antithrombotic agent [28]. An earthworm known in Chinese medicine as "Di Long" has long been used in the form of dried powder in the treatment of diseases, and a fibrinolytic enzyme called lumbrokinase has been purified from the earthworm [29].

In this study, a plasmin-like marine protease was isolated and purified from Annelida (phylum), *P. aibuhitensis*, named FELP. It was purified to homogeneity by using two column chromatography steps with a purification of 10.61-fold, which demonstrates that the protease is a microcomponent in *P. aibuhitensis*. Compared with the traditional purification of fibrinolytic enzymes [30,31], the target protease with fibrinolytic activity could be purified in only two steps, which greatly improved the purification efficiency and had a wide range of application prospects. Moreover, in the purification of FELP with activity monitoring, the fractions are collected from the first peak of G-50 to the base regression level, and only one tube has a protein band, indicating that fraction i is single. Our results show that the molecular mass of the purified enzyme is estimated to be 28.9 kDa with SDS-PAGE, which is within the molecular weight range of most fibrinolytic enzymes [25]. The MW of the purified enzyme is similar to the fibrinolytic protein from annelids, such as *Pheretima vulgaris* [27], and snake venom [32]. Few proteases with fibrinolytic activity have been isolated and purified from marine beach organisms, demonstrating that FELP is a novel fibrinolytic enzyme and can be a potential source for the development of therapeutic agents for the clinical treatment of thrombosis.

Based on the mechanism of action, fibrinolytic enzymes are classified as serine proteases, metalloproteinases, and serine metalloproteinases; the inhibitor of the enzyme is crucial for studying the types of enzymes. To further explore the physicochemical properties of FELP, corresponding inhibitors were used to examine their effect on FELP activity. As shown in Figure 3, the activity of FELP is correlated with SBTI and PMSF; however, the activity of FELP had not been affected by EACA and EDTA. PMSF, known as a serine protease inhibitor, can be used to identify fibrinolytic enzymes of the serine protease group [33] by sulphonate essential serine residues in the active site of the protease, resulting in a complete loss of enzyme activity [34]. As we all know, t-PA and uPA are the only serine proteases currently approved by the US Food and Drug Administration. Most of the fibrinolytic proteases from the sandworm are serine proteases [35–37], while SBTI is a specific inhibitor for trypsin. The above results clarify that FELP is a trypsin-like serine protease.

As shown in Figures 4 and 5, FELP is most active at pH 9.0 and can maintain good stability in an alkaline environment, suggesting that FELP may be an alkaline protease. Moreover, the optimum pH for FELP is higher than the protease from terrestrial organisms [27,38]. It was observed that FELP is stable at 30–60 °C and can still maintain more than 60% activity after incubation for 2 h, exhibiting excellent thermal stability. Its optimum temperature is 50 °C, which is higher than that of the NJP isolated from Neanthes japonica (Iznka) [35]. Furthermore, FELP has excellent fibrinolytic activity at 37 °C and neutral pH, which indicates that the enzyme can retain its fibrinolytic activity in the human body and has application prospects.

Due to the information provided by Uniprot, B8Y626 has serine-type endopeptidase activity. Also, all six peptide fragments have a protein group of one, indicating that these peptides are unique for this protein. The sequence homology results also show that the purified enzyme may belong to serine protease (Figure 6). The above studies have been cross-checked to indicate that FELP is a trypsin-like serine protease. The peptides obtained are as follows:

IVGGQESRPNEFPWQVSMQSSFGSHYCGAIIINRNWIMTAAHCTAGDSASDLYLMVGEHDR; TAVVSGWGTLRSGGPCCPQILQYVQVPVISNNECNTIDYPGDITDGMICAGNRLSTDACQGDSGGPLVVK; VSTYMNWIGL

The purified enzyme can be observed as a distinctly transparent circle on fibrin plates. As illustrated in Figure 7A, both FELP and UK exhibited strong fibrinolytic activity in plasminogen-rich plates; additionally, we used plasminogen-free plates. However, UK could not cleave plasminogen to formative plasmin to achieve fibrinolytic activity; as expected, it did not obtain a transparent circle in Figure 7B. Nevertheless, FELP also showed hydrolyzing activity in the plate without plasminogen. Therefore, we believe that FELP can not only directly hydrolyze fibrin but also convert plasminogen to plasmin; this suggests that FELP shows a bi-functional manner in hydrolyzing fibrin, as documented in the reports on a fibrinolytic protein from *Pheretima vulgaris* [27], a fibrinolytic enzyme from the marine-derived fungus *Aspergillus versicolor* ZLH-1 [17], and an antithrombotic protease from *Sipunculus nudus* [21]. The present study shows that FELP exhibits excellent fibrinolytic activity.

In addition, FELP can exert its fibrinolytic activity by degrading fibrinogen, and it shows a dose and time dependency. The fibrinogenolysis starts with the Aα-chain, followed by the Bβ-chain and the γ-chain. This pattern is similar to that observed with fibrinolytic enzymes from most annelids, such as hirudo [39] and *Pheretima vulgaris* [27]. The γ-chain is the most difficult to degrade and was not completely degraded after 5 h of incubation at the sample concentration of 50 mg/mL. The mixture of fibrinogen and FELP was incubated at 37 °C for 24 h, and the γ-chain was finally completely degraded. The fibrinogen without the addition of FELP did not show degradation with incubation at 37 °C for 24 h (Figure 8), suggesting that the degradation of the three chains of fibrinogen was entirely due to the addition of FELP. From the above discussion, it can be concluded that FELP may show strong fibrinolytic activity by degrading fibrinogen.

4. Materials and Methods

4.1. Chemicals and Reagents

Ammonium sulfate $(NH_4)_2SO_4$, Tris (hydroxymethyl) aminomethane, agarose, and ethylene diamine tetraacetic acid (EDTA) were purchased from Sinopharm Chemical

Reagent Co., Ltd. (Shanghai, China). Urokinase was purchased from Shanghai Macklin Biochemical Technology Co., Ltd. (Shanghai, China). Fibrinogen was purchased from Beijing Solarbio Science & Technology Co., Ltd. (Beijing, China). Thrombin was purchased from Abmole (Houston, TX, USA). An Omni-EasyTM One-step PAGE Gel Fast Preparation Kit (12.5%, Catalog No. PG213) was purchased from Shanghai Epizyme Biomedical Technology Co., Ltd. (Shanghai, China). A 10× Tris/Glycine/SDS Buffer (Catalog 1610732), 4× Laemmli Sample Buffer (Catalog No. 1610747) and Precision Plus Protein Dual Color Standards with MW of 10–250 kDa (Catalog 1610374) were purchased from Bio-Rad Laboratories Inc. (Hercules, CA, USA). The bicinchoninic acid (BCA) protein quantitation kit (Catalog PA115-01) was purchased from Tiangen Biotech (Beijing, China) Co., Ltd. (Beijing, China). DEAE-Sepharose FF, Sephadex G-50, soybean trypsin inhibitor (SBTI), and phenyl methane sulfonyl fluoride (PMSF) were purchased from Shanghai yuanye Bio-Technology Co., Ltd. (Shanghai, China). Epsilon amino caproic acid (EACA) was purchased from Shanghai Aladdin Biochemical Technology Co., Ltd. (Shanghai, China). All reagents used were of analytical grade unless otherwise stated.

4.2. Preparation of Crude Extracts of FELP from P. aibuhitensis

P. aibuhitensis was provided by Yancheng Fengyueyuan Fishing Bait Co., Ltd. (Huangshagang, China). The isolation of FELP from *P. aibuhitensis* was based on the method of Zhihui Deng et al. (2010) with modifications [35]. All operations were carried out at 4 °C. For specific operating procedures, refer to Ge et al. (2022) [40]. The 500 mg dried sample was immersed in 100 mL PBS for 3 h and centrifuged at 9900× g for 20 min at 4 °C using a Himac CR 21G high-speed floor centrifuge (Hitachi, Tokyo, Japan). Ammonium sulfate was stirred into the supernatant until dissolved, reaching 30 to 90% saturation, and then left for 2 h. The precipitates collected with centrifugation at 15,400× g for 30 min were resuspended in PBS (pH 7.4) and dialyzed using dialysis membranes (MWCO: 10 kDa) against 0.02 M Tris-HCl (pH 7.4) for 48 to 72 h. The dialyzed sample was pre-cooled at −80 °C for 4 h and lyophilized using a freeze-dryer (Labconco Freezone 2.5 L, Kansas City, MO, USA). The fibrinolytic activity and protein content of the samples taken at each ammonium sulphate saturation level were measured to calculate the specific activity.

4.3. The Fibrin-Plate Method

The fibrin-plate assay was used to study the fibrinolytic activity of FELP, according to Astrup and Müllertz [41] with slight modifications. Both fibrinogen-free and fibrinogen-rich plates were used. To prepare the plasminogen-rich fibrin plates, specifically speaking, 10 mL of a 0.2% (w/v) fibrinogen solution in saline (medicine) was mixed with 10 mL of a 1.5% (w/v) agarose solution and 1 mL of a thrombin solution (20 U/mL) in a Petri dish and then kept at ambient temperature for 1 h to form a fibrin clot layer. A total of 10 µL of sample solutions were carefully placed onto the pre-punched holes of the fibrin plate and incubated at 37 °C for 18 h. The fibrinogen-free fibrin plates were prepared by placing the fibrin plates at 80 °C for an additional 2 h to extinguish the fibrinogen. To determine fibrinolytic activity, FELP (50 mg/mL) was prepared; urokinase (1000 U) was used as a positive control, and saline (0.9% NaCl) was used as a negative control. The activity was quantified by measuring the area of fibrinolysis on the plate.

4.4. Protein Concentration

Protein concentration was measured with the BCA Protein Assay Kit. The principle is that the peptide bond structure in proteins can generate complexes with Cu^{2+} and reduce Cu^{2+} to Cu^+ under an alkaline environment, and the BCA reagent can specifically bind to Cu^+ to form a colored complex with maximum absorbance at 562 nm. The 96-well plate was spiked with 20 µL of sample; then, 200 µL of BCA working solution was added and incubated for 30 min at 37 °C. The absorbance at 562 nm was measured, wherein bovine serum albumin (BSA) was used as the standard.

4.5. Enzyme Purification

The crude enzyme (200 mg) was applied onto a DEAE Sepharose FF column (diameter: 2.6 cm, height: 20 cm) and equilibrated with 20 mM Tris-HCl buffer (pH 7.4). The bound proteins were eluted with 0.1 to 0.5 M NaCl in the 20 mM Tris-HCl buffer (pH 7.4) at a flow rate of 1 mL/min and were monitored with HD-3 (Shanghai Huxi Analysis Instrument Factory Co., Ltd., Shanghai, China) with an ultraviolet detector at 280 nm. The activity of the individual fractions was detected using the fibrin-plate assay. The active fractions (1 g) were pooled and further purified with Sephadex G-50 (diameter: 1.6 cm, height: 60 cm) and equilibrated with 20 mM Tris-HCl buffer (pH 7.4) at a flow rate of 0.8 mL/min with one tube collected every 3 min. The fraction with fibrinolytic activity was collected and lyophilized as the purified enzyme preparation.

4.6. SDS-PAGE

The molecular pattern of the FELP from *P. aibuhitensis* was determined by using SDS-PAGE (separating gel of 12.5% polyacrylamide with a stacking gel of 4.5% polyacrylamide) according to Laemmli's method [42]. The mixture of the sample (50 mg/mL) and the 4× Laemmli Sample Buffer was boiled for 5 min with a palm-sized drive lock incubator, standard type (Bio Medical Science Inc., Tokyo, Japan) and then briefly centrifuged at 1800× *g* using an S1010E mini-centrifuge (SCILOGEX, Rocky Hill, CT, USA). The samples were placed at room temperature, and the Precision Plus Protein Dual Color Standards were loaded onto the lanes of the gel and then electrophoresed at a constant voltage of 180 V with 1× Tris/Glycine/SDS Buffer for 45 min using a Mini-PROTEAN Tetra Cell (Bio-Rad Laboratories Inc., Richmond, CA, USA). After the gel was discolored in a solution prepared with 0.25% (*w*/*v*) Coomassie Brilliant Blue R250 for 20 min, it was transferred to the decolorizing fluid (Ethanol:Acetic acid:H_2O = 2:1:7) on a shaker with 80 rpm speed until clear protein bands were observed. Then, the gel was imaged with the GenoSens 2100 (T) Clinx Gel Documentation System (Clinx Science Instruments Co., Ltd., Shanghai, China).

4.7. Analysis of FELP from P. aibuhitensis

The sample was obtained from a clearly visible SDS-PAGE protein band and was analyzed with liquid chromatography–tandem mass spectrometry (LC–MS/MS). Specifically, the gel strip was cut after reduction and alkylation treatment and digested with trypsin at 37 °C for 20 h. The enzyme digestion products were desalted, lyophilized, and re-dissolved in 0.1% FA solution. The column was equilibrated with 95% liquid A (liquid A was an aqueous solution of 0.1% formic acid, and liquid B was an aqueous solution of 0.1% formic acid in acetonitrile (84%)). The mixture of peptides was loaded onto the trap column by the autosampler and separated with Easy-nLC 1000 (Thermo Fisher Scientific; Waltham, MA, USA). The peptides with high abundance were analyzed with a Q Exactive mass spectrometer (Thermo Fisher Scientific; Waltham, MA, USA); the primary mass resolution was 70,000 at 200 *m/z*, secondary mass spectral resolution was 17,500 at 200 *m/z*, normalized collision energy was 27 eV, and underfill was 0.1%. The data obtained from the secondary mass spectrometry were compared with the data retrieved from the corresponding database (Uniprotkb_Perinereis_245_2023_08_20) using the search engine Proteome Discoverer 2.5 to obtain the identified proteins. The three-dimensional structural homology modeling of FELP was projected with the SWISS-MODEL (https://swissmodel.expasy.org/, accessed on 22 January 2024) based on the amino acid sequence. The secondary structure of the peptides was predicted with the Protein Structure Prediction Server (PSIPRED) (http://bioinf.cs.ucl.ac.uk/psipred/, accessed on 22 January 2024).

4.8. Effect of Protease Inhibitors on Fibrinolytic Activity

FELP was incubated with PMSF (5 mM), EDTA (5 mM), SBTI (5 mM), and EACA (10 mM) at 37 °C for 2 h; a total of 10 μL of the mixture was removed to the already configured fibrin plate (the plate with a diameter of 4 cm) and incubated for 18 h to measure the two vertical diameters of the transparent circle to calculate the activities. The relative activity was calculated by dividing the enzyme activity under each condition by the enzyme activity under the condition without added inhibitors. The activity of FELP without inhibitors was considered to be 100%. Three parallel experiments were performed for each set of conditions.

4.9. Effect of Temperature on Fibrinolytic Activity and Thermal Stability

The influence of temperature on fibrinolytic activity was determined with the fibrin-plate assay. FELP was placed on the prepared fibrin plate, incubated at 30 to 65 °C for 18 h, and the vertical diameter of the transparent circle was measured to calculate the activities. The relative activity was calculated by dividing the activity for each condition by the maximum activity. FELP was incubated at temperatures of 30, 40, 50, 60, 70 and 80 °C; the 10 µL samples were collected at 0 min, 20 min, 40 min, 60 min, 80 min, 100 min, and 120 min to assess the thermal stability of the protease. The enzyme activity before holding was defined as 100%; the residual enzyme activity under the other conditions was calculated. Three parallel experiments were performed at each gradient.

4.10. Effect of pH on Fibrinolytic Activity and pH Stability of FELP

The effect of pH on fibrinolytic activity was recorded after incubation of FELP at a pH of 3, 4, 5, 6, 7, 8, 9, 10, and 11. The buffers were 0.1 M citric acid –sodium citrate buffer (pH 3–5), 0.1 M phosphate-buffered saline (pH 6–7), 0.1 M Tris-HCl (pH 8–9), and 0.1 M sodium carbonate–bicarbonate buffer (pH 10–11). FELP was redissolved in buffers of different pH; a total of 10 µL of each gradient was added to fibrin plates prepared with a different pH and incubated for 18 h at 37 °C. The relative activity was calculated by dividing the activity measured in each condition by the maximum activity. The pH stability of FELP was evaluated by incubating the enzyme in different buffers at intervals of 0 h, 2 h, 4 h, 6 h, 8 h, and 10 h. The enzyme activity before incubation was defined as 100%, and the residual enzyme activity under the other conditions was calculated. Three parallel experiments were performed at each gradient.

4.11. Degradation of Fibrinogen In Vitro

4.11.1. Dose-Effect Evaluation

Fibrinogen degradation with FELP in a dose-manner was analyzed with SDS-PAGE. Briefly, 1% fibrinogen was mixed with different sample concentrations (1.56 mg/mL, 3.12 mg/mL, 6.24 mg/mL, 12.5 mg/mL, 25 mg/mL, and 50 mg/mL) of fibrinolytic enzymes and incubated at 37 °C for 5 h. The concentration of proteins was determined with the BCA Protein kit. Equal amounts of total proteins were resuspended in loading buffer and separated with 12.5% SDS-PAGE. Each gradient was repeated three times in independent experiments.

4.11.2. Time-Effect Evaluation

The degradation pattern of fibrinogen by FELP was also analyzed with SDS-PAGE. Briefly, 100 µL of 1% fibrinogen was incubated with 100 µL (50 mg/mL) of FELP for 1 h, 2 h, 4 h, 8 h, 16 h, and 24 h, respectively. Each dosage was repeated in triplicate, and independent experiments were performed. After treatment, 30 µL of the samples was quantified with a BCA assay kit. Equivalent amounts of proteins were removed and mixed with 4× Laemmli sample buffer to stop the reactions. The samples with the buffer were boiled at 100 °C for 5 min, brought to room temperature, and stored at 4 °C to standby. The products were separated with 12.5% SDS-PAGE.

4.12. Statistic Analysis

Statistical analysis was performed using GraphPad Prism 9 software (GraphPad Inc, San Diego, CA, USA) using two-way ANOVA with Fisher's LSD test multiple comparison analysis. Data were presented as means ± SD. The values identified as outliers were excluded from the statistical analysis. The results were considered statistically significant if the p-value < 0.05.

5. Conclusions

In this study, FELP from *P. aibuhitensis* was purified, and its physicochemical properties and activity in vitro were studied. The molecular weight of FELP was found to be 28.9 kDa. Fibrin-plate assays showed the enzyme was a fibrinolytic protease, which can exert fibrinolytic activity by directly acting on fibrin or through activation of fibrinogen. Inhibition of fibrinolytic activity by the standard serine protease inhibitors PMSF and SBTI confirmed it to be a trypsin-like serine protease. The peptide fragments were characterized with LC–MS/MS. The enzyme showed maximum fibrinolytic activity at pH 9 and temperature 50 °C and has excellent stability at pH 7–11 or 30–60 °C. FELP exhibited higher fibrinolytic activity than urokinase (1000 U) in fibrin plates and not only directly dissolved fibrin but also indirectly exerted fibrinolytic activity through the activation of fibrinogen. The gel electrophoresis analysis results of the fibrinogenolytic mechanism showed that the degradation of the subunit in fibrinogen demonstrated dose and time dependency, which was in the order chain A-α, chain B-β, and chain γ, and three chains were nearly thoroughly degraded after 24 h. Collectively, our results identified a marine-derived enzyme. We were surprised to find that it has shown stable fibrinolytic activity, but its thrombolytic mechanism needs to be further studied and verified.

Author Contributions: Conceptualization, T.J. and W.W.; Methodology, W.W.; Software, T.J., H.Z., M.W. and Y.S.; Validation, T.J. and B.Z.; Formal Analysis, T.J.; Investigation, T.J. and S.Y.; Resources, T.J.; Data Curation, T.J. and M.W.; Writing—Original Draft Preparation, T.J.; Writing—Review and Editing, B.Z. and T.S.; Visualization, T.J.; Supervision, W.W. and Y.Z.; Project Administration, W.W.; Funding Acquisition, W.W. All authors have read and agreed to the published version of the manuscript.

Funding: This research work was financially supported by the National Natural Science Foundation of China (No. 82173731), the Natural Science Foundation of Shanghai (No. 21ZR1427300), and the Shanghai Innovation Action Plan (No. 19440741200).

Institutional Review Board Statement: Not applicable.

Data Availability Statement: The original data presented in the study are included in the article; further inquiries can be directed to the corresponding author.

Acknowledgments: We are thankful and acknowledge the College of Food Science and Technology, Shanghai Ocean University, China for providing the proper facilities to carry out this work.

Conflicts of Interest: The authors declare no conflicts of interest.

References

1. Figueiredo Sena Macedo, M.W.; da Cunha, N.B.; Carneiro, J.A.; da Costa, R.A.; de Alencar, S.A.; Cardoso, M.H.; Franco, O.L.; Dias, S.C. Marine Organisms as a Rich Source of Biologically Active Peptides. *Front. Mar. Sci.* **2021**, *8*, 667764. [CrossRef]
2. Karthikeyan, A.; Joseph, A.; Nair, B.G. Promising bioactive compounds from the marine environment and their potential effects on various diseases. *J. Genet. Eng. Biotechnol.* **2022**, *20*, 14. [CrossRef]
3. Peters, M.K.; Astafyeva, Y.; Han, Y.; Macdonald, J.F.H.; Indenbirken, D.; Nakel, J.; Virdi, S.; Westhoff, G.; Streit, W.R.; Krohn, I. Novel marine metalloprotease-new approaches for inhibition of biofilm formation of *Stenotrophomonas maltophilia*. *Appl. Microbiol. Biotechnol.* **2023**, *107*, 7119–7134. [CrossRef]
4. Sharma, C.; Osmolovskiy, A.; Singh, R. Microbial Fibrinolytic Enzymes as Anti-Thrombotics: Production, Characterisation and Prodigious Biopharmaceutical Applications. *Pharmaceutics* **2021**, *13*, 1880. [CrossRef] [PubMed]
5. Daniotti, S.; Re, I. Marine Biotechnology: Challenges and Development Market Trends for the Enhancement of Biotic Resources in Industrial Pharmaceutical and Food Applications. A Statistical Analysis of Scientific Literature and Business Models. *Mar. Drugs* **2021**, *19*, 61. [CrossRef] [PubMed]
6. Guo, S.; Zhang, Z.; Xu, X.; Cai, J.; Wang, W.; Guo, L. Antagonistic activity and mode of action of trypacidin from marine-derived *Aspergillus fumigatus* against *Vibrio parahaemolyticus*. *3 Biotech* **2022**, *12*, 131. [CrossRef] [PubMed]
7. Syhapanha, K.S.; Russo, D.A.; Deng, Y.; Meyer, N.; Poulin, R.X.; Pohnert, G. Transcriptomics-guided identification of an algicidal protease of the marine bacterium Kordia algicida OT-1. *MicrobiologyOpen* **2023**, *12*, e1387. [CrossRef] [PubMed]

8. Barzkar, N. Marine microbial alkaline protease: An efficient and essential tool for various industrial applications. *Int. J. Biol. Macromol.* **2020**, *161*, 1216–1229. [CrossRef] [PubMed]
9. Zhang, H.; Li, H.; Liu, H.; Lang, D.A.; Xu, H.; Zhu, H. The application of a halotolerant metalloprotease from marine bacterium *Vibrio* sp. LA-05 in liquid detergent formulations. *Int. Biodeterior. Biodegrad.* **2019**, *142*, 18–25. [CrossRef]
10. Wang, Y.; Liu, B.-X.; Cheng, J.-H.; Su, H.-N.; Sun, H.-M.; Li, C.-Y.; Yang, L.; Shen, Q.-T.; Zhang, Y.-Z.; Zhang, X.; et al. Characterization of a New M4 Metalloprotease with Collagen-Swelling Ability from Marine *Vibrio pomeroyi* Strain 12613. *Front. Microbiol.* **2020**, *11*, 1868. [CrossRef]
11. Nguyen, T.N.T.; Chataway, T.; Araujo, R.; Puri, M.; Franco, C.M.M. Purification and Characterization of a Novel Alginate Lyase from a Marine *Streptomyces* Species Isolated from Seaweed. *Mar. Drugs* **2021**, *19*, 590. [CrossRef] [PubMed]
12. Barzkar, N.; Sohail, M. An overview on marine cellulolytic enzymes and their potential applications. *Appl. Microbiol. Biotechnol.* **2020**, *104*, 6873–6892. [CrossRef] [PubMed]
13. Perera, E.; Rodriguez-Viera, L.; Montero-Alejo, V.; Perdomo-Morales, R. Crustacean Proteases and Their Application in Debridement. *Trop. Life Sci. Res.* **2020**, *31*, 187–209. [CrossRef]
14. Leite, A.H.P.; da Silva, I.H.A.; Pastrana, L.; Nascimento, T.P.; da Silva Telles, A.M.; Porto, A.L.F. Purification, biochemical characterization and fibrinolytic potential of proteases produced by bacteria of the genus *Bacillus*: A systematic literature review. *Arch. Microbiol.* **2022**, *204*, 503. [CrossRef] [PubMed]
15. Syahbanu, F.; Giriwono, P.E.; Tjandrawinata, R.R.; Suhartono, M.T. Molecular analysis of a fibrin-degrading enzyme from *Bacillus subtilis* K2 isolated from the Indonesian soybean-based fermented food moromi. *Mol. Biol. Rep.* **2020**, *47*, 8553–8563. [CrossRef] [PubMed]
16. Popova, E.A.; Kreyer, V.G.; Komarevtsev, S.K.; Shabunin, S.V.; Osmolovskiy, A.A. Properties of Extracellular Proteinase of the Micromycete *Aspergillus ustus* 1 and Its High Activity during Fibrillary-Proteins Hydrolysis. *Appl. Biochem. Microbiol.* **2021**, *57*, 200–205. [CrossRef]
17. Zhao, L.; Lin, X.; Fu, J.; Zhang, J.; Tang, W.; He, Z. A Novel Bi-Functional Fibrinolytic Enzyme with Anticoagulant and Thrombolytic Activities from a Marine-Derived Fungus *Aspergillus versicolor* ZLH-1. *Mar. Drugs* **2022**, *20*, 356. [CrossRef]
18. Chimbekujwo, K.I.; Ja'afaru, M.I.; Adeyemo, O.M. Purification, characterization and optimization conditions of protease produced by Aspergillus brasiliensis strain BCW2. *Sci. Afr.* **2020**, *8*, e00398. [CrossRef]
19. Che, Z.; Cao, X.; Chen, G.; Liang, Z. An effective combination of codon optimization, gene dosage, and process optimization for high-level production of fibrinolytic enzyme in *Komagataella phaffii* (*Pichia pastoris*). *BMC Biotechnol.* **2020**, *20*, 63. [CrossRef]
20. Bi, Q.; Chu, J.; Feng, Y.; Jiang, Z.; Han, B.; Liu, W. Purification and Characterization of a New Serine Protease with Fibrinolytic Activity from the Marine Invertebrate, *Urechis unicinctus*. *Appl. Biochem. Biotechnol.* **2013**, *170*, 525–540. [CrossRef]
21. Ge, Y.-H.; Chen, Y.-Y.; Zhou, G.-S.; Liu, X.; Tang, Y.-P.; Liu, R.; Liu, P.; Li, N.; Yang, J.; Wang, J.; et al. A Novel Antithrombotic Protease from Marine Worm *Sipunculus Nudus*. *Int. J. Mol. Sci.* **2018**, *19*, 3023. [CrossRef]
22. Yang, M.; Zeng, C.; Xia, J.; Liu, Q.; Fang, J.; Zhang, Q. Disinfection of *Perinereis aibuhitensis* eggs with peroxymonosulfate to eliminate covert mortality nodavirus (CMNV). *Aquaculture* **2023**, *572*, 739539. [CrossRef]
23. Cong, Y.; Lou, Y.; Zhao, H.; Li, Z.; Zhang, M.; Jin, F.; Wang, Y.; Wang, J. Polystyrene microplastics alter bioaccumulation, and physiological and histopathological toxicities of cadmium in the polychaete *Perinereis aibuhitensis*. *Front. Mar. Sci.* **2022**, *9*, 939530. [CrossRef]
24. Yang, L.; Jing, L.; Tianhong, L.; Ying, W.; Zhongzheng, Z.; Feng, C.; Chao, F.; Xiaojie, C.; Hongjun, L.; Xiguang, C. Preparation and antithrombotic activity identification of Perinereis aibuhitensis extract: A high temperature and wide pH range stable biological agent. *Food Funct.* **2017**, *8*, 3533–3541. [CrossRef]
25. Moula Ali, M.; Bindu Bavisetty, S.C. Purification, physicochemical properties, and statistical optimization of fibrinolytic enzymes especially from fermented foods: A comprehensive review. *Int. J. Biol. Macromol.* **2020**, *163*, 1498–1517. [CrossRef]
26. Yang, H.R.; Hwang, D.H.; Prakash, R.L.M.; Kim, J.-H.; Hong, I.-H.; Kim, S.; Kim, E.; Kang, C. Exploring the Fibrin(ogen)olytic, Anticoagulant, and Antithrombotic Activities of Natural Cysteine Protease (Ficin) with the κ-Carrageenan-Induced Rat Tail Thrombosis Model. *Nutrients* **2022**, *14*, 3552. [CrossRef] [PubMed]
27. Liu, H.; Yang, J.; Li, Y.; Ma, Y.; Wang, W.; Zhong, W.; Li, P.; Du, S. A Novel Fibrinolytic Protein from *Pheretima vulgaris*: Purification, Identification, Antithrombotic Evaluation, and Mechanisms Investigation. *Front. Mol. Biosci.* **2022**, *8*, 772419. [CrossRef] [PubMed]
28. Wu, Y.; Hu, S.; Ma, Y.; Zhao, B.; Yang, W.; Lu, Y.; Li, P.; Du, S. Novel *Pheretima guillelmi*-derived antithrombotic protein DPf3: Identification, characterization, in vitro evaluation and antithrombotic mechanisms investigation. *Int. J. Biol. Macromol.* **2020**, *154*, 545–556. [CrossRef] [PubMed]
29. Zhao, J.; Li, L.; Wu, C.; He, R.Q. Hydrolysis of fibrinogen and plasminogen by immobilized earthworm fibrinolytic enzyme II from *Eisenia fetida*. *Int. J. Biol. Macromol.* **2003**, *32*, 165–171. [CrossRef] [PubMed]
30. Deng, Y.; Liu, X.; Katrolia, P.; Kopparapu, N.K.; Zheng, X. A dual-function chymotrypsin-like serine protease with plasminogen activation and fibrinolytic activities from the GRAS fungus, *Neurospora sitophila*. *Int. J. Biol. Macromol.* **2018**, *109*, 1338–1343. [CrossRef] [PubMed]
31. Zhang, Y.; Yang, R.; Wang, L.; Li, Y.; Han, J.; Yang, Y.; Zheng, H.; Lu, M.; Shen, Y.; Yang, H. Purification and characterization of a novel thermostable anticoagulant protein from medicinal leech *Whitmania pigra* Whitman. *J. Ethnopharmacol.* **2022**, *288*, 114990. [CrossRef] [PubMed]

32. Sanchez, E.F.; Richardson, M.; Gremski, L.H.; Veiga, S.S.; Yarleque, A.; Niland, S.; Lima, A.M.; Estevao-Costa, M.I.; Eble, J.A. A novel fibrinolytic metalloproteinase, barnettlysin-I from *Bothrops barnetti* (Barnett's pitviper) snake venom with anti-platelet properties. *Biochim. Biophys. Acta Gen. Subj.* **2016**, *1860*, 542–556. [CrossRef]
33. Sekar, V.; Hageman, J.H. Specificity of the serine protease inhibitor, phenylmethylsulfonyl fluoride. *Biochem. Biophys. Res. Commun.* **1979**, *89*, 474–478. [CrossRef] [PubMed]
34. Gold, A.M.; Fahrney, D. Sulfonyl Fluorides as Inhibitors of Esterases. II. Formation and Reactions of Phenylmethanesulfonyl alpha-chymotrypsin. *Biochemistry* **1964**, *3*, 783–791. [CrossRef]
35. Deng, Z.; Wang, S.; Li, Q.; Ji, X.; Zhang, L.; Hong, M. Purification and characterization of a novel fibrinolytic enzyme from the polychaete, *Neanthes japonica* (Iznka). *Bioresour. Technol.* **2010**, *101*, 1954–1960. [CrossRef] [PubMed]
36. Wang, S.; Deng, Z.; Li, Q.; Ge, X.; Bo, Q.; Liu, J.; Cui, J.; Jiang, X.; Liu, J.; Zhang, L.; et al. A novel alkaline serine protease with fibrinolytic activity from the polychaete, *Neanthes japonica*. *Comp. Biochem. Physiol. B Biochem. Mol. Biol.* **2011**, *159*, 18–25. [CrossRef]
37. Kim, H.J.; Shim, K.H.; Yeon, S.J.; Shin, H.S. A Novel Thrombolytic and Anticoagulant Serine Protease from Polychaeta, *Diopatra sugokai*. *J. Microbiol. Biotechnol.* **2018**, *28*, 275–283. [CrossRef]
38. Wu, J.; Lan, G.; He, N.; He, L.; Li, C.; Wang, X.; Zeng, X. Purification of fibrinolytic enzyme from *Bacillus amyloliquefaciens* GUTU06 and properties of the enzyme. *Food Chem. X* **2023**, *20*, 100896. [CrossRef]
39. Chu, F.; Wang, X.; Sun, Q.; Liang, H.; Wang, S.; An, D.; Cui, C.; Chai, Y.; Li, S.; Song, S.; et al. Purification and characterization of a novel fibrinolytic enzyme from *Whitmania pigra* Whitman. *Clin. Exp. Hypertens.* **2016**, *38*, 594–601. [CrossRef]
40. Ge, B.; Hou, C.; Bao, B.; Pan, Z.; Mate Sanchez de Val, J.E.; Elango, J.; Wu, W. Comparison of Physicochemical and Structural Properties of Acid-Soluble and Pepsin-Soluble Collagens from Blacktip Reef Shark Skin. *Mar. Drugs* **2022**, *20*, 376. [CrossRef]
41. Astrup, T.; Mullertz, S. The fibrin plate method for estimating fibrinolytic activity. *Arch. Biochem. Biophys.* **1952**, *40*, 346–351. [CrossRef] [PubMed]
42. Laemmli, U.K. Cleavage of structural proteins during the assembly of the head of bacteriophage T4. *Nature* **1970**, *227*, 680–685. [CrossRef] [PubMed]

Disclaimer/Publisher's Note: The statements, opinions and data contained in all publications are solely those of the individual author(s) and contributor(s) and not of MDPI and/or the editor(s). MDPI and/or the editor(s) disclaim responsibility for any injury to people or property resulting from any ideas, methods, instructions or products referred to in the content.

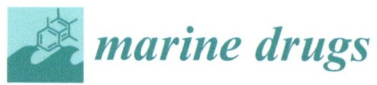

Article

Carneusones A-F, Benzophenone Derivatives from Sponge-Derived Fungus *Aspergillus carneus* GXIMD00543

Chun-Ju Lu [†], Li-Fen Liang [†], Geng-Si Zhang, Hai-Yan Li, Chun-Qing Fu, Qin Yu, Dong-Mei Zhou, Zhi-Wei Su, Kai Liu, Cheng-Hai Gao, Xin-Ya Xu *, and Yong-Hong Liu *

Guangxi Key Laboratory of Marine Drugs, Institute of Marine Drugs, Guangxi University of Chinese Medicine, Nanning 530200, China; luchunjv@163.com (C.-J.L.); 15277833592@163.com (L.-F.L.); 15534445495@163.com (G.-S.Z.); lihaiyan12368@163.com (H.-Y.L.); 18378464907@163.com (C.-Q.F.); 19862354152@163.com (Q.Y.); zhoudm@gxtcmu.edu.cn (D.-M.Z.); suzw1454@126.com (Z.-W.S.); liuk@gxtcmu.edu.cn (K.L.); gaoch@gxtcmu.edu.cn (C.-H.G.)

* Correspondence: xyxu@gxtcmu.edu.cn (X.-Y.X.); yonghongliu@scsio.ac.cn (Y.-H.L.)
† These authors contributed equally to this work.

Abstract: Six benzophenone derivatives, carneusones A–F (**1–6**), along with seven known compounds (**7–13**) were isolated from a strain of sponge-derived marine fungus *Aspergillus carneus* GXIMD00543. Their chemical structures were elucidated by detailed spectroscopic data and quantum chemical calculations. Compounds **5**, **6**, and **8** exhibited moderate anti-inflammatory activity on NO secretion using lipopolysaccharide (LPS)-induced RAW 264.7 cells with EC_{50} values of 34.6 ± 0.9, 20.2 ± 1.8, and 26.8 ± 1.7 μM, while **11** showed potent effect with an EC_{50} value of 2.9 ± 0.1 μM.

Keywords: marine fungus; anti-inflammatory activity; *Aspergillus carneus*; benzophenone; Beibu gulf

1. Introduction

Marine microorganisms, including fungi, are widely distributed in various marine environments, such as the deep sea, polar regions, even in the body of the host organisms including marine animals and plants [1]. As a result of their long-term existence in extreme survival environments, marine fungi have evolved unique metabolic methods and could produce abundant structurally diverse secondary metabolites [2,3]. Compounds isolated from marine fungi have also attracted considerable attention for their broad range of biological activities and have become important sources of novel drugs [4]. In the last five years, over one third of bioactive natural marine products were obtained from marine fungi and mangrove fungi [5].

Natural benzophenone derivatives, or dipenyl ketone analogues, are a class of compounds widely distributed in nature with a phenol–carbonyl–phenol skeleton. More than 300 benzophenone derivatives have been isolated from plants and fungi. They exhibit great structural diversity, which is attributed to protons replaced by hydroxyl, alkyl, alkyloxy groups, or halogen atoms [6,7]. Owing to their variable substituents, many benzophenone derivatives show a range of biological activities including anticancer, anti-inflammatory, antimicrobial, and antiviral effects [8].

Aspergillus is an important fungal genera producing benzophenones derivatives. Four xanthones oxisterigmatocystins A–C, and 5-methoxysterigmatocystin were isolated from one strain of deep-sea-derived fungus *Aspergillus versicolor*. 5-Methoxysterigmatocystin exhibited moderate cytotoxicities against the A-549 and HL-60 cell lines with IC_{50} values of 3.86 and 5.32 μM [9]. New benzophenone derivatives versixanthones A–F were retrieved from a mangrove endophyte *Aspergillus versicolor* HDN1009. They exhibited cytotoxicities against seven cancer cell lines (HL-60, K562, A549, H1945, 803, HO-8910, and HCT-116) with IC_{50} values ranging from 0.7 to 20.8 μM. Compound versixanthone F showed potent cytotoxicity against HCT-116 cells with an IC_{50} value of 0.7 μM [10]. Compounds monochlorsulochrin, dihydrogeodin, methyl-(2-chloro-1,6-dihydroxy-3-methylxanthone)-8-carboxylate, and methyl-(4- chloro-1,6-dihydroxy-3-methylxanthone)-8-carboxylate) were isolated from the extract of a strain of *Aspergillus flavipes* DL-11. They exhibited antibacterial activities against six pathogenic Gram-positive bacteria *Staphylococcus aureus* (ATCC43300), *Staphylococcus aureus* (ATCC29213), *Staphylococcus aureus* (ATCC33591), *Staphylococcus aureus* (ATCC25923), *Enterococcus faecalis* (ATCC51299), and *Enterococcus faecium* (ATCC35667) with MIC values ranging from 1.56 to 50 μg/mL [11].

As part of our ongoing search for bioactive compounds from marine fungi, *Aspergillus carneus* GXIMD00543, which is associated with sponge sample obtained from Weizhou Island, Beibu Gulf, was selected for further studies. Chemical investigation of the fungal extract led to the isolation of six benzophenone derivatives (**1–6**), along with seven known compounds (**7–13**) (Figure 1). The anti-inflammatory potential of the compounds was assayed. Herein, we reported the details of the isolation, structural elucidation, and determination of the anti-inflammatory effect of those compounds.

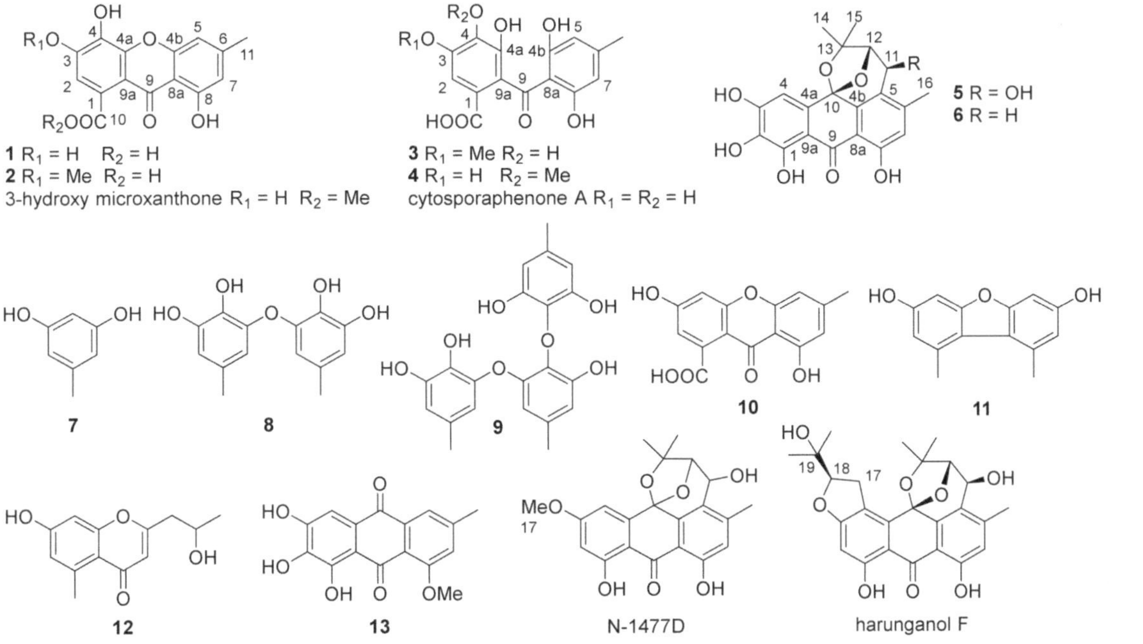

Figure 1. The chemical structures of compounds **1–13**, 3-hydroxy microxanthone [9], cytosporaphenone A [10], N-1477D [11], and harunganol F [12].

2. Results and Discussion

2.1. Strain Isolation and Species Identification

The fungus was identified as *Aspergillus carneus* based on its morphological features and the sequence analysis of the ITS region of the rRNA gene (Figure S1), which exhibited 99.81% similarity with fungal strain *A. carneus*, with GenBank accession number MH777426.1.

2.2. Elucidation of Chemical Structures

Compound **1** was obtained as yellowish powder. The molecular formula was determined to be $C_{15}H_{10}O_7$ according to the HRESIMS peaks at m/z 303.0510 ([M + H]$^+$, calcd. 303.0499) and 325.0330 ([M + Na]$^+$, calcd. 325.0319). The ^{1}H NMR spectrum of **1** exhibited signals of three aromatic protons at δ_H 6.81 (1H, s, H-2), 6.87 (1H, s, H-5), and 6.61 (1H, s, H-7), one methyl proton at δ_H 2.39 (3H, s, H-11), and one hydroxyl group signal at the low field region δ_H 12.57 (1H, br s, OH-8), which formed an intramolecular hydrogen bond with the carbonyl group at C-9 (Table 1). The ^{13}C NMR and HSQC spectra of **1** exposed the presence of one methyl group at δ_C 22.0 (C-11), three aromatic methines at δ_C 107.3 (C-5), 110.9 (C-7), and 111.9 (C-2), eleven quaternary carbons, including nine aromatic carbons, at δ_C 105.6 (C-8a), 109.1 (C-9a), 126.6 (C-1), 133.3 (C-4), 145.9 (C-3), 148.4 (C-6), 152.3 (C-4a), 155.3 (C-4b), and 160.7 (C-8), and two carbonyl carbons at δ_C 170.1 (C-10) and 179.8 (C-9) (Table 2). The HMBC spectrum showed correlations from H-2 to C-1, C-3, C-4, C-9a, and C-10, from H-5 to C-4b, C-7, C-8a, C-9, and C-11, from H-7 to C-5, C-8, C-9, and C-11, and from CH$_3$-11 to C-5, C-6, and C-7 (Figure 2). All these data exhibited close similarity with compound 3-hydroxy microxanthone [12] except for the absence of the methoxy group at C-10. Thus **1** was determined to be 3,4,8-trihydroxy-6-methyl-9-oxo-9*H*-xanthene-1-carboxylic acid and trivially named carneusone A.

Table 1. ^{1}H NMR data for compounds **1–4**, 3-hydroxy microxanthone and cytosporaphenone A (*J* in Hz, δ in ppm).

No.	**1** [a]	**2** [a]	**3** [a]	**4** [a]	3-Hydroxy Microxanthone [b]	Cytosporaphenone A [c]
2	6.81, s	6.87, s	7.00, s	6.93, s	6.90, s	7.18, s
5	6.87, s	6.95, s	6.07, s	6.07, s	6.90, s	6.18, s
7	6.61, s	6.65, s	6.07, s	6.07, s	6.64, s	6.18, s
11	2.39, s	2.39, s	2.15, s	2.14, s	2.40, s	2.19, s
12		3.91, s	3.83, s	3.74, s	3.82, s	
OH-8	12.57, br s	12.43, br s				

[a] Measured at 500 MHz in DMSO-d_6; [b] measured in DMSO-d_6 [12]; [c] measured in CD$_3$OD [13].

Table 2. ^{13}C NMR data for compounds **1–4**, 3-hydroxy microxanthone and cytosporaphenone A (*J* in Hz, δ in ppm).

	1 [a]	**2** [a]	**3** [a]	**4** [a]	3-Hydroxy Microxanthone [b]	Cytosporaphenone A [c]
No.	δ_C, Type	δ_C, Type	δ_C, Type	δ_C, Type	δ_C, Type	δ_C, Type
1	126.6, C	131.4, C	128.1, C	126.0, C	123.8, C	127.1, C
2	111.9, CH	112.5, CH	104.1, CH	108.6, CH	112.1, CH	109.8, CH
3	145.9, C	156.9, C	146.0, C	149.5, C	146.0, C	144.2, C
4	133.3, C	134.7, C	137.7, C	138.6, C	133.8, C	137.3, C
4a	152.3, C	150.6, C	141.9, C	146.6, C	151.3, C	142.1, C
4b	155.3, C	155.1, C	161.6, C	161.7, C	155.3, C	162.1, C
5	107.3, CH	107.5, CH	107.5, CH	107.5, CH	107.5, CH	107.9, CH
6	148.4, C	148.6, C	146.7, C	146.8, C	148.7, C	147.1, C
7	110.9, CH	111.2, CH	107.5, CH	107.5, CH	110.0, CH	107.9, CH
8	160.7, C	160.6, C	161.6, C	161.7, C	160.5, C	162.1, C
8a	105.6, C	105.6, C	109.8, C	109.6, C	105.6, C	109.1, C
9	179.8, C	179.4, C	200.6, C	200.2, C	179.7, C	200.0, C
9a	109.1, C	109.2, C	119.4, C	123.7, C	110.0, C	118.4, C
10	170.1, C	169.5, C	167.6, C	167.1, C	168.8, C	166.5, C
11	22.0, CH$_3$	21.9, CH$_3$	21.6, CH$_3$	21.6, CH$_3$	22.0, CH$_3$	21.0, CH$_3$
12		60.8, CH$_3$	55.9, CH$_3$	60.0, CH$_3$	52.5, CH$_3$	

[a] Measured at 125 MHz in DMSO-d_6; [b] measured in DMSO-d_6 [12]; [c] measured in CD$_3$OD [13].

Compound **2** was a yellowish powder with a molecular formula C$_{16}$H$_{12}$O$_7$ based on the HRESIMS peaks at *m*/*z* 317.0661 ([M + H]$^+$, calcd. 317.0656) and 339.0481 ([M + Na]$^+$, calcd. 339.0475). The NMR data of **2** showed great similarity with **1** except for the presence of an extra methoxy group signal at δ_H 3.91 (3H, H-12) and δ_C 60.8 (C-12), respectively (Tables 1 and 2). One hydroxyl group at δ_H 12.43 (1H, br s, OH-8) indicated the formation of an intramolecular hydrogen bond with the carbonyl group. The HMBC correlations from H-2 to C-3, C-4, C-9a, C-10, and from OCH$_3$-12 to C-4 suggested the methoxy group was attached at C-4 of compound **2** (Figure 2). All the data confirmed

2 as 3,8-dihydroxy-4-methoxy-6-methyl-9-oxo-9H-xanthene-1-carboxylic acid and it was trivially named carneusone B.

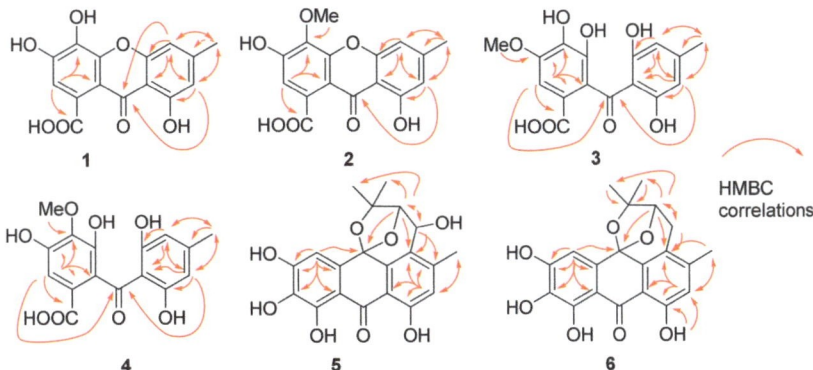

Figure 2. The key HMBC correlations of **1–6**.

Compound **3** was isolated as a yellowish powder, and its molecular formula was determined to be $C_{16}H_{14}O_8$ from the HRESIMS peak at m/z 357.0588 ([M + Na]$^+$, calcd. 357.0581). The ^{1}H NMR spectrum of **3** displayed the signals of three aromatic protons at δ_H 6.07 (2H, s, H-5 and H-7), 7.00 (1H, s, H-2), one methoxy group proton at δ_H 3.83 (3H, H-12), and one methyl proton at δ_H 2.15 (3H, s, H-11) (Table 1). The ^{13}C NMR and HSQC spectra of **3** indicated the presence of one methyl group at δ_C 21.6 (C-11), three aromatic methines at δ_C 107.5 (C-5 and C-7), 104.1 (C-2), eleven quaternary carbons including nine aromatic carbons at δ_C 109.8 (C-8a), 119.4 (C-9a), 128.1 (C-1), 137.7 (C-4), 141.9 (C-4a), 146.7 (C-6), 146.8 (C-3), and 161.6 (C-4b and C-8), and two carbonyl carbons at δ_C 167.6 (C-11), 200.6 (C-9) (Table 2). The HMBC spectrum showed correlations from H-2 to C-1, C-3, C-4, C-9, and C-9a, from H-5/H-7 to C-4b, C-6, C-8, C-9, and C-11, from CH$_3$-11 to C-5, C-6, and C-7, and from OCH$_3$-12 to C-4 (Figure 2). The data were similar to benzophenone-derivative cytosporaphenone A [13], except for extra methoxy group signals at δ_H 3.83 (3H, H-12) and δ_C 55.9 (C-12). The HMBC correlations from OCH$_3$-12 to C-3 indicated the methoxy group was attached at the C-3 of compound **3** (Figure 2). Thus, **3** was elucidated as 2-(2,6-dihydroxy-4-methylbenzoyl)-3,4-dihydroxy-5-methoxybenzoic acid and trivially named carneusone C.

Compound **4** had the same molecular formula, $C_{16}H_{14}O_8$, as **3** based on the HRESIMS peaks at m/z 335.0767 ([M + H]$^+$, calcd. 335.0761), and 357.0593 ([M + Na]$^+$, calcd. 357.0581). The NMR data of **4** also exhibited great similarity with **3** except the HMBC correlations were from OCH$_3$-12 to C-4 instead of from OCH$_3$-12 to C-3 as in **3** (Tables 1 and 2). Thus, **4** was determined as 2-(2,6-dihydroxy-4-methylbenzoyl)-3,5-dihydroxy-4-methoxybenzoic acid and trivially named carneusone D.

Compound **5** yielded as a brown amorphous powder. The molecular formula was determined to be $C_{20}H_{18}O_8$ by the HRESIMS peak at m/z 387.1085 ([M + H]$^+$, calcd. 387.1074). The ^{1}H NMR spectrum of **5** displayed two aromatic protons at δ_H 6.83 (1H, H-7), 6.91 (1H, H-4), and two oxy-methine protons at δ_H 4.52 (1H, H-11) and 4.57 (1H, H-12), and three methyl protons at δ_H 1.06 (3H, H-15), 1.38 (3H, H-14), and 2.41 (3H, H-16) (Table 3). One hydroxyl group signal was observed at δ_H 11.96 (1H, br s, OH-8). The ^{13}C NMR and HSQC spectra signals of **5** implied the presence of three methyl groups at δ_C 18.5 (C-16), 23.1 (C-15), and 29.9 (C-14), two oxy-methines at δ_C 61.7 (C-11) and 87.1 (C-12), two aromatic methines at δ_C 107.4 (C-4) and 118.6 (C-7), and thirteen quaternary carbons at δ_C 78.4 (C-13), 97.2 (C-10), 107.4 (C-4), 107.8 (C-9a), 108.9 (C-8a), 123.5 (C-5), 130.2 (C-4a), 133.5 (C-2), 139.2 (C-4b), 149.0 (C-6), 151.5 (C-1), 153.7 (C-3), 160.4 (C-8), and 189.7 (C-9). The HMBC spectrum exposed correlations from H-4 to C-2, C-3, C-4a, C-9a, and C-10, from H-7 to C-5, C-6, C-8, C-8a, and C-16, from H-11 to C-4b, C-5, C-6, and

C-12, from H-12 to C-5, C-10, C-11, C-13, and C-14, and from CH$_3$-14/CH$_3$-15 to C-12, C-13. All these data showed great similarity with compound N-1447D [14] except for the absence of methoxy group at C-3 and an extra hydroxyl group at C-2 (Table 3). The relative configurations of H-11 and H-12 were proposed as α-orientations on the basis of NOESY correlations CH$_3$-15 with H-11 and H-12, which was consistent with prenylated anthranol harunganol F (Table 3) [15]. The result was confirmed by the quantum chemical calculation of NMR data (qccNMR). A molecular Merck force field (MMFF) conformational search of four configurations, (10S,11S,12S)-**5a**, (10R,11R,12R)-**5b**, (10S,11R,12S)-**5c**, and (10R,11S,12R)-**5d**, was performed with CONFLEX 8.5 (Conflex Corp., Tokyo, Japan). Each isomer only gave one energy minimum with a 10 kcal/mol energy window, which was optimized using the DFT method at a B3LYP/6-31G(d) level with the Gaussian16 program package (Gaussian Inc., Wallingford, CT, USA). Gauge-independent atomic orbital (GIAO) calculations of the optimized conformers were performed at mPW1PW91/6-311+G(d,p) level in a DMSO solution. The sum of (10S,11S,12S)-**5a** and (10R,11R,12R)-**5b** isomers have 100% DP4+ probability (Figure S36), which confirmed that H-11 and H-12 were on the same side of the tetrahydropyran moiety of **5** [16]. The most probable absolute configuration was further determined as (10S,11S,12S) based on the comparison of calculated ECD curves of (10S,11S,12S)-**5** with the experimental CD spectrum (Figure 3).

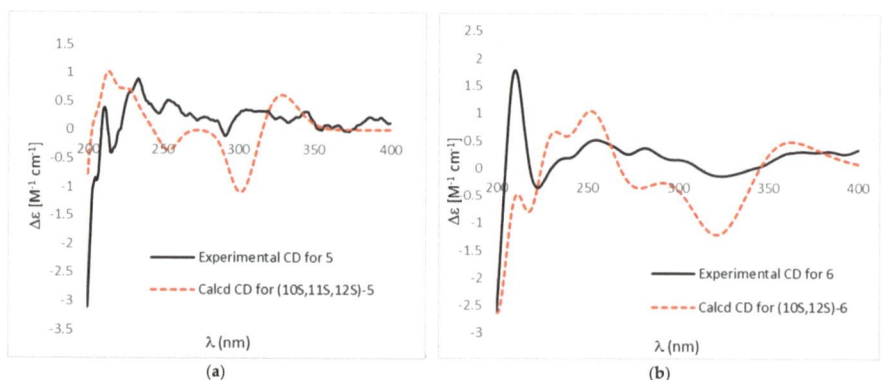

Figure 3. (**a**) Comparison of calculated ECD spectra of (10S,11S,12S)-**5** (red) in MeOH and experimental CD (black). σ = 0.16 eV, UV shift = 0 nm; (**b**) comparison of calculated ECD spectra of (10S, 12S)-**6** (red) in MeOH and experimental CD (black). σ = 0.30 eV, UV shift = 20 nm.

Table 3. ^{1}H and ^{13}C NMR data for compounds **5**, **6**, N-1447D and harunganol F (J in Hz, δ in ppm).

No.	5 [a]		6 [a]		N-1447D [b]		Harunganol F [c]	
	δ$_C$, Type	δ$_H$	δ$_C$, Type	δ$_H$	δ$_C$, Type	δ$_H$	δ$_C$, Type	δ$_H$
1	151.5, C		151.6, C				166.3, C	
2	133.5, C		133.5, C				99.5, CH	6.36, s
3	153.7, C		153.5, C		102.2, 106.9, 109.1, 109.7, 119.9, 122.2, 138.9, 140.2, 148.8, 162.1, 165.5, 166.9, 190.0, not assigned	6.97, s	168.0, C	
4	107.4, CH	6.91, s	107.4, CH	6.92, s			119.7, C	
4a	130.2, C		130.5, C				132.9, C	
4b	139.2, C		139.3, C					
5	123.5, C		121.0, C				121.9, C	
6	149.0, C		147.1, C				148.2, C	
7	118.6, CH	6.83, s	117.9, CH	6.80, s		6.81, s	120.0, CH	6.77, s
8	160.4, C		159.2, C				162.0, C	
8a	108.9, C		109.4, C				109.8, C	

Table 3. Cont.

No.	5 [a] δ_C, Type	δ_H	6 [a] δ_C, Type	δ_H	N-1447D [b] δ_C, Type	δ_H	Harunganol F [c] δ_C, Type	δ_H
9	189.7, C		189.8, C				189.6, C	
9a	107.8, C		108.1, C				108.9, C	
10	97.2, C		97.2, C		98.1, C		99.4, C	
11	61.7, CH	4.52, s	27.1, CH$_2$	2.78, d, (17.4) 3.04, dd, (17.4, 5.4)	63.9, CH	4.58, s	63.6, CH	4.48, br d (10.0)
12	87.1, CH	4.57, s	81.1, CH	4.75, d, (5.4)	87.9, CH	4.72, s	87.6, CH	4.67, overlapped
13	78.4, C		82.1, C		79.2, C		78.3, C	
14	29.9, CH$_3$	1.38, s	29.6, CH$_3$	1.37, s	30.2, CH$_3$	1.50, s	29.9, CH$_3$	1.46, s
15	23.1, CH$_3$	1.06, s	23.6, CH$_3$	1.15, s	23.2, CH$_3$	1.17, s	23.4, CH$_3$	1.09, s
16	18.5, CH$_3$	2.41, s	19.1, CH$_3$	2.24, s	18.9, CH$_3$	2.47, s	18.7, CH$_3$	2.40, s
17					55.9, CH$_3$	3.90, s	29.8, CH$_2$	3.50, dd, (7.2, 16.7) 3.37 dd, (9.5, 16.7)
18							91.3, CH	4.71, dd, (7.2, 9.5)
19							71.9, C	
20							24.5, CH$_3$	1.23, s
21							25.7, CH$_3$	1.35, s
OH-1				12.05, br s				
OH-8		11.96, br s		11.68, br s				

[a] Measured in DMSO-d_6; [b] Measured in CDCl$_3$ [14]; [c] Measured in CDCl$_3$ [15].

Compound **6** was obtained as a brown amorphous powder with molecular formula C$_{20}$H$_{18}$O$_7$ by the HRESIMS peaks at m/z 371.1140 ([M + H]$^+$, calcd. 371.1125) and m/z 393.0958 ([M + Na]$^+$, calcd. 393.0945). Compound **6** has very similar NMR data to **5** except there was a ^{13}C NMR upfield shift from δ_C 61.7 (C-11) in **5** to 27.1 (C-11) in **6** (Table 3). The HSQC spectrum and HMBC correlations from H-11 to C-4b, C-5, C-12, and C-13, from H-12 to C-10, C-5, C-11, C-13, and C-14, and from OH-8 to C-7 and C-8, indicated the hydroxyl group at C-11 in **5** was missing in **6**. The absolute configuration was identified as (10*S*, 12*S*) based on the comparison of calculated ECD curves with the experimental CD spectrum (Figure 3).

The known compounds were elucidated as orcinol (**7**) [17], cordyol C (**8**) [18], aspergilol C (**9**) [19], calyxanthone (**10**) [20], 3,7-dihydroxy-1,9-dimethyldibenzofuran (**11**) [21], 2-(2′-hydroxypropyl)-5-methyl-7-hydroxychromone (**12**) [22], and evariquinone (**13**) [23] by comparing NMR data with those previously published in the literature.

2.3. Anti-Inflammatory Activity Test

All the compounds were determined for inhibition on NO secretion using LPS induced RAW 264.7 cells. Compounds **5**, **6**, and **8** exhibited a moderate effect with EC$_{50}$ values of 34.6 ± 0.9, 20.2 ± 1.8, and 26.8 ± 1.7 µM, while **11** showed a potent effect with an EC$_{50}$ value of 2.9 ± 0.1 µM. The positive control dexamethasone had an EC$_{50}$ value of 2.9 ± 0.1 µM (Figure 4).

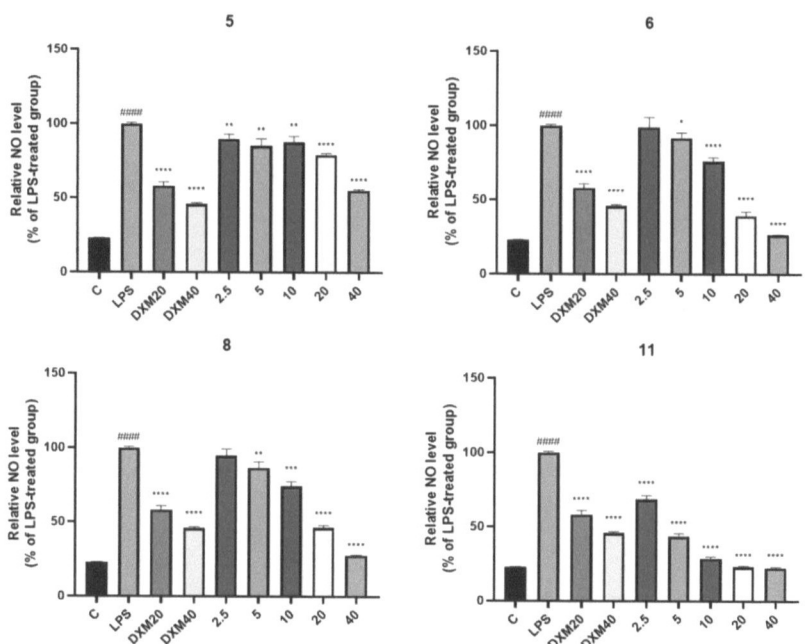

Figure 4. The inhibition of NO secretion in the RAW 264.7 cell line by the compounds **5, 6, 8,** and **11**. The inhibitory rate of NO in RAW 264.7 cells with different concentrations of compounds. Data were presented as mean ± SD of the experiments (n = 3). #### $p < 0.0001$ compared with the blank control. * $p < 0.05$, ** $p < 0.01$, *** $p < 0.001$ and **** $p < 0.0001$ compared with the LPS model group. No cytotoxicity of compounds on RAW 264.7 cells was observed at 40 µM.

3. Materials and Methods

3.1. General Experimental Procedures

The optical rotation was analyzed using a InsMark IP-digi3 polarimeter (InsMark, Shanghai, China). Circular dichroism was measured with a JASCO J-1500 circular dichroism spectrophotometer (JASCO, Easton, PA, USA). ^{1}H-NMR, ^{13}C-NMR, and 2D NMR spectra were recorded on a Bruker Ascend 500 spectrometer (Bruker, Billerica, MA, USA) with TMS as a reference. High-resolution TOFESIMS was performed on a WATERS Xevo G2-S Qtof Quadrupole Time of Flight Mass Spectrometry (Waters, Milford, MA, USA). Analysis and semi-preparative reversed-phase HPLC were performed on a Shimadzu LC-2030 liquid chromatograph (Shimadzu, Kyoto, Japan) with YMC-Pack ODS-A column 250 × 10 mm i.d., S-5 µm × 12 nm. Column chromatography (CC) was performed on a silica gel (200–300 mesh, Jiangyou Silica Gel Co., Ltd., Yantai, China) or CHROMATOREX C18 silica (Fuji Silysia Chemical Ltd., Kozoji-cho, Kasugai Aichi, Japan).

3.2. Isolation and Species Identification of Marine Fungus

The fungal strain GXIMD00543 was isolated from a sponge tissue sample that was collected from the Weizhou islands coral reef, Beibu Gulf, in December 2019. The sponge was collected and identified as *Haliclona* sp. by Dr. Xin-Ming Liu, Institute of Marine Drugs, Guangxi University of Chinese Medicine (Nanning, China) (Figure S1).

The strain was deposited in the Institute of Marine Drugs, Guangxi University of Chinese Medicine, Nanning, China. The fungus was identified by its morphological features and the sequence analysis of the internally transcribed spacer (ITS) region of the rRNA gene. The ITS sequence was amplified from the genome DNA via PCR with primers (ITS1: 5′TCCGTAGGTGAACCTGCGG3′ and ITS4: 5′TCCTCCGCTTATTGATATGC3′). ITS sequences (see Supplementary Materials) were then uploaded to the National Center of Biotechnology Information (NCBI) for BLAST analysis (GenBank accession number: OR501447).

3.3. Fungal Fermentation

The fungal strain was statically cultivated in one hundred and fifty 1000 mL Erlenmeyer flasks, each containing modified solid rice medium (80 g of rice, 0.4 g of yeast extract, 0.4 g of glucose, 3.6 g of artificial sea salt, and 120 mL of H_2O) for 35 days at room temperature. Then, the fermented cultures were extracted with EtOAc three times and concentrated *in vacuo* to obtain extract (230 g).

3.4. Extration and Isolation

The extract (230 g) was subjected to a silica gel column (1000 g) and eluted with CH_2Cl_2/MeOH (100:0–80:20, v/v) to yield 9 fractions (Fr. 1–9).

Fraction 5 was separated using a silica gel column and eluted with CH_2Cl_2/EtOAc (98:2–50:50, v/v) to give 18 sub-fractions (sFr. 5-1–5-18). sFr. 5-8 was separated using an ODS silica gel column and eluted with CH_3CN/H_2O (20:80–80:20, v/v) to give 20 sub-fractions (sFr. 5-8-1–5-8-20). sFr. 5-8-12 was subjected to a semi-preparation of HPLC (42% CH_3CN/H_2O) at a flow rate of 3 mL/min to obtain **6** (12 mg, t_R 27.2 min) and **11** (6 mg, t_R 33.4 min). sFr. 5-9 was separated using an ODS silica gel column and eluted with CH_3CN/H_2O (25:75–65:35, v/v) to give 22 sub-fractions (sFr. 5-9-1–5-9-22). sFr. 5-9-9 was subjected to a semi-preparation of HPLC (42% CH_3CN/H_2O) at a flow rate of 3 mL/min to obtain **2** (11 mg, t_R 36.3 min), **7** (28 mg, t_R 39.7 min), and **9** (13 mg, t_R 49.6 min). sFr. 5-9-10 was subjected to Sephedex (LH-20) and a further semi-preparation of HPLC (28% CH_3CN/H_2O) at a flow rate of 3 mL/min to obtain **8** (14 mg, t_R 19.5 min). sFr. 5-10 was separated using an ODS silica gel column and eluted with CH_3CN/H_2O (25:75–65:35, v/v) to give 21 sub-fractions (sFr. 5-10-1–5-10-21). sFr. 5-10-9 was subjected to a semi-preparation of HPLC (33% CH_3CN/H_2O) at a flow rate of 3 mL/min to obtain **12** (14 mg, t_R 22.9 min). sFr. 5-10-11 was subjected to a semi-preparation of HPLC (34% CH_3CN/H_2O) at a flow rate of 3 mL/min to obtain **5** (16 mg, t_R 25.4 min). sFr. 5-10-16 was recrystallized by CH_2Cl_2/MeOH to obtain **13** (28 mg).

Fraction 6 was separated by ODS silica gel column and eluted with CH_3CN/H_2O (20:80–80:20, v/v) to give 19 sub-fractions (sFr. 6-1–6-19). sFr. 6-8 was subjected to a semi-preparation of HPLC (24% CH_3CN/H_2O) at a flow rate of 3 mL/min to give 4 sub-fractions (sFr. 6-8-1–6-8-4). sFr. 6-8-1 was subjected to a semi-preparation of HPLC (17% CH_3CN/H_2O) at a flow rate of 3 mL/min to obtain **3** (15 mg, t_R 31.0 min) and **4** (26 mg, t_R 36.7 min). sFr. 6-11 was subjected to a semi-preparation of HPLC (37% CH_3CN/H_2O) at a flow rate of 3 mL/min to obtain **1** (10 mg, t_R 12.4 min) and **10** (15 mg, t_R 27.6 min).

3.5. Spectroscopic and Spectrometric Data

Carneusone A (**1**): Yellowish powder; UV (MeOH): λ_{max} (log ε) 204 (3.18), 253 (3.44), 327 (2.98) nm; ^{1}H and ^{13}C NMR data, see Tables 1 and 2; HRESIMS m/z 303.0510 ([M + H]$^+$, calcd. 303.0499) and 325.0330 ([M + Na]$^+$, calcd. 325.0319).

Carneusone B (**2**): Yellowish powder; UV (MeOH): λ_{max} (log ε) 205 (3.33), 244 (3.53), 312 (3.16) nm; ^{1}H and ^{13}C NMR data, see Tables 1 and 2; HRESIMS m/z 317.0661 ([M + H]$^+$, calcd. 317.0656) and 339.0481 ([M + Na]$^+$, calcd. 339.0475).

Carneusone C (**3**): Yellowish powder; UV (MeOH): λ_{max} (log ε) 214 (3.31), 277 (3.06) nm; ^{1}H and ^{13}C NMR data, see Tables 1 and 2; HRESIMS m/z 357.0588 ([M + Na]$^+$, calcd. 357.0581).

Carneusone D (**4**): Yellowish powder; UV (MeOH): λ_{max} (log ε) 213 (3.28), 277 (2.90) nm; ^{1}H and ^{13}C NMR data, see Tables 1 and 2; HRESIMS m/z 335.0767 ([M + H]$^+$, calcd. 335.0761), and 357.0593 ([M + Na]$^+$, calcd. 357.0581).

Carneusone E (**5**): Brown amorphous powder; $[\alpha]_D^{21}$ = +8.5 (c 0.9, MeOH); UV (MeOH): λ_{max} (log ε) 202 (3.28), 261 (2.81), 280 (2.67), 296 (2.31), 368 (2.75) nm; CD (MeOH) λ_{max} ($\Delta\varepsilon$): 211 (+0.39), 216 (−0.41), 234 (+0.89), 247 (+0.28), 253 (+0.52), 291 (−0.11), 305

(+0.35), 344 (+0.32) nm; ^{1}H and ^{13}C NMR data, see Table 3; HRESIMS m/z 387.1085 ([M + H]$^+$, calcd. 387.1074).

Carneusone F (**6**): Brown amorphous powder; $[\alpha]_D^{21}$ = +35.5 (c 0.5, MeOH); UV (MeOH): λ_{max} (log ε) 200 (3.43), 261 (2.98), 280 (2.88), 294 (2.44), 374 (2.94) nm; CD (MeOH) λ_{max} (Δε): 210 (+1.79), 223 (−0.36), 255 (+0.52), 272 (+0.26), 282 (+0.37), 324 (−0.14) nm; ^{1}H and ^{13}C NMR data, see Table 3; HRESIMS m/z 371.1140 ([M + H]$^+$, calcd. 371.1125) and m/z 393.0958 ([M + Na]$^+$, calcd. 393.0945).

3.6. Computational Methods

MMFF and DFT/TDDFT calculations were performed with CONFLEX 8.5 (Conflex Corp., Tokyo, Japan) and Gaussian16 program package (Gaussian Inc., Wallingford, CT, USA), respectively. The MMFF94s conformational search-generated low-energy conformers within a 10 kcal/mol energy window were subjected to further geometry optimization and frequency calculation using the B3LYP/6-31G(d) method. The single-point energy of the optimized conformers was recalculated at the M06-2X/def2TZVP level. Thus, the Gibbs free energy, obtained by the sum of the single-point energy and the thermal correction was used for the relative thermal free energy (DG) calculation and following Boltzmann population analysis at 298.15 K. The TDDFT-calculated conformers were performed using the cam-B3LYP functional with def2TZVP basis set. The number of excited states per each molecule was set to 20. The CD spectra were generated by the program SpecDis V1.71 [24] using a Gaussian band shape from dipole-length dipolar and rotational strengths. The calculated spectra were finally generated from the Boltzmann weighting of each conformer. The Grimme's dispersion (D3 version) was used for empirical dispersion correction. Solvent effects (in MeOH) were taken into account by using the default SCRF method integral equation formalism variant (IEFPCM) for the whole calculation.

The B3LYP/6-31G(d) optimized geometries of **5** were adopted for further NMR computation. GIAO calculations of the ^{1}H and ^{13}C NMR chemical shifts were accomplished by DFT at the mPW1PW91/6-311+G(d,p) level in DMSO solution. The calculated NMR spectroscopic data were averaged according to the Boltzmann distribution by the program Multiwfn 3.7 [25].

3.7. Anti-Inflammatory Activity Test

The inhibition of the NO production assay was performed according to the reported procedures [26]. The mouse macrophage RAW264.7 cell lines used in this study were purchased from the American Type Culture Collection (ATCC, Manassas, VA, USA) and maintained in Dulbecco's Modified Eagle Medium (DMEM) containing 10% fetal bovine serum (FBS), 100 ug/L of streptomycin, and 100 IU/mL of penicillin at 37 °C and 5% CO_2 atmosphere (PHCbi, Minato-ku, Tokyo, Japan). The viability of the RAW264.7 cells was determined by MTT assay. The RAW264.7 cells were seeded at a density of 5×10^5 cells/well in 96-well plates and incubated for 24 h at 37 °C and 5% CO_2. Then, the media in each well was replaced using fresh FBS-free DMEM media. Different concentrations of compounds (2.5, 5, 10, 20, 40 μM) were prepared in FBS-free DMEM to give a total volume of 100 μL in each well of a microtiter plate. After 1 h of treatment, the cells were stimulated with 1 μg/mL of LPS for 24 h. The presence of nitrite was determined in the cell culture media using a commercial Griess reagent kit (Thermo Fisher Scientific, Waltham, MA, USA). Protocols supplied with assay kit were used for the application of the assay procedure. Briefly, 100 μL of cell culture medium with an equal volume of Griess reagent in a 96-well plate was incubated at room temperature for 10 min. Then, the absorbance was measured at 540 nm in a microplate reader (PerkinElmer, Waltham, MA, USA). The amount of nitrite in the media was calculated from the standard curve of sodium nitrite ($NaNO_2$). Dexamethasone (DXM) was used as a positive control.

4. Conclusions

In summary, six benzophenone derivatives (**1–6**) and seven known compounds were obtained from sponge-derived fungus *Aspergillus carneus* GXIMD00543. Compounds **5**, **6**, **8**, and **11** exhibited anti-inflammatory effects by inhibiting NO secretion using LPS induced RAW 264.7 cells.

Supplementary Materials: The following supporting information can be downloaded at: https://www.mdpi.com/article/10.3390/md22020063/s1, Figure S1: The sponge *Haliclona* sp., colonies and the ITS rRNA sequences of sponge-derived fungus *Aspergillus carneus* GXIMD00543; Figures S2–S34: ^{1}H NMR, ^{13}C NMR, HSQC, HMBC, NOESY, HRESIMS of compounds **1–6**; Figures S35 and S36, Tables S1–S4: The quantum chemical calculation for compound **5**; Figure S37, Table S5: The quantum chemical calculation for compound **6**; The NMR data for known compounds **7–13**.

Author Contributions: Conceptualization, X.-Y.X. and Y.-H.L.; methodology, C.-J.L. and L.-F.L.; software, K.L.; validation, C.-Q.F. and Q.Y.; investigation, G.-S.Z., H.-Y.L., and Z.-W.S.; resources, G.-S.Z., H.-Y.L., and Z.-W.S.; Data curation, C.-J.L. and L.-F.L.; Writing—original draft, C.-J.L. and L.-F.L.; Writing—review and editing, X.-Y.X. and Y.-H.L.; Supervision, D.-M.Z. and C.-H.G. All authors have read and agreed to the published version of the manuscript.

Funding: This research was funded by the Guangxi Natural Science Foundation (2020GXNS-FGA297002, 2021GXNSFDA075010), the National Natural Science Foundation of China (42066006, U20A20101, 32060098), the Special Fund for Bagui Scholars of Guangxi (05019055); The Scientific Research Foundation of GXUCM (2022C011, 2022A007); Guangxi First-class Discipline: Chinese Materia Medica (Scientific Research of Guangxi Education Department [2022] No. 1), Innovation Project of Guangxi Graduate Education (YCSW2023381, JGY2022181).

Institutional Review Board Statement: Not applicable.

Data Availability Statement: The original data presented in the study are included in the article/Supplementary Materials; further inquiries can be directed to the corresponding author.

Acknowledgments: We would like to thank Hu-Mu Lu, Xian-Qiang Chen, and Xiao Lin from Institute of Marine Drugs, Guangxi University of Chinese Medicine, for the collection of NMR and MS spectral data. We also thank Xin-Ming Liu, from the Institute of Marine Drugs, Guangxi University of Chinese Medicine, for the collection and identification of sponge samples.

Conflicts of Interest: The authors declare no conflicts of interest.

References

1. Gonçalves, M.F.M.; Esteves, A.C.; Alves, A. Marine fungi: Opportunities and challenges. *Encyclopedia* **2022**, *2*, 559–577. [CrossRef]
2. Sebak, M.; Molham, F.; Greco, C.; Tammam, M.A.; Sobeh, M.; El-Demerdash, A. Chemical diversity, medicinal potentialities, biosynthesis, and pharmacokinetics of anthraquinones and their congeners derived from marine fungi: A comprehensive update. *RSC Adv.* **2022**, *12*, 24887–24921. [CrossRef]
3. Shabana, S.; Lakshmi, K.R.; Satya, A.K. An updated review of secondary metabolites from marine fungi. *Mini-Rev. Med. Chem.* **2021**, *21*, 602–642. [CrossRef]
4. Jimenez, C. Marine natural products in medicinal chemistry. *ACS Med. Chem. Lett.* **2018**, *9*, 959–961. [CrossRef]
5. Carroll, A.R.; Copp, B.R.; Davis, R.A.; Keyzers, R.A.; Prinsep, M.R. Marine natural products. *Nat. Prod. Rep.* **2023**, *40*, 275–325. [CrossRef]
6. Marinov, T.; Kokanova-Nedialkova, Z.; Nedialkov, P.T. Naturally occurring simple oxygenated benzophenones: Structural diversity, distribution, and biological properties. *Diversity* **2023**, *15*, 1030. [CrossRef]
7. Wu, S.B.; Long, C.; Kennelly, E.J. Structural diversity and bioactivities of natural benzophenones. *Nat. Prod. Rep.* **2014**, *31*, 1158–1174. [CrossRef] [PubMed]
8. Surana, K.; Chaudhary, B.; Diwaker, M.; Sharma, S. Benzophenone: A ubiquitous scaffold in medicinal chemistry. *MedChemComm* **2018**, *9*, 1803–1817. [CrossRef] [PubMed]
9. Cai, S.; Zhu, T.; Du, L.; Zhao, B.; Li, D.; Gu, Q. Sterigmatocystins from the deep-sea-derived fungus *Aspergillus versicolor*. *J. Antibiot.* **2011**, *64*, 193–196. [CrossRef]
10. Wu, G.; Yu, G.; Kurtán, T.; Mándi, A.; Peng, J.; Mo, X.; Liu, M.; Li, H.; Sun, X.; Li, J.; et al. Versixanthones A–F, cytotoxic xanthone–chromanone dimers from the marine-derived fungus *Aspergillus versicolor* HDN1009. *J. Nat. Prod.* **2015**, *78*, 2691–2698. [CrossRef] [PubMed]
11. Ji, Y.B.; Chen, W.J.; Shan, T.Z.; Sun, B.Y.; Yan, P.C.; Jiang, W. Antibacterial diphenyl ether, benzophenone and xanthone derivatives from *Aspergillus flavipes*. *Chem. Biodivers.* **2020**, *17*, e1900640. [CrossRef]

12. Jin, Y.; Qin, S.; Gao, H.; Zhu, G.; Wang, W.; Zhu, W.; Wang, Y. An anti-HBV anthraquinone from aciduric fungus *Penicillium* sp. OUCMDZ-4736 under low pH stress. *Extremophiles* **2018**, *22*, 39–45. [CrossRef]
13. Liu, H.X.; Tan, H.B.; Liu, Y.; Chen, Y.C.; Li, S.N.; Sun, Z.H.; Li, H.H.; Qiu, S.X.; Zhang, W.M. Three new highly-oxygenated metabolites from the endophytic fungus *Cytospora rhizophorae* A761. *Fitoterapia* **2017**, *117*, 1–5. [CrossRef] [PubMed]
14. Nishino, T.; Tagawa, M.; Osawa, H.; Seki, T. Agrochemical N-1477 Manufacture with *Aspergillus*. Japan Patent JP2001261610, 26 September 2001.
15. Johnson, O.O.; Zhao, M.; Gunn, J.; Santarsiero, B.D.; Yin, Z.Q.; Ayoola, G.A.; Coker, H.A.; Che, C.T. Alpha-Glucosidase inhibitory prenylated anthranols from *Harungana madagascariensis*. *J. Nat. Prod.* **2016**, *79*, 224–229. [CrossRef] [PubMed]
16. Zanardi, M.M.; Sarotti, A.M. Sensitivity analysis of DP4+ with the probability distribution terms: Development of a universal and customizable method. *J. Org. Chem.* **2021**, *86*, 8544–8548. [CrossRef] [PubMed]
17. Rojas, I.S.; Lotina-Hennsen, B.; Mata, R. Effect of lichen metabolites on thylakoid electron transport and photophosphorylation in isolated spinach chloroplasts. *J. Nat. Prod.* **2000**, *63*, 1396–1399. [CrossRef] [PubMed]
18. Bunyapaiboonsri, T.; Yoiprommarat, S.; Intereya, K.; Kocharin, K.; National, C.F.G.E. New diphenyl ethers from the insect pathogenic fungus *Cordyceps* sp. BCC 1861. *Chem. Pharm. Bull.* **2007**, *55*, 304–307. [CrossRef] [PubMed]
19. Wu, Z.; Wang, Y.; Liu, D.; Proksch, P.; Yu, S.; Lin, W. Antioxidative phenolic compounds from a marine-derived fungus *Aspergillus versicolor*. *Tetrahedron* **2016**, *72*, 50–57. [CrossRef]
20. Zhou, Y.J.; Xu, S.X.; Wang, X.W.; Wang, H.Y.; Wang, Z.X.; Gu, X.H.; Liu, S.Z. Two new minor compounds with inhibitory effect on K562 cells from *Ventilago leiocarpa* Benth. *J. Herb. Pharmacother.* **2001**, *1*, 35–41. [CrossRef]
21. Tanahashi, T.; Takenaka, Y.; Nagakura, N.; Hamada, N. Dibenzofurans from the cultured lichen mycobionts of *Lecanora cinereocarnea*. *Phytochemistry* **2001**, *58*, 1129–1134. [CrossRef]
22. Gao, L.; Xu, X.; Yang, J. Chemical constituents of the roots of Rheum officinale. *Chem. Nat. Compd.* **2013**, *49*, 603–605. [CrossRef]
23. Bringmann, G.; Lang, G.; Steffens, S.; Gunther, E.; Schaumann, K. Evariquinone, isoemericellin, and stromemycin from a sponge derived strain of the fungus *Emericella variecolor*. *Phytochemistry* **2003**, *63*, 437–443. [CrossRef]
24. Bruhn, T.; Schaumloffel, A.; Hemberger, Y.; Bringmann, G. SpecDis: Quantifying the comparison of calculated and experimental electronic circular dichroism spectra. *Chirality* **2013**, *25*, 243–249. [CrossRef]
25. Lu, T.; Chen, F. Multiwfn: A multifunctional wavefunction analyzer. *J. Comput. Chem.* **2012**, *33*, 580–592. [CrossRef] [PubMed]
26. Lee, H.S.; Kwon, Y.J.; Seo, E.B.; Kim, S.K.; Lee, H.; Lee, J.T.; Chang, P.S.; Choi, Y.J.; Lee, S.H.; Ye, S.K. Anti-inflammatory effects of *Allium cepa* L. peel extracts via inhibition of JAK-STAT pathway in LPS-stimulated RAW264.7 cells. *J. Ethnopharmacol.* **2023**, *317*, 116851. [CrossRef] [PubMed]

Disclaimer/Publisher's Note: The statements, opinions and data contained in all publications are solely those of the individual author(s) and contributor(s) and not of MDPI and/or the editor(s). MDPI and/or the editor(s) disclaim responsibility for any injury to people or property resulting from any ideas, methods, instructions or products referred to in the content.

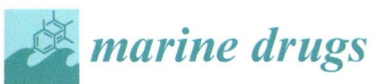 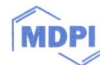

Article

New Polyene Macrolide Compounds from Mangrove-Derived Strain *Streptomyces hiroshimensis* GXIMD 06359: Isolation, Antifungal Activity, and Mechanism against *Talaromyces marneffei*

Zhou Wang [1,2,†], Jianglin Yin [1,2,3,†], Meng Bai [1,2], Jie Yang [1,2], Cuiping Jiang [1,2], Xiangxi Yi [2], Yonghong Liu [1,2,*] and Chenghai Gao [1,2,*]

1. Institute of Marine Drugs, Guangxi University of Chinese Medicine, Nanning 530200, China; wangzhou2021@stu.gxtcmu.edu.cn (Z.W.); yinjianglin@126.com (J.Y.); xxbai2014@163.com (M.B.); jieyang202312@163.com (J.Y.); ping990120@foxmail.com (C.J.)
2. Guangxi Key Laboratory of Marine Drugs, Guangxi University of Chinese Medicine, Nanning 530200, China; yixiangxi2017@163.com
3. Guangxi Scientific Research Center of Traditional Chinese Medicine, Nanning 530200, China
* Correspondence: yonghongliu@scsio.ac.cn (Y.L.); gaoch@gxtcmu.edu.cn (C.G.)
† These authors contributed equally to this work.

Abstract: Mangrove-derived actinomycetes represent a rich source of novel bioactive natural products in drug discovery. In this study, four new polyene macrolide antibiotics antifungalmycin B-E (**1–4**), along with seven known analogs (**5–11**), were isolated from the fermentation broth of the mangrove strain *Streptomyces hiroshimensis* GXIMD 06359. All compounds from this strain were purified using semi-preparative HPLC and Sephadex LH-20 gel filtration while following an antifungal activity-guided fractionation. Their structures were elucidated through spectroscopic techniques including UV, HR-ESI-MS, and NMR. These compounds exhibited broad-spectrum antifungal activity against *Talaromyces marneffei* with minimum inhibitory concentration (MIC) values being in the range of 2–128 μg/mL except compound **2**. This is the first report of polyene derivatives produced by *S. hiroshimensis* as bioactive compounds against *T. marneffei*. In vitro studies showed that compound **1** exerted a significantly stronger antifungal activity against *T. marneffei* than other new compounds, and the antifungal mechanism of compound **1** may be related to the disrupted cell membrane, which causes mitochondrial dysfunction, resulting in leakage of intracellular biological components, and subsequently, cell death. Taken together, this study provides a basis for compound **1** preventing and controlling talaromycosis.

Keywords: actinomycetes; polyene macrolide; *Streptomyces hiroshimensis*; antifungal activity; antifungal mechanism; *Talaromyces marneffei*

1. Introduction

Talaromyces (*Penicillium*) *marneffei* causes a life-threatening mycosis—Talaromycosis, an endemic invasive mycosis found primarily in tropical and subtropical Southeast Asia [1–3]. In recent years, some drugs have been reported to encounter antifungal resistance for *T. marneffei*, especially fluconazole [4–9]. Moreover, the disease is being recognized with an increasing frequency well beyond the original endemic areas [10–16]. Therefore, the discovery of new antifungal drugs is necessary to cover the shifting challenges of this and other fungal infections.

Mangroves are ecologically significant plants in marine habitats that inhabit the coastlines of many countries [17]. Being a highly productive and diverse ecosystem, mangroves are rich in numerous classes of actinomycete that are of great importance in the field of antibiotics [18]. Furthermore, about 200 compounds, such as salinosporamide A (to be processed for clinical trials for cancer treatment), xiamycins, rifamycins, and antimycin A were discovered from mangrove actinobacteria, which have become an important source of novel bioactive compounds [19–23].

In our preliminary study, *Streptomyces hiroshimensis* GXIMD 06359 was isolated from mangrove in the west coast of Hainan [24], which was identified as the potential strain to produce antimicrobial active metabolites against *T. marneffei* in Am2ab medium. The scaled-up fermentation and extensive chromatographic separation of the EtOAc extract resulted in the isolation of four new metabolites, namely antifungalmycins B-E (**1–4**), together with seven known compounds (**5–11**). Herein, we report the isolation and structural determination of these compounds (Figure 1) along with the antifungal activities. Then the mechanism of compound **1** inhibiting *T. marneffei* was studied, with the aim of finding potential new drugs for the precision treatment of talaromycosis.

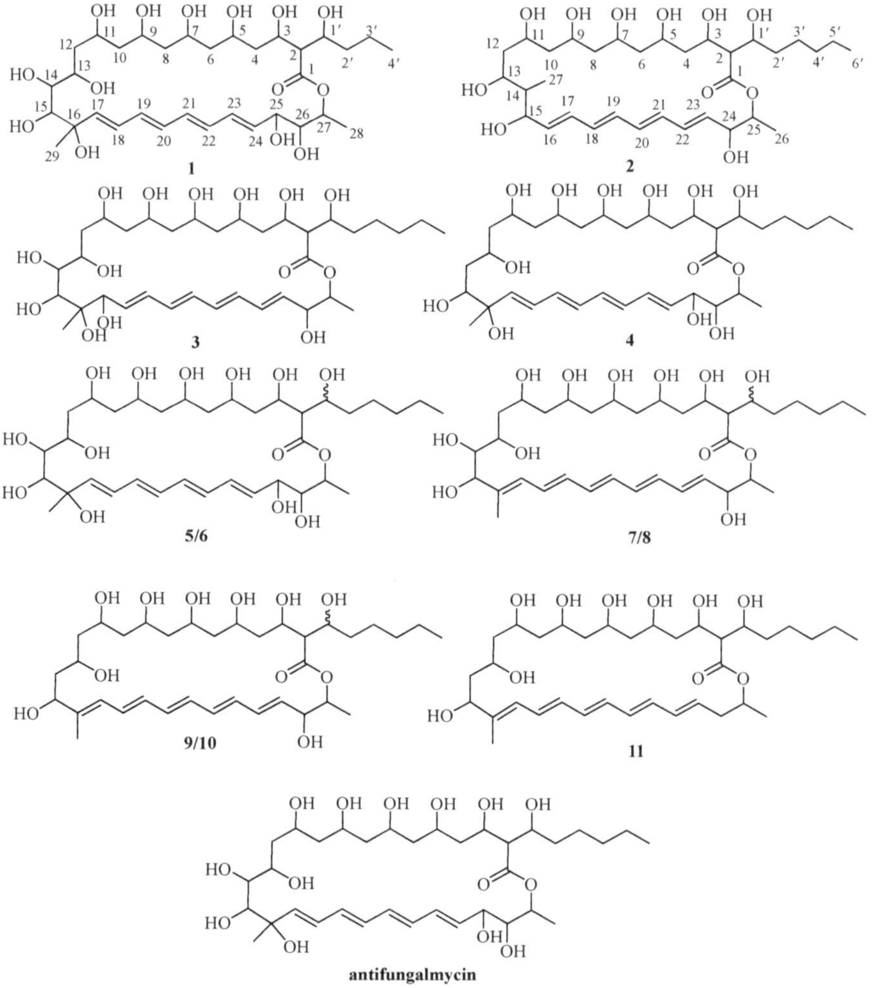

Figure 1. Chemical structures of compounds **1–11** and antifungalmycin.

2. Results

2.1. Structural Elucidation

Compound **1** was obtained as a light-yellow amorphous powder. Its HR-ESI-MS spectrum showed a characteristic [M − H]⁻ ion peak at *m/z* 675.3578 (calcd for 675.3592), which is consistent with the molecular formula of $C_{33}H_{56}O_{14}$, indicating 6 degrees of unsaturation. The ^1H NMR spectrum (Figure S1) shows resonances for three methyl protons δ_H 1.14 (3H, d, J = 6.2 Hz, H_3-28), 1.06 (3H, s, H_3-29), and 0.84 (3H, t, J = 6.2 Hz, H_3-6′); seven methylene protons δ_H 1.71 (1H, m, H-10a), 1.25 (1H, m, H-10b), 1.62 (2H, m, H_2-12), δ_H 1.54 (2H, m, H_2-6), 1.52 (2H, m, H_2-4), 1.47 (2H, m, H_2-8), 1.44 (1H, m, H-3′a), 1.25 (1H, m, H-3′b), 1.29 (1H, m, H-2′a), and 1.24 (1H, m, H-2′b); thirteen methine protons δ_H 4.71 (1H, m, H-27), 4.24 (1H, dd, J = 5.7, 2.3 Hz, H-25), 4.02 (1H, m, H-3), 3.97 (1H, m, H-9), 3.90 (1H, m, H-5), 3.90 (1H, m, H-7), 3.90 (1H, m, H-11), 3.68 (1H, m, H-1′), 3.65 (1H, m, H-15), 3.51 (1H, dd, J = 7.2, 2.6 Hz, H-26), 3.34 (1H, m, H-14), 3.29 (1H, m, H-13), and 2.46 (1H, dd, J = 8.6, 6.8 Hz, H-2); and eight olefinic protons δ_H 6.28 (1H, m, H-21), 6.28 (1H, m, H-22), 6.28 (1H, m, H-23), 6.26 (1H, m, H-20), 6.24 (1H, m, H-19), 6.15 (1H, dd, J = 15.1, 9.4 Hz, H-18), 5.72 (1H, d, J = 15.0 Hz, H-17), and 5.67 (1H, dd, J = 14.6, 5.8 Hz, H-24). The ^{13}C NMR and DEPT 135 spectra (Figures S2 and S3) displayed thirty-three signals for carbon, including one carbonyl carbon δ_C 171.6 (C-1); one quaternary carbon δ_C 82.0 (C-16); eight olefinic carbons δ_C 138.9 (C-17), 134.1 (C-24), 133.5 (C-22), 133.2 (C-20), 131.5 (C-19), 131.2 (C-21), 130.4 (C-23), and 126.3 (C-18); thirteen methine carbons δ_C 82.7 (C-15), 82.3 (C-14), 75.7 (C-26), 75.2 (C-13), 72.0 (C-25), 70.3 (C-27), 69.6 (C-3), 69.2 (C-9), 69.2 (C-1′), 68.5 (C-7), 67.8 (C-5), 67.8 (C-11), and 58.3 (C-2); seven methylene carbons δ_C 44.5 (C-8), 44.3 (C-6), 42.2 (C-10), 41.6 (C-12), 40.9 (C-4), 36.7 (C-2′), and 18.2 (C-3′); and three methyl carbons δ_C 22.9 (C-29), 17.4 (C-28), and 14.0 (C-1′).

Careful analysis of the ^1H and ^{13}C NMR data (Table 1) of 1 showed they were very similar to antifungalmycin [25,26], which possesses the same lactone ring. The main difference was that the signals for two methylene groups [(δ_H 1.24, δ_C 31.3, CH_2-4′) and (δ_H 1.25, δ_C 22.1, CH_2-5′)] at the side chain in the NMR spectra of antifungalmycin were absent in compound 1. Those were supported by the ^1H-^1H COSY and HMBC correlations (Figure 2). In the ^1H-^1H COSY spectrum of compound 1, correlations were observed for H-2/H-3/H-1′/H-2′/H-3′/H-4′, H-10/H-11/H-12/H-13/H-14/H-15, and H-24/H-25/H-26/H-27. The HMBC spectrum shows correlations of H-2 to C-1/C-4/C-1′/C-2′, H-14 to C-12/C-13/C-15, H-15 to C-16/C-17/C-29, H-25 to C-23/C-24/C-25, H-26 to C27/C-28, and H-27 to C-1. Thus, the planar structure of 1 was determined. In the NOESY spectrum, the correlations of H-3/H-1′, H-13/H-15, H-25/H-26 (Figure 3) were not enough to elucidate the compound 1 relative configuration. Consequently, compound 1's relative configuration has not been elucidated, and is named antifungalmycin B.

Compound 2, isolated as a light-yellow amorphous powder. The molecular formula was deduced to be $C_{33}H_{56}O_{11}$ by the HR-ESI-MS peak at m/z 627.3743 [M−H]$^-$ (calcd for 627.3744), indicating 6 degrees of unsaturation. The ^1H NMR spectrum (Figure S10) shows resonances for three methyl protons δ_H 1.19 (3H, d, J = 6.3 Hz, H_3-26), 0.84 (3H, m, H_3-27), and 0.84 (3H, t, J = 6.9 Hz, H_3-6′); eight methylene protons δ_H 1.92 (1H, m, H-12a), 1.52 (1H, m, H-12b), 1.50 (2H, m, H_2-8), 1.42 (1H, m, H-3′a), 1.24 (1H, m, H-3′b), 1.38 (2H, m, H_2-4), 1.40 (2H, m, H_2-6), 1.70 (1H, m, H-10a), 1.25 (1H, m, H-10b), 1.34 (1H, m, H-2′a), 1.23 (1H, m, H-2′b), 1.24 (2H, m, H_2-4′), and 1.24 (2H, m, H_2-5′); twelve methine protons δ_H 4.62 (1H, m, H-25), 4.05 (1H, m, H-3), 3.93 (1H, m, H-5), 3.93 (1H, m, H-7), 3.93 (1H, m, H-9), 3.93 (1H, m, H-11), 3.82 (1H, m, H-24), 3.72 (1H, m, H-1′), 3.63 (1H, m, H-15), 3.21 (1H, m, H-13), 2.87 (1H, m, H-14), and 2.38 (1H, t, J = 8.0 Hz, H-2); and eight olefinic protons δ_H 6.28 (1H, m, H-19), 6.26 (1H, m, H-20), 6.23 (1H, m, H-21), 6.20 (1H, m, H-17), 6.20 (1H, m, H-22), 6.18 (1H, m, H-18), 5.89 (1H, dd, J = 14.0, 3.1 Hz, H-16), and 5.79 (1H, dd, J = 14.7, 6.8 Hz, H-23). The ^{13}C NMR and DEPT 135 spectra (Figures S11 and S12) displayed thirty-three signals for carbon, including one carbonyl carbon δ_C 171.2 (C-1); eight olefinic carbons δ_C 135.9 (C-23), 133.8 (C-22), 133.3 (C-17), 131.4 (C-19), 131.1 (C-21), 130.7 (C-20), 130.4 (C-18), and 129.5 (C-16); twelve methine carbons δ_C 80.5 (C-13), 76.1 (C-14), 73.3 (C-26), 73.0 (C-13), 72.0 (C-25), 70.3 (C-27), 70.2 (C-3), 69.8 (C-9), 69.7 (C-1′), 69.6 (C-7), 66.7 (C-5), and 58.5 (C-2); seven methylene carbons δ_C 44.0 (C-6), 43.7 (C-8), 43.3 (C-10), 40.9 (C-4), 38.5 (C-12), 33.9 (C-2′), 24.4 (C-3′), 31.3 (C-4′), and 22.1 (C-5′); and three methyl carbons δ_C 17.8 (C-26), 15.6 (C-27), and 14.0 (C-1′).

Table 1. ^{1}H NMR and ^{13}C NMR data for compounds **1-4** in DMSO-d_6.

NO.	1[a] δ$_H$ (J in Hz)	1[a] δ$_C$	2[a] δ$_H$ (J in Hz)	2[a] δ$_C$	3[b] δ$_H$ (J in Hz)	3[b] δ$_C$	4[b] δ$_H$ (J in Hz)	4[b] δ$_C$
1	-	171.6, C	-	171.2, C	-	171.3, C	-	171.7, C
2	2.46, dd (8.6, 6.8)	58.3, CH	2.38, t (8.0)	58.5, CH	2.48, m	58.2, CH	2.46, dd (8.8, 6.6)	58.2, CH
3	4.02, m	69.6, CH	4.05, m	69.7, CH	4.05, m	70.0, CH	4.03, m	69.4, CH
4	1.52, m	40.9, CH$_2$	1.38, m	40.9, CH$_2$	1.45, m	43.3, CH$_2$	1.50, m	40.9, CH$_2$
5	3.90, m	67.8, CH	3.93, m	70.2, CH	3.93, m	68.2, CH	3.92, m	69.4, CH
6	1.54, m	44.3, CH$_2$	1.40, m	44.0, CH$_2$	1.45, m	45.4, CH$_2$	1.50, m	44.1, CH
7	3.90, m	68.5, CH	3.93, m	70.3, CH	3.98, m	69.0, CH	3.92, m	68.2, CH
8	1.47, m	44.5, CH$_2$	1.50, m	43.7, CH$_2$	1.46, m	46.3, CH$_2$	1.50, m	44.6, CH$_2$
9	3.97, m	69.2, CH	3.93, m	69.8, CH	3.93, m	67.0, CH	3.97, m	68.2, CH
10	1.71, m; 1.25, m	42.2, CH$_2$	1.70, m; 1.25, m	42.9, CH$_2$	1.76, m; 1.45, m	43.6, CH$_2$	1.76, m; 1.53, m	41.4, CH$_2$
11	3.90, m	67.8, CH	3.93, m	66.7, CH	3.93, m	66.9, CH	3.87, m	67.5, CH
12	1.62, m	41.6, CH$_2$	1.92, m; 1.52, m	38.5, CH$_2$	3.33, m	63.1, CH$_2$	1.74, m; 1.50, m	44.4, CH$_2$
13	3.29, m	75.2, CH	3.21, m	80.5, CH	3.46, m	66.0, CH	3.65, m	71.2, CH
14	3.34, m	82.3, CH	2.87, m	73.0, CH	3.80, m	84.6, CH	2.16, m	41.9, CH$_2$
15	3.65, d (5.4)	82.7, CH	3.63, m	80.5, CH	3.71, d	78.6, CH	3.90, m	76.0, CH
16	-	82.0, C	5.89, dd (14.0, 3.1)	129.5, CH	-	80.0, C	-	84.5, CH
17	5.72, d (15.0)	138.9, CH	6.20, m	133.3, CH	4.18, d (4.4)	83.4, CH	5.65, d (15.0)	137.8, C
18	6.15, dd (15.1, 9.4)	126.3, CH	6.18, m	130.4, CH	5.72, dd (14.5, 4.3)	129.1, CH	6.15, dd (14.5, 6.2)	127.4, CH
19	6.24, m	131.5, CH	6.28, m	131.4, CH	6.31, m	131.1, CH	6.22, m	130.8, CH
20	6.26, m	133.2, CH	6.26, m	130.7, CH	6.26, m	130.4, CH	6.21, m	131.1, CH
21	6.28, m	131.2, CH	6.23, m	131.1, CH	6.31, m	131.5, CH	6.21, m	133.5, CH
22	6.28, m	133.5, CH	6.20, m	133.8, CH	6.26, m	131.2, CH	6.32, m	134.0, CH
23	6.28, m	130.4, CH	5.79, dd (14.7, 6.8)	135.9, CH	6.23, m	133.1, CH	6.25, m	130.3, CH
24	5.67, dd (14.6, 5.8)	134.1, CH	3.82, m	73.3, CH	6.36, m	133.9, CH	5.68, dd (14.6, 6.1)	134.4, CH
25	4.24, dd (5.7, 2.3)	72.0, CH	4.62, m	72.0, CH	5.99, dd (15.1, 5.1)	136.1, CH	4.23, m	72.1, CH
26	3.51, dd (7.2, 2.6)	75.7, CH	1.19, d (6.3)	17.8, CH$_3$	3.87, m	72.4, CH	3.50, m	75.5, CH
27	4.71, m	70.3, CH	0.84, m	15.6, CH$_3$	4.57, dd (8.9, 6.3)	72.5, CH	4.77, m	70.2, CH
28	1.14, d (6.2)	17.4, CH$_3$	-	-	1.21, d (6.2)	17.9, CH$_3$	1.14, d (6.3)	17.5, CH$_3$
29	1.06, s (7.1)	22.9, CH$_3$	-	-	1.20, s	19.6, CH$_3$	1.10, s	22.2, CH$_3$
1'	3.68, m	69.2, CH	3.72, m	69.6, CH	3.68, m	69.7, CH	3.65, m	69.2, CH
2'	1.29, m; 1.24, m	36.7, CH$_2$	1.34, m; 1.23, m	33.9, CH$_2$	1.45, m; 1.25, m	34.3, CH$_2$	1.33, m; 1.24, m	34.5, CH$_2$
3'	1.44, m; 1.25, m	18.2, CH$_2$	1.42, m; 1.24, m	24.4, CH$_2$	1.45, m; 1.25, m	24.6, CH$_2$	1.42, m; 1.24, m	24.5, CH$_2$
4'	0.83, t (7.0)	14.0, CH$_3$	1.24, m	31.3, CH$_2$	1.24, m	31.3, CH$_2$	1.24, m	31.3, CH$_2$
5'	-	-	1.24, m	22.1, CH$_2$	1.25, m	22.1, CH$_2$	1.25, m	22.1, CH$_2$
6'	-	-	0.84, t (6.9)	14.0, CH$_3$	0.85, t (6.9)	14.0, CH$_3$	0.85, t (7.1)	14.0, CH$_3$

Table 1. *Cont.*

NO.	1 [a] δ_H (J in Hz)	1 [a] δ_C	2 [a] δ_H (J in Hz)	2 [a] δ_C	3 [b] δ_H (J in Hz)	3 [b] δ_C	4 [b] δ_H (J in Hz)	4 [b] δ_C
3-OH	5.12, s	-	5.06, m	-	5.23, d	-	5.10, d	-
5-OH	4.85, m	-	4.90, d	-	4.94, d	-	4.88, m	-
7-OH	4.85, m	-	5.04, m	-	4.82, d	-	4.88, m	-
9-OH	4.90, m	-	5.07, m	-	4.32, d	-	4.86, m	-
11-OH	4.85, m	-	4.56, d	-	4.40, d	-	4.68, d	-
13-OH	-	-	4.78, d	-	4.71, m	-	4.80, m	-
14-OH	-	-	-	-	4.65, d	-	-	-
15-OH	-	-	4.78, m	-	4.92, d	-	4.88, m	-
16-OH	-	-	-	-	4.48, d	-	-	-
17-OH	-	-	-	-	5.00, m	-	-	-
24-OH	-	-	5.26, d	-	-	-	4.86, m	-
25-OH	-	-	-	-	-	-	4.91, d	-
26-OH	-	-	-	-	5.29, d	-	-	-
1'-OH	4.85, m	-	4.82, d	-	4.85, d	-	4.80, m	-

[a] The ^{1}H NMR measured at 500 MHz and ^{13}C NMR measured at 175 MHz. [b] The ^{1}H NMR measured at 700 MHz and ^{13}C NMR measured at 175 MHz.

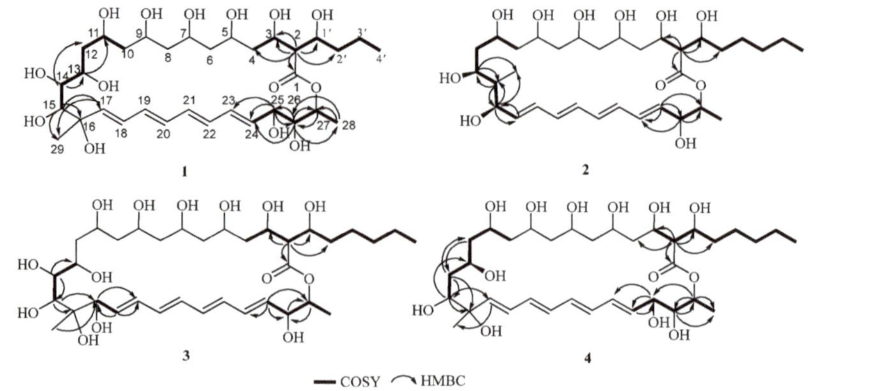

Figure 2. The key ^{1}H-^{1}H COSY, HMBC correlations of compounds **1–4**.

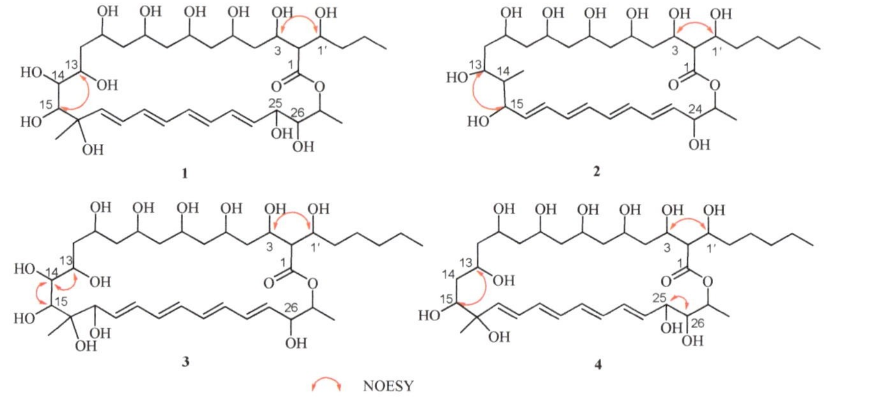

Figure 3. The key NOESY correlations of compounds **1–4**.

The ^{1}H and ^{13}C NMR data (Table 1) of **2** suggested that it was similar to antifungalmycin [25,26]. Combined with analyzing the ^{1}H–^{1}H COSY and HMBC spectra, it was revealed that compound **2** was a 26-membered macrocyclic lactone ring. Compared with antifungalmycin, the signals for one-quarter carbon (δ_C 82.0) and one methylene were absent in the lactone ring in compound **2**. In the COSY spectrum, correlations were observed for H-2/H-3/H-4/H-1′/H-2′/H-3′/H-4′/H-5′/H-6′, H-10/H-11/H-12/H-13/H-14/H-15/H-16, and H-23/H-24/H-25/H-26 (Figure 2). The HMBC spectrum shows correlations of H-13 to C-14/C-27, H-15 to C-14/C-16/C-27, H-23 to C-22/C-23/C-24, H-24 to C-22/C-25, and H-25 to C-1. Thus, the planner structure of **2** was confirmed. In the NOESY spectrum, the correlations of H-3/H-1′ and H-13/H-15 (Figure 3) were not enough to elucidate its relative configuration. Compound **2's** relative configuration has not been elucidated, and is named antifungalmycin C.

Compound **3** was obtained as a light-yellow amorphous powder. Its HR-ESI-MS data ([M + H]$^+$, 705.4088; calcd for $C_{35}H_{61}O_{14}$, 705.4061) possessed the molecular formula of $C_{35}H_{60}O_{14}$ (6 degrees of unsaturation). The ^{1}H NMR spectrum (Figure S19) shows resonances for three methyl protons δ_H 1.21 (3H, d, J = 6.2 Hz, H$_3$-28), 1.20 (3H, s, H$_3$-29), and 0.85 (3H, t, J = 6.9 Hz, H$_3$-6′); eight methylene protons δ_H 3.33 (2H, m, H$_2$-12), 1.76 (1H, m, H-10a),1.45 (1H, m, H-10b), 1.46 (2H, m, H$_2$-8), 1.45 (2H, m, H$_2$-6), 1.45 (2H, m, H$_2$-4), 1.45 (1H, m, H-2′a), 1.25 (1H, m, H-2′b), 1.45 (1H, m, H-3′a), 1.25 (1H, m, H-3′b), 1.25 (2H, m, H$_2$-5′), and 1.24 (2H, m, H$_2$-4′); twelve methine protons δ_H 4.57 (1H, dd, J = 5.1, 2.7 Hz, H-27), 4.05 (1H, m, H-3), 3.98 (1H, m, H-7), 3.93 (1H, m, H-5), 3.93 (1H, m, H-9), 3.93 (1H, m,

H-11), 3.87 (1H, m, H-26), 3.80 (1H, m, H-14), 3.71 (1H, dd, J = 5.1, 2.7 Hz, H-15), 3.68 (1H, m, H-1′), 3.46 (1H, m, H-13), and 2.48 (1H, m, H-2); and eight olefinic protons δ_H 6.36 (1H, m, H-24), 6.31 (1H, m, H-19), 6.31 (1H, m, H-21), 6.26 (1H, m, H-20), 6.26 (1H, m, H-22), 6.23 (1H, m, H-23), 5.99 (1H, dd, J = 15.1, 5.1 Hz, H-23), and 5.72 (1H, dd, J = 14.5, 4.3 Hz, H-18). The ^{13}C NMR (Figure S20) displayed thirty-five signals for carbon, including one carbonyl carbon δ_C 171.3 (C-1); one quaternary carbon δ_C 80.0 (C-16); eight olefinic carbons δ_C 129.1 (C-18), 131.1 (C-19), 130.4 (C-20), 131.5 (C-21), 131.2 (C-22), 133.1 (C-23), 133.9 (C-24), and 136.1 (C-25); twelve methine carbons δ_C 84.6 (C-14), 83.4 (C-17), 78.6 (C-15), 72.5 (C-27), 72.4 (C-26), 70.0 (C-3), 69.7 (C-1′), 69.0 (C-7), 68.2 (C-5), 67.0 (C-9), 66.9 (C-11), and 58.2 (C-2); eight methylene carbons δ_C 46.3 (C-8), 45.4 (C-6), 43.6 (C-10) 43.3 (C-4), 63.1 (C-12), 34.3 (C-2′), 24.6 (C-3′), 31.3 (C-4′), and 22.1 (C-5′); and three methyl carbons δ_C 17.9 (C-28), 19.6 (C-29), and 14.0 (C-1′).

The NMR data (Table 1) of 3 suggested that it was similar to antifungalmycin [25,26]. Detailed analysis of the ^{1}H–^{1}H COSY and HMBC spectra revealed that the main differences between them were the positions of conjugated double bonds. The conjugated double bonds of 3 were in C-18 to C-25, but in antifungalmycin were in C-17 to C-24. In the COSY spectrum, correlations were observed for H-2/H-3/H-4/H-1′/H-2′/H-3′/H-4′/H-5′/H-6′, H-13/H-14/H-15, H-17/H-18, and H-25/H-26/H-27/H-28 (Figure 2). The HMBC spectrum shows correlations of H-2 to C-1/C-3/C-1′/C-2′, H-14 to C-13/C-14, H-15 to C-16/C-17, H-17 to C-19, H-18 to C-17/C-19, H-25 to C-24/C-26/C-27, and H-29 to C-17 (Figure 2). Thus, the planar structure of 3 was determined. In the NOESY spectrum, the correlations of H-3/H-1′, H-13/H-14/H-15 (Figure 3) were not enough to elucidate the compound 3 relative configuration. Consequently, compound 3's relative configuration has not been elucidated, and is named antifungalmycin D.

Compound 4 was obtained as a light-yellow amorphous powder. The molecular formula was determined as $C_{35}H_{60}O_{13}$ (five degrees of unsaturation) via HR-ESI-MS (m/z 687.3975, [M − H]$^−$, ($C_{35}H_{59}O_{13}$ calcd. 687.3956)). The ^{1}H NMR spectrum (Figure S27) shows resonances for three methyl protons δ_H 1.14 (3H, d, J = 6.3 Hz, H$_3$-28), 1.10 (3H,s, H$_3$-29), and 0.84 (3H, t, J = 7.1 Hz, H$_3$-6′); seven methylene protons δ_H 1.76 (1H, m, H-10a), 1.53 (1H, m, H-10b), 1.74 (1H, m, H-12a),1.50 (1H, m, H-12b), 1.50 (2H, m, H$_2$-4), 1.50 (2H, m, H$_2$-6), 1.50 (2H, m, H$_2$-8), 1.42 (1H, m, H-3′a), 1.24 (1H, m, H-3′b), 1.33 (1H, m, H-2′a), 1.24 (1H, m, H-2′b), 1.25 (2H, m, H$_2$-5′), and 1.24 (2H, m, H$_2$-4′); thirteen methine protons δ_H 4.77 (1H, m, H-27), 4.23 (1H, dd, J = 5.7, 2.3 Hz, H-25), 4.03 (1H, m, H-3), 3.97 (1H, m, H-9), 3.92 (1H, m, H-5), 3.92 (1H, m, H-7), 3.90 (1H, m, H-15), 3.87 (1H, m, H-11), 3.65 (1H, m, H-13), 3.65 (1H, m, H-1′), 3.50,(1H, m, H-26), 2.46 (1H, dd, J = 8.8, 6.6 Hz, H-2), and 2.16 (1H, m, H-14); and eight olefinic protons δ_H 6.32 (1H, m, H-22), 6.25 (1H, m, H-23), 6.22 (1H, m, H-19), 6.21 (1H, m, H-20), 6.21 (1H, m, H-21), 6.15 (1H, dd, J = 14.5, 6.2 Hz, H-18), 5.68 (1H, dd, J = 14.6, 6.1 Hz, H-24), and 5.65 (1H, d, J = 15.0 Hz, H-17). The ^{13}C NMR and DEPT 135 spectra (Figures S28 and S29) displayed thirty-five signals for carbon, including one carbonyl carbon δ_C 171.7 (C-1); one quaternary carbon δ_C 84.5 (C-16); eight olefinic carbons δ_C 137.8 (C-17), 134.4 (C-24), 134.0 (C-22), 133.5 (C-21), 131.1 (C-20), 130.8 (C-19), 130.3 (C-23), and 127.4 (C-18); eleven methine carbons δ_C 76.0 (C-15), 75.5 (C-26), 72.1 (C-25), 71.2 (C-13), 70.2 (C-27), 69.4 (C-3), 69.4 (C-5), 69.2 (C-1′), 68.2 (C-7), 67.5 (C-11), and 58.3 (C-2); seven methylene carbons δ_C 44.6 (C-8), 44.4 (C-12), 44.1 (C-6), 41.9 (C-14), 41.4 (C-10), 40.9 (C-4), 34.5 (C-2′), 24.5 (C-3′), 31.3 (C-4′), and 22.1 (C-5′); and three methyl carbons δ_C 22.2 (C-29), 17.5 (C-28), and 14.0 (C-1′).

The ^{1}H and ^{13}C NMR data (Table 1) of compound 4 were very similar to antifungalmycin [25,26]. Detailed analysis of the ^{1}H–^{1}H COSY and HMBC spectra revealed that compound 4 has no hydroxyl substitution in the C-14 (δ_H 2.16/δ_C 41.9). In the COSY spectrum, correlations were observed for H-2/H-3/H-1′/H-2′/H-3′/H-4′/H-5′/H-6′, H-10/H-11/H-12/H-13/H-14/H-15, and H-24/H-25/H-26/H-27/H-28 (Figure 2). The HMBC spectrum shows correlations of H-2 to C-1/C-3/C-4/C-1′/C-2′, H-15 to C-13/C-16/C-17, H-25 to C-22/C-23/C-24, and H-27 to C-1/C-25/C-26/C-28 (Figure 2). On the basis of the evidence, the planar structure of 4 was confirmed. In the NOESY spectrum, the correlations of H-3/H-1′, H-13/H-15, and H-25/H-26 (Figure 3) were not enough to elucidate the compound **4**'s relative configuration. Consequently, compound **4**'s relative configuration has not been elucidated, and is named antifungalmycin E.

The known compounds **5** and **6** had the same molecular formula of $C_{35}H_{59}O_{14}$ as determined by HR-ESI-MS. The ^1H and ^{13}C NMR data of compounds **5** and **6** revealed that they were similar to the previously reported antifungalmycin [25,26]. The differences between **5** and **6** were in the positions C-1 (δ_C 171.8 vs. 171.1), C-2 (δ_C 57.5 vs. 58.2), C-3 (δ_C 69.7 vs. 69.2), C-1′ (δ_C 69.5 vs. 68.2), 2-H (δ_H 2.46 vs. 2.32), and 1′-OH (δ_H 4.81 vs. 4.45). The above difference in chemical shift may be caused by the different stereoscopic configuration of C-3 and C-1′. Thus, compound **5** was named antifungalmycin a_1 and compound **6** was named antifungalmycin a_2.

The molecular formulas of compounds **7** and **8** were determined to be $C_{35}H_{58}O_{12}$ by HR-ESI-MS. They were identified as fungichromin [27], by comparing NMR and HR-ESI-MS data with reported values. The differences between **7** and **8** were in the positions C-1 (δ_C 171.1 vs. 170.5), C-2 (δ_C 58.7 vs. 57.8), C-3 (δ_C 70.0 vs. 69.4), C-1′ (δ_C 69.6 vs. 68.2), 2-H (δ_H 2.46 vs. 2.31), and 1′-OH (δ_H 4.81 vs. 4.38). The difference in chemical shift may be caused by the different stereoscopic configuration of C-3 and C-1′. Thus, compound **7** was named fungichromin a_1 and compound **8** was named fungichromin a_2.

The known compounds **9** and **10** were identified as filipin III by comparing their NMR and HR-ESI-MS data with those previously reported [28]. The differences between **9** and **10** were in the positions C-1 (δ_C 171.1 vs. 170.5), C-2 (δ_C 58.7 vs. 57.8), C-3 (δ_C 70.0 vs. 69.7), C-1′ (δ_C 69.6 vs. 67.9), 2-H (δ_H 2.46 vs. 2.29), and 1′-OH (δ_H 4.89 vs. 4.42). The above difference in chemical shift may be caused by the different stereoscopic configuration of C-3 and C-1′. Thus, compound **9** was named filipin III a_1 and compound **10** was named filipin III a_2.

The known compound **11** was obtained as a light-yellow amorphous powder. It was identified as filipin I [29], by comparing ^1H-NMR, ^{13}C-NMR, and HR-ESI-MS data with that reported.

2.2. Antifungal Activity of the Compounds

The antifungal potency of the compounds against *T. marneffei* was evaluated by MIC and MFC values; the results are shown in Table 2. In our experiment, most of the compounds exhibited antifungal activity except compound **2**, which has an MIC value of more than 128 µg/mL. In addition, compound **9** exhibited the best antifungal activity against *T. marneffei*, with MIC and MFC values of 2 and 4 µg/mL, respectively. Moreover, compound **1** showed the lowest MIC and MBC values, which represented the best antifungal activity of all the new compounds. So, we further explore the antifungal mechanism of compound **1** in the next experiment.

Table 2. MIC and MFC of the compounds.

Compounds	MIC (µg/mL)	MFC (µg/mL)
1	16	64
2	>128	——
3	128	——
4	32	——
5	32	64
6	128	——
7	4	8
8	16	16
9	2	4
10	32	128
11	32	——
FLC *	16	64
AMB *	0.5	1

* FLC and AMB serve as positive controls. FLC, Fluconazole; AMB, Amphotericin B. "——" means compounds is not enough to support the experiment, no detection.

2.3. Compound 1 Inhibited the Growth of T. marneffei

To further analyze the growth-inhibiting characteristics of compound **1**, the time course of *T. marneffei* growth in the presence of **1** at different concentrations was plotted. *T. marneffei* exhibited rapid growth in the control group, and the logarithmic growth stage was achieved within 40 h of incubation, then entered a stabilization phase after 60 h of incubation (Figure 4A). However, the growth of *T. marneffei* after treatment with **1** at 1/2 MIC and 1 MIC showed a substantially lower growth rate than that of the control. Moreover, before 60 h of incubation, no further growth of *T. marneffei* was observed in 1/2 MIC and 1 MIC compound **1**-treated groups. But after 60 h of incubation, *T. marneffei* with **1** continued to grow, though at a lower rate than control, and the fungi growth rate of group compound **1** at 1 MIC was lower than group compound **1** at 1/2 MIC. Overall, these results confirmed that **1** had an inhibitory effect on *T. marneffei* growth, and was shown to be concentration-dependent and time-limited.

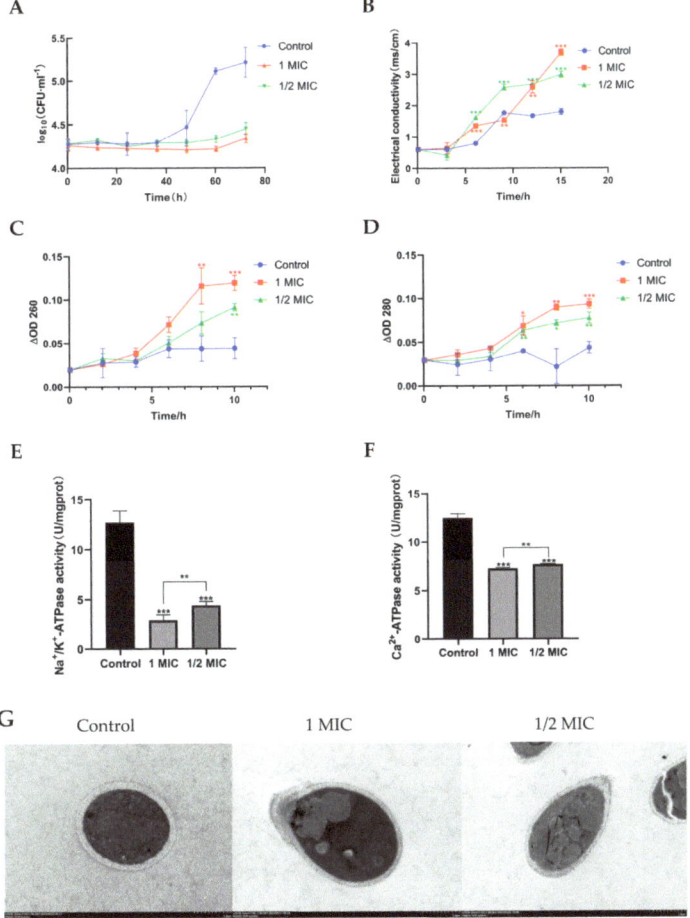

Figure 4. (**A**) Time-kill curve of compound **1** against *T. marneffei*. (**B**) The effect of compound **1** on the extracellular conductivity of *T. marneffei*. (**C**) The effect of compound **1** on the extracellular nucleic acids of *T. marneffei*. (**D**) The effect of compound **1** on the extracellular proteins of *T. marneffei*. (**E**) The effect of compound **1** on Na^+/K^+-ATPase activity against *T. marneffei*. (**F**) The effect of compound **1** on Ca^{2+}-ATPase activity against *T. marneffei*. (**G**) TEM of *T. marneffei* treated with compound **1** for 72 h. Data are shown as mean ± S.D. * $p < 0.05$, ** $p < 0.01$, and *** $p < 0.001$; Student's *t* test, $n = 3$.

*2.4. Compound **1** Disrupted the Cell Membrane of T. marneffei*

The membrane integrity of the fungi was investigated to verify the ability of compound **1** to damage the fungal cell membrane. The electric conductivity of the cell suspensions implied the permeability of the cell membrane. Electrolytes are charged molecules such as sodium chloride and potassium chloride, and they are essential for fungal metabolism and growth [30]. Thus, their leakage can lead to fungal inhibition or death. Compared with the control, compound **1** resulted in a significant increase in conductivity. The conductivity of *T. marneffei* increased significantly from 1.80 for the control to 2.99 and 3.69 in the presence of compound **1** at the levels of 1/2 MIC and 1 MIC after 15 h, respectively (Figure 4B). Moreover, after 9 h exposure to the 1/2 MIC of compound **1**, the extracellular conductivity entered a steady stage. However, for the group of 1 MIC, the extracellular conductivity continued to increase. This indicates that compound **1** has a destructive effect on the cell membrane of *T. marneffei*, and shows a concentration dependence consistent with the growth-inhibiting results.

In order to further determine the degree of cell membrane damage by compound **1**, in the current work, nucleic acids and proteins released from the cytoplasm were monitored by the detection of absorbance at 260 nm and 280 nm, respectively. As the previous work reported, nucleic acid and protein play important roles in bacterial metabolism as they dominate the genetic information and cellular structure [31]. Leakage of cellular materials was analyzed by detecting 260 nm and 280 nm absorbing materials. Therefore, the absorbance of the material and proteins at 260 nm and 280 nm wavelengths can be used as an indicator of damage to the cell wall and membrane, which causes leakage of the cellular materials into the surroundings [32]. As shown in Figure 4C,D, both cell constituents were released rapidly from *T. marneffei* into cell suspensions and their amounts increased multi-fold after treatment with compound **1**. In addition, there was a progressive release of proteins and nucleic acids from *T. marneffei* after exposure to compound **1** for 4 h, followed by a steady state. Moreover, the leakage of nucleic acids and proteins in the group treated with 1 MIC compound **1** was larger than the control and 1/2 MIC compound **1** group. Compound **1** dose-dependently destroyed the cell membrane of *T. marneffei*, which was consistent with the previous results. Similar results have also been reported for the crude methanolic extract of *Myrtus communis* roots and leaves when tested against *Candida glabrata*, showing increased absorbance at a wavelength of 260 nm [33]. In this study, compound **1** was efficacious in inhibiting or killing the fungi by damaging their cell membranes, resulting in the leakage of the 260 nm and 280 nm absorbing materials, such as DNA, RNA, and proteins, which are essential for fungal growth.

To further investigate the mechanisms underlying compound **1**'s disruption of the cell membrane in *T. marneffei* cells, the Na^+/K^+-ATPase and Ca^{2+}-ATPase activities of T. marneffei cells were detected. Na^+/K^+-ATPase is a carrier protein that exists in the phospholipid bilayer of cells. It mainly controls the transmembrane transport of Na^+ and K^+. It can release energy by decomposing ATP, and uses this energy to transport Na^+ and K^+ [34]. Ca^{2+}-ATPase is a membrane transport protein ubiquitously found in the endoplasmic reticulum of all eukaryotic cells. As a calcium transporter, Ca^{2+}-ATPase maintains a low cytosolic calcium level that enables a vast array of signaling pathways and physiological processes [35]. Na^+/K^+-ATPase and Ca^{2+}-ATPase are important components of cell membrane transport. The $Na+/K^+$-ATPase and Ca^{2+}-ATPase activities of *T. marneffei* cells are shown in Figure 4E,F. Compared with the control group without **1**, the Na^+/K^+-ATPase and Ca^{2+}-ATPase activities of the experimental group with compound **1** were significantly decreased. Among them, the experimental group with **1** at the levels of 1 MIC had the largest decrease. This showed that compound **1** had a certain inhibitory effect on the Na^+/K^+-ATPase and Ca^{2+}-ATPase activities of *T. marneffei*, which is consistent with the above results.

These results indicated that the antibacterial action mode of compound **1** against *T. marneffei* probably involved the alteration of the structure of cell wall and membrane, causing the loss of cell viability.

2.5. Effect of Compound 1 on Morphology of T. marneffe

The morphological and ultrastructural changes in *T. marneffei* treated with compound **1** for 72 h were observed by SEM and TEM to better understand the antifungal mode of action of compound **1**. For *T. marneffei* cells, deformation was the most significant feature, which was apparent in the SEM image (Figure 5). The *T. marneffei* cells treated with compound **1** at 1/2 MIC displayed distorted membrane morphology, disruption of cell membrane, and leakage of cellular contents; and those treated with 1 MIC displayed distorted membrane morphology. Furthermore, a proportion of *T. marneffei* cells treated with compound **1** showed abnormalities in the TEM images, including the disappearance of cell wall, disruption of cell membrane, thinning of cytoplasm, distortion of cells, heterogeneous distribution of melanin, and leakage of intracellular materials (Figure 4G). S.K.P. Lau et al. reported that *T. marneffei* in yeast form can cause infections, and produce melanin as well, which plays an important role in the pathogenicity of *T. marneffei* [36]. Therefore, the decrease in intracellular melanin may also be the pathway of compound 1 inhibiting *T. marneffei*. These findings supported the results of the leakage of extracellular conductivity, nucleic acids and proteins leakage analysis, and Na^+/K^+-ATPase and Ca^{2+}-ATPase activities in the present study.

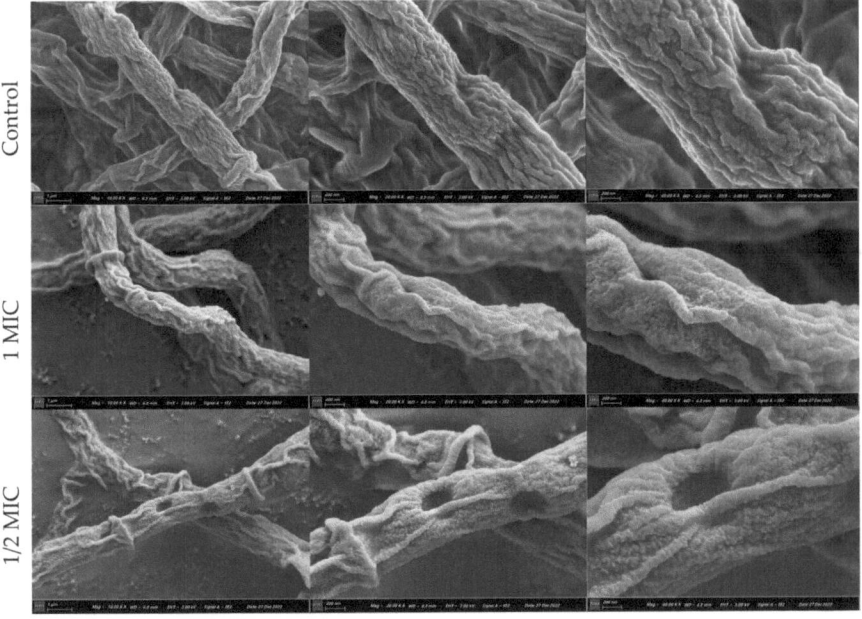

Figure 5. SEM of *T. marneffei* treated with compound **1** for 72 h.

2.6. Effects of Compound 1 on Mitochondrial Function

Mitochondria are key energy and metabolic regulatory centers within cells and also play an important role in maintaining cell growth and survival in mycelial cells. The core function of mitochondria is to synthesize ATP through oxidative phosphorylation. Therefore, the normal conduct of mitochondrial oxidative phosphorylation and the TCA cycle, especially the activities of related enzymes, is essential for maintaining cell survival. ATPase has an important role in energy metabolism [37]. The results of ATPase content in *T. marneffei* cells are shown in Figure 6A. The ATP content of the control group was 23,693.5 μmol/gprot. After treatment with 1 MIC compound **1**, the intracellular ATP level reduced to 8151.1 μmol/gprot, which was a 65.6% reduction ($p < 0.05$). In addition, after treatment with 1/2 MIC compound **1**, the intracellular ATP level reduced to 16,213.2 μmol/gprot, which was a 31.6% reduction ($p < 0.05$). ATPase content was significantly decreased after compound **1** treatment. These results indicated that the antifungal activity of compound **1** against *T. marneffei* can be attributed to disruption of the respiratory chain.

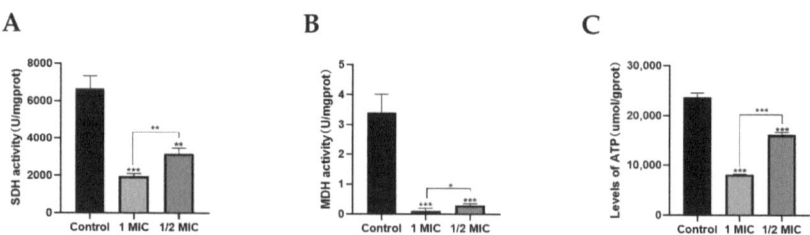

Figure 6. (**A**) The effect of compound **1** on ATPase content against *T. marneffei*. (**B**) The effect of compound **1** on SDH activity against *T. marneffei*. (**C**) The effect of compound **1** on MDH activity against *T. marneffei*. Data are shown as mean ± S.D. * $p < 0.05$, ** $p < 0.01$, and *** $p < 0.001$; Student's *t* test, $n = 3$.

SDH (Succinate dehydrogenase) is a part of the respiratory chain (complex II). SDH catalyzes the oxidation of succinate to fumaric acid and FADH2. Therefore, it connects the TCA cycle with the respiratory chain, and the generated FADH2 does not dissociate from the enzyme, which directly uses the electrons to reduce the coenzyme Q, and then passes it to the complex III [38]. MDH (Malate dehydrogenase) can catalyze the reversible conversion between malic acid and oxaloacetate, and is also an important enzyme in mitochondrial function, which is mainly involved in some metabolic pathways such as photosynthesis, TCA cycle, and C4 cycle. Compared with the control, compound **1** resulted in a reduction in the activity of SDH and MDH. The SDH activity of compound **1** at the levels of 1/2 MIC and 1 MIC was significantly reduced compared with the control ($p < 0.05$) (Figure 6B), and the MDH activity of compound **1** at the levels of 1/2 MIC and 1 MIC was considerably lower than that of the control ($p < 0.05$) (Figure 6C). The above experimental results showed that MDH and SDH activities decreased with increasing compound **1** concentration in *T. marneffei* (Figure 6A,B), which suggested that compound **1** disrupts mitochondrial function by affecting MDH and SDH activities.

The above results suggested that compound **1** blocked the respiratory chain and energy metabolism, thereby killing the fungi.

3. Discussion

Polyene macrolide antibiotics are a significant group of antibiotics and have an important role in the treatment of fungal infections [39]. For example, amphotericin B, pimamycin, and nystatin have been widely used in clinical treatment [40]. Many researchers suggest that most polyene macrolides are bioactive compounds with a wide range of antifungal activity. However, the high hemolytic toxicity, poor water solubility, and unstable exposure to light limit the development of some compounds with good antifungal activity into clinical drugs. For a long time, researchers have been committed to chemical derivation, structural modification, genetic engineering, combined biosynthesis, and other methods to improve the antibacterial activity and solubility of these compounds and reduce the hemolytic toxicity. This has made certain research progress, but far from enough. Extensive research has shown that some bioactive secondary metabolites of marine microbial origin with strong antibacterial and antifungal activities are being intensely used as antibiotics and may be effective against infectious diseases [41]. In our study, four new compounds—tetrene macrolide compounds (**1**–**4**), and seven known polyene macrolide antibiotics, were isolated from the fermentation broth of the mangrove strain *S. hiroshimensis* GXIMD 06359. Their structures, including their relative configurations, were determined by HR-ESI-MS and NMR spectra. The antifungal activity of the compounds against *T. marneffei* was measured by detection of MIC and MBC in the present study. The results demonstrated that

all compounds except compound 2 exhibit antifungal and fungicidal properties against
T. marneffei. Moreover, the lowest MIC and MFC of the new compounds was compound
1. To further analyze the antifungal activity of 1, the time course of *T. marneffei* growth
in the presence of 1 at different concentrations was plotted. These results demonstrated
that 1 can significantly inhibit the growth of *T. marneffei*. Therefore, compound 1 could be
considered an effective antibacterial agent; we further explore the mechanism of compound
1 inhibiting *T. marneffei*.

Cell membranes have important physiological functions, including maintaining the
stability of the intracellular environment, signal transduction, and material transportation [42]. The integrity of cell membranes is crucial for cell viability, and membrane damage
can lead to high cytotoxicity. Numerous studies have shown that the cell membrane of fungi
is a target for inhibiting fungal growth and reproduction [43]. The previous studies have
reported that the antifungal mechanism of action of polyene macrolides is binding to the
fungal surface, which produces membrane breakdown, resulting in leakage of protein and
vital nutrients and, ultimately, cell death [44–46]. In this study, it was found that compound
1 caused significant damage to cell membranes. Compound 1 irreversibly damaged the
plasma membrane of *T. marneffei* cells. Its treatment increased extracellular conductivity,
proteins, and nucleic acids in *T. marneffei* cultures, suggesting electrolyte leakage due to
reduced membrane integrity of *T. marneffei* cells. Moreover, the decrease in Na^+/K^+-ATPase
and Ca^{2+}-ATPase activities confirmed the destruction of cell membrane function. SEM and
TEM results confirmed that compound 1 treatment disrupted the integrity of *T. marneffei* cell
walls and membranes. Cell wall and membrane integrity are critical for maintaining fungal
viability. Kamble, M. T. et al. reported that SGF disrupted the bacterial cell membrane,
resulting in leakage of intracellular biological components, and subsequently, cell death, in
Vibrio parahaemolyticus and *Vibrio harveyi*, which is similar to our results [47].

In addition to destroying the cell membrane, mitochondrial dysfunction plays an
important role in the potential mechanisms of antifungal drugs [48]. Xin et al. reported that
antofine against *P. digitatum* is related to the cell membrane integrity and energy metabolism
by affecting intracellular ATP content [49]. Pristimerin has been reported to exert antifungal
activity; it caused mitochondrial membrane damage and affected mitochondria structure
and functions, then oxidative phosphorylation and TCA cycle were inhibited, and energy
metabolism was blocked in *S. sclerotiorum* [50]. In this study, we also investigated the role of
mitochondrial function pathways against *T. marneffei*. Our results indicated that compound
1 caused a significant decrease in intracellular ATP levels and a significant decrease in the
activities of MDH and SDH, and this was shown to be concentration-dependent. These
results indicated that the antifungal activity of compound 1 against *T. marneffei* can be
attributed to disruption of the respiratory chain. Therefore, the death of *T. marneffei* may
be caused by mitochondrial dysfunction, in turn caused by the destruction of cytoplasmic
membrane permeability and integrity.

This study showed that compound 1 effectively prevented *T. marneffei* growth. Compound 1 disrupts cytoplasmic membrane permeability and integrity, causes mitochondrial
dysfunction, and *T. marneffei* metabolic disorders. We speculate that the antifungal mechanism of compound 1 on *T. marneffei* is through the destruction of *T. marneffei* cell membrane
integrity and mitochondrial function to induce apoptosis. Compound 1 showed promising
potential as a drug against *T. marneffei*. But the detailed role of compound 1 in bacterial
membranes is unclear and needs further investigation.

4. Materials and Methods

4.1. General Experimental Procedures

TLC analyses were conducted on silica gel 60 F254-precoated plates. Silica gel 60
(200–300 mesh) were used for column chromatography (CC). For the HPLC analysis and
purification, we used YMC C18 column (250 mm × 4.6 mm, 5 μm) and (250 mm × 10 mm,
5 μm). NMR spectra were recorded on Bruker AVANCE 500/125 spectrometer (Bruker,

Fällanden, Switzerland) and Bruker AVANCE 700/175 spectrometer (Bruker, Hong Kong, China) with TMS as the internal standard.

4.2. Actinomycete Material

The strain *S. hiroshimensis* GXIMD 06359 was isolated from mangrove in the west coast of Hainan [24]. This strain is stored at Institute of Marine Drugs, Guangxi University of Chinese Medicine.

4.3. Fermentation, Extraction, and Isolation

After activation, *S. hiroshimensis* GXIMD 06359 was inoculated into 1 L flapper conical flask (containing 300 mL Am2ab medium, sterilized) and fermented in a constant temperature shaking table at 28 °C and 180 r/min for 10 days. After fermentation, the fermentation solution was filtered, and the bacterial solution and bacteria were separated. The bacterial solution was extracted with equal volume ethyl acetate three times, and the bacteria were soaked in equal volume acetone and extracted by ultrasound for 20 min until nearly colorless. The ethyl acetate phase and acetone phase fermentation crude extracts were obtained after concentration under reduced pressure. The crude extract (200.2 g) was subjected to normal phase silica gel column chromatography and gradient elution was performed with chloroform/acetone system (10:0, 10:2, 10:4, 10:8) and chloroform/methanol system (10:1, 10:2, 10:4, 0:10). The collected fractions were analyzed by thin layer chromatography (TLC) and HPLC. A total of 13 fractions (Fr. A1–A13) were obtained.

Fr. A10 (8.82 g) was separated by medium pressure preparative chromatography with ODS self-loaded column and gradient elution with methanol/water system at the flow rate of 15 mL/min. After the fraction was collected and analyzed by HPLC, a total of nine fractions (Fr. B1–Fr. B9) were obtained from the combined samples. Fr. B3 (0.2490 g) was separated by gel column chromatography, and three fractions (Fr. D1–D3) were obtained. Fr. D1 was separated and purified by semi-preparative HPLC. The mobile phase of Fr. D1 was methanol/water system [0–30 min: 42% methanol, 35–60 min: 55% methanol, compound **1** (3.6 mg, t_R = 36.85 min) and compound **6** (2.2 mg, t_R = 53.58 min) were obtained at the flow rate of 3 mL/min]. Compound **2** (1.5 mg, t_R = 63.45 min) was purified by semi-preparative HPLC from Fr. B4 (0.1772 g) by semi-preparative HPLC (48% methanol iso-degree elution for 40 min, flow rate 3 mL/min). Fr. B5 (2.7342 g) was isolated and purified by semi-preparative HPLC (0–30 min: 52% methanol, 35–60 min: 58% methanol, 65–100 min: 70% methanol, compound **5** (9.0 mg, t_R = 30.83 min), compound **3** (1.8 mg, t_R = 42.85 min), compound **4** (5.3 mg, t_R = 36.44 min), compound **7** (36.8 mg, t_R = 47.59 min), compound **8** (3.3 mg, t_R = 58.93 min), compound **9** (7.9 mg, t_R = 63.27 min), and compound **10** (1.6 mg, t_R = 71.65 min) were obtained at rate of 3 mL/min. Compound **11** (2 mg, t_R = 30.66 min) was purified by semi-preparative HPLC from Fr.B9 (82% methanol iso-degree elution for 40 min, flow rate 3 mL/min).

4.4. Microbial Strains OriginA and Culture Conditions

Reference strains (*Talaromyces marneffei* ATCC) were from YE Li from Guangxi Medical University (Guangxi Key Laboratory of AIDS Prevention and Control, School of Public Health, Guangxi Medical University). Seven-day-old pure culture of the yeast form grown on brain-heart infusion (BHI) agar was used in all reactions. The colonies of *T. marneffei* were flooded with Phosphate buffer saline (PBS) and the number of fungi was counted with a hemocytometer after washing three times. The cells were suspended in PBS and thoroughly vortexed. The suspensions were added to RPMI 1640 medium to obtain a stock of $1–5 \times 10^6$ CFU/mL that was then diluted 1:100, resulting in a working stock of $1–5 \times 10^4$ CFU/mL.

4.5. Antifungal Activity

Antifungal susceptibility testing was performed using the microdilution method according to CLSI protocol M27-A3 (Clinical and Laboratory Standards Institute) with minor modifications [51]. *Candida parpsilosis* ATCC 22019 was included as quality control through for all experiments. Wells containing inoculum alone and inoculum with DMSO were used as negative controls. AMB and FLC were used as a positive control. The minimum inhibitory concentration (MIC) was defined as the lowest concentration resulting in 100% inhibition of visible fungal growth after incubation at 37 °C for 72 h.

4.6. Determination of Minimal Fungicidal Concentration (MFC)

The MFCs of compounds were determined according to the methods of Mbah et al. [52]. Briefly, 10 µL from wells corresponding to 1, 2, 3, and 4-fold of the MIC, were placed on a Sabouraud Dextrose Agar (SDA) and incubated at optimal temperatures for 72 h. MFC was defined as the lowest concentration with no fungal growth.

4.7. Mode of Action of Compound **1**

4.7.1. Time-Kill Curve

Exponentially growing yeast cells were harvested and resuspended in RPMI-1640 to obtain a final concentration of $1\text{–}5 \times 10^4$ CFU/mL. Different concentrations of compound **1** were added to the cells. Cells were incubated under shaking 180 rpm at 37 °C, and 10 µL from suspensions were placed on SDA and incubated at optimal temperatures for 72 h, then measured at the indicated time points after incubation (0, 12, 24, 36, 48, 60, and 72 h). The same volumes of solvents (DMSO) were added to the untreated controls. Three independent experiments were performed for optimal results.

4.7.2. Scanning Electron Microscopy (SEM) and Transmission Electron Microscopy (TEM)

SEM was used to observe the morphological changes of compound **1**-treated *T. marneffei*. The fungal cells obtained from the logarithmic growth phase were treated with the compound **1** at 1/2 and 1-fold of the MIC value at 37 °C for 72 h. Then, the suspensions were centrifuged at 12,000 rpm/min for 10 min. The sediments were washed with 0.1 M PBS, (pH = 7.2) and fixed with 2.5% glutaraldehyde in PBS for 2 h at 4 °C. The cells were washed in the same buffer and were post-fixed for 30 min with osmium tetroxide. After harvesting, the cells were further dehydrated via graded ethanol concentrations (30%, 50%, 70%, 90%, and 100%) for 10 min each. Untreated cells were similarly processed and used as control. Then, cells were fixed on SEM support and observed by SEM (Sigma300, Zeiss), Wuhan, Hubei, China.

The pretreatment of fungal cells for transmission electron microscopy (TEM) were the same as that for scanning electron microscopy (SEM, Wuhan, Hubei, China). After being fixed with 2.5% glutaraldehyde, post-fixed by 1% osmic acid, dehydrated using alcohol, permeated using white resin, and embedded by roasting at 55 °C, the samples were cut into thin sections to perform TEM (HITACHI HT 7800 120 kv, Wuhan, Hubei, China).

4.7.3. Leakage of Extracellular Conductivity

Fungal membrane permeability was determined and expressed as the electric conductivity according to the method by Maliehe, T. S. et al. [53]. Fungal cells were cultivated at 37 °C to mid-exponential stage and collected by centrifugation (8000 rpm for 15 min). Cells were washed twice in 0.1 M PBS. The different concentrations compound **1** were added into the isotonic fungal suspensions (1×10^4 CFU/mL) and incubated at 37 °C for 15 h. Thereafter, their conductivities were measured and recorded as A_1 (0, 3, 6, 9, 12, 15 h). The conductivities of the fungi in 0.1 M PBS treated with boiling water for 5 min were used as the control and marked as A_0. The cell membrane permeability was then calculated using the formula: Electric conductivity = $A_1 - A_0$.

4.7.4. Leakage of 260 nm and 280 nm Absorbing Material

Fungal strains were cultured in RPMI-1640 and incubated at 37 °C for 12 h. The most active compound **1** were added to the fungal suspensions at 1-fold and 1/2-fold of the MIC values. Suspensions were incubated at 37 °C and samples were removed at times 0, 2,

4, 6, 8, and 10 h and centrifuged at 10,000× g for 10 min at 4 °C. 200 µL of supernatants from each condition were added to a 96-well plate. Wells and absorbance values at 260 nm and 280 nm were recorded using a UV spectrophotometer. The following controls were included: a fungal suspension in RPMI-1640 without antimicrobial agents as the negative control; a fungal suspension with AMB as the positive controls.

4.7.5. Detection of Na^+/K^+-ATPase and Ca^{2+}-ATPase

The fungal cells obtained from the logarithmic growth phase were treated with the compound **1** at $\frac{1}{2}$ and 1-fold of the MIC value at 37 °C for 72 h. Drug-treated fungal solutions were rinsed with sterile PBS and resuspended (1×10^4 cells mL^{-1}). The activities of Na^+/K^+-ATPase and Ca^{2+}-ATPase were analyzed using commercial kits (NanJing JianCheng, Nanjing, China) according to the instructions.

4.7.6. Measurement of Intracellular ATPase Concentration

The fungal cells obtained from the logarithmic growth phase were treated with the compound **1** at $\frac{1}{2}$ and 1-fold of the MIC value at 37 °C for 72 h. Drug-treated fungal solutions were rinsed with sterile PBS and resuspended (1×10^4 cells mL^{-1}). The intracellular ATPase concentration was determined using the ATP assay kit (NanJing JianCheng, Nanjing, China).

4.7.7. Detection of MDH and SDH

The fungal cells obtained from the logarithmic growth phase were treated with the compound **1** at $\frac{1}{2}$ and 1-fold of the MIC value at 37 °C for 72 h. Drug-treated fungal solutions were rinsed with sterile PBS and resuspended (1×10^4 cells mL^{-1}). The activities of MDH and SDH were analyzed using commercial kits (NanJing JianCheng, Nanjing, China) according to the instructions.

Supplementary Materials: The following supporting information can be downloaded at: https://www.mdpi.com/article/10.3390/md22010038/s1. Figures S1–S35: NMR, HR-ESI-MS and UV spectra for compounds **1–4**.

Author Contributions: Conceptualization, C.G. and Y.L.; methodology, Z.W., J.Y. (Jianglin Yin), J.Y. (Jie Yang) and C.J. validation, M.B.; formal analysis, Z.W., J.Y. (Jianglin Yin) and M.B.; investigation, Z.W., J.Y. (Jianglin Yin) and J.Y. (Jie Yang); resources, C.G. and Y.L.; data curation, Z.W. and J.Y. (Jianglin Yin); Writing—review and editing, Z.W., J.Y. (Jianglin Yin), M.B., C.J., X.Y., Y.L. and C.G.; visualization, Z.W., J.Y. (Jianglin Yin) and M.B.; supervision, C.G. and Y.L.; project administration, Y.L. and C.G.; funding acquisition, Y.L. and C.G. All authors have read and agreed to the published version of the manuscript.

Funding: This study was supported by the National Natural Science Foundation of China (82060640), Natural Science Foundation of Guangxi (2020GXNSFGA297002), National Natural Science Foundation (U20A20101), Special Fund for Bagui Scholars of Guangxi (Yonghong Liu), Guangxi University of Chinese Medicine "Guipai Traditional Chinese Medicine Inheritance and Innovation Team" Project (2022A007), High-level Talent of Guangxi Traditional Chinese Medicine (2022C008), and The scientific Research Foundation of Institute of Marine Drugs, GXUCM (2018ZD005-C03).

Data Availability Statement: The data presented in this study are available upon request from the corresponding author.

Conflicts of Interest: The authors declare no conflict of interest.

References

1. Hu, Y.; Zhang, J.; Li, X.; Yang, Y.; Zhang, Y.; Ma, J.; Xi, L. *Penicillium marneffei* infection: An emerging disease in mainland China. *Mycopathologia* **2013**, *175*, 57–67. [CrossRef]
2. Imwidthaya, P. Update of *Penicillosis marneffei* in Thailand. *Mycopathologia* **1994**, *127*, 135–137. [CrossRef] [PubMed]
3. Tsang, C.C.; Lau, S.K.; Woo, P.C. Sixty years from Segretain's description: What have we learned and should learn about the basic mycology of *Talaromyces marneffei*? *Mycopathologia* **2019**, *184*, 721–729. [CrossRef] [PubMed]

4. Lau, S.K.; Lo, G.C.; Lam, C.S.; Chow, W.N.; Ngan, A.H.; Wu, A.K. In vitro activity of posaconazole against *Talaromyces marneffei* by broth microdilution and Etest methods and comparison to itraconazole, voriconazole, and anidulafungin. *Antimicrob. Agents Chemother.* **2017**, *61*, e01480-16. [CrossRef] [PubMed]
5. Liu, D.; Liang, L.; Chen, J. In vitro antifungal drug susceptibilities of *Penicillium marneffei* from China. *J. Infect. Chemother.* **2013**, *19*, 776–778. [CrossRef]
6. Supparatpinyo, K.; Schlamm, H.T. Voriconazole as therapy for systemic *Penicillium marneffei* infections in AIDS patients. *Am. J. Trop. Med. Hyg.* **2007**, *77*, 350–353. [CrossRef]
7. Wu, T.C.; Chan, J.W.; Ng, C.K.; Tsang, D.N.; Lee, M.P.; Li, P.C. Clinical presentations and outcomes of *Penicillium marneffei* infections: A series from 1994 to 2004. *Hong Kong Med. J.* **2008**, *14*, 103.
8. Larsson, M.; Nguyen, L.H.T.; Wertheim, H.F.; Dao, T.T.; Taylor, W.; Horby, P. Clinical characteristics and outcome of *Penicillium marneffei* infection among HIV-infected patients in northern Vietnam. *AIDS Res. Ther.* **2012**, *9*, 24. [CrossRef]
9. Son, V.T.; Khue, P.M.; Strobel, M. Penicilliosis and AIDS in Haiphong, Vietnam: Evolution and predictive factors of death. *Med. Mal. Infect.* **2014**, *44*, 495–501. [CrossRef]
10. Antinori, S.; Gianelli, E.; Bonaccorso, C.; Ridolfo, A.L.; Croce, F.; Sollima, S.; Parravicini, C. Disseminated *Penicillium marneffei* infection in an HIV-positive Italian patient and a review of cases reported outside endemic regions. *J. Travel Med.* **2006**, *13*, 181–188. [CrossRef]
11. Castro-Lainez, M.T.; Sierra-Hoffman, M.; LLompart-Zeno, J.; Adams, R.; Howell, A.; Hoffman-Roberts, H. *Talaromyces marneffei* infection in a non-HIV non-endemic population. *IDCases* **2018**, *12*, 21–24. [CrossRef]
12. Julander, I.; Petrini, B. *Penicillium marneffei* infection in a Swedish HIV-infected immunodeficient narcotic addict. *Scand. J. Infect. Dis.* **1997**, *29*, 320–322. [CrossRef]
13. De Monte, A.; Risso, K.; Normand, A.C.; Boyer, G.; L'Ollivier, C.; Marty, P.; Gari-Toussaint, M. Chronic pulmonary penicilliosis due to *Penicillium marneffei*: Late presentation in a french traveler. *J. Travel Med.* **2014**, *21*, 292–294. [CrossRef] [PubMed]
14. Patassi, A.A.; Saka, B.; Landoh, D.E.; Kotosso, A.; Mawu, K.; Halatoko, W.A. First observation in a non-endemic country (Togo) of *Penicillium marneffei* infection in a human immunodeficiency virus-infected patient: A case report. *BMC Res. Notes* **2013**, *6*, 506. [CrossRef] [PubMed]
15. Pautler, K.B.; Padhye, A.; Ajello, L. Imported *Penicilliosis marneffei* in the United States: Report of a second human infection. *Sabouraudia* **1984**, *22*, 433–438. [CrossRef] [PubMed]
16. Li, L.; Chen, K.; Dhungana, N.; Jang, Y.; Chaturvedi, V.; Desmond, E. Characterization of clinical isolates of *Talaromyces marneffei* and related species, California, USA. *Emerg. Infect. Dis.* **2019**, *25*, 1765. [CrossRef] [PubMed]
17. Kalasuba, K.; Miranti, M.; Rahayuningsih, S.R.; Safriansyah, W.; Syamsuri, R.R.P.; Farabi, K.; Oktavia, D.; Alhasnawi, A.N.; Doni, F. Red Mangrove (*Rhizophora stylosa* Griff.)-A Review of Its Botany, Phytochemistry, Pharmacological Activities, and Prospects. *Plants* **2023**, *12*, 2196. [CrossRef]
18. Ye, J.J.; Zou, R.J.; Zhou, D.D.; Deng, X.L.; Wu, N.L.; Chen, D.D.; Xu, J. Insights into the phylogenetic diversity, biological activities, and biosynthetic potential of mangrove rhizosphere Actinobacteria from Hainan Island. *Front. Microbiol.* **2023**, *14*, 1157601. [CrossRef]
19. Xu, J. Biomolecules produced by mangrove-associated microbes. *Curr. Med. Chem.* **2011**, *18*, 5224–5266. [CrossRef]
20. Xu, J. Bioactive natural products derived from mangrove-associated microbes. *RSC Adv.* **2015**, *5*, 841–892. [CrossRef]
21. Jiang, Z.K.; Tuo, L.; Huang, D.L.; Osterman, I.A.; Tyurin, A.P.; Liu, S.W. Diversity, novelty, and antimicrobial activity of endophytic actinobacteria from mangrove plants in Beilun Estuary National Nature Reserve of Guangxi, China. *Front. Microbiol.* **2018**, *9*, 868. [CrossRef] [PubMed]
22. Li, K.; Chen, S.; Pang, X.; Cai, J.; Zhang, X.; Liu, Y. Natural products from mangrove sediments-derived microbes: Structural diversity, bioactivities, biosynthesis, and total synthesis. *Eur. J. Med. Chem.* **2022**, *230*, 114117. [CrossRef] [PubMed]
23. Tian, X.; Zhang, S.; Li, W. Advance in marine actinobacterial research--A review. *Wei Sheng Wu Xue Bao = Acta Microbiol. Sin.* **2011**, *51*, 161–169.
24. Jiang, S.; Li, M.; Hou, S.; Han, M.; Yin, J.; Gao, C. Diversity and anti-aging activity of endophytic actinobacteria from true mangrove plants collected from the west coast of Hainan. *Guihaia* **2020**, *40*, 320–326.
25. Wang, Y.F.; Wei, S.J.; Zhang, Z.P.; Zhan, T.H.; Tu, G.Q. Antifungalmycin, an antifungal macrolide from *Streptomyces padanus* 702. *Nat. Prod. Bioprospecting* **2012**, *2*, 41–45. [CrossRef]
26. Xiong, Z.Q.; Tu, X.R.; Wei, S.J.; Huang, L.; Li, X.H.; Lu, H.; Tu, G.Q. The mechanism of antifungal action of a new polyene macrolide antibiotic antifungalmycin 702 from *Streptomyces padanus* JAU4234 on the rice sheath blight pathogen *Rhizoctonia solani*. *PLoS ONE* **2013**, *8*, e73884. [CrossRef] [PubMed]
27. Song, X.; Jiang, X.; Sun, J.; Zhang, C.; Zhang, Y.; Lu, L.; Ju, J. Antibacterial secondary metabolites produced by mangrove-derived Actinomycete Stremptmeces costaricanus SCSIO ZS0073. *Nat. Prod. Res. Dev.* **2017**, *29*, 410.
28. Rochet, P.; Lancelin, J.M. Revised ^{1}H and ^{13}C NMR assignments of the polyene antibiotic filipin III. *Magn. Reson. Chem.* **1997**, *35*, 538–542. [CrossRef]
29. Barreales, E.G.; Rumbero, Á.; Payero, T.D.; de Pedro, A.; Jambrina, E.; Aparicio, J.F. Structural and bioactivity characterization of filipin derivatives from engineered *Streptomyces filipinensis* strains reveals clues for reduced haemolytic action. *Antibiotics* **2020**, *9*, 413. [CrossRef]

30. Cai, R.; Hu, M.; Zhang, Y.; Niu, C.; Yue, T.; Yuan, Y.; Wang, Z. Antifungal activity and mechanism of citral, limonene and eugenol against *Zygosaccharomyces rouxii*. *LWT* **2019**, *106*, 50–56. [CrossRef]
31. Kohanski, M.A.; Dwyer, D.J.; Collins, J.J. How antibiotics kill bacteria: From targets to networks. *Nat. Rev. Microbiol.* **2010**, *8*, 423–435. [CrossRef] [PubMed]
32. Zhang, J.; Ye, K.P.; Zhang, X.; Pan, D.D.; Sun, Y.Y.; Cao, J.X. Antibacterial activity and mechanism of action of black pepper essential oil on meat-borne Escherichia coli. *Front. Microbiol.* **2017**, *7*, 2094. [CrossRef] [PubMed]
33. Alyousef, A.A. Antifungal Activity and Mechanism of Action of Different Parts of Myrtus communis Growing in Saudi Arabia against *Candida* Spp. *J. Nanomater.* **2021**, *2021*, 3484125. [CrossRef]
34. Zhang, J.; Cui, X.; Zhang, M.; Bai, B.; Yang, Y.; Fan, S. The antibacterial mechanism of perilla rosmarinic acid. *Biotechnol. Appl. Biochem.* **2022**, *69*, 1757–1764. [CrossRef]
35. Primeau, J.O.; Armanious, G.P.; Fisher, M.L.E.; Young, H.S. The sarcoendoplasmic reticulum calcium ATPase. *Membr. Protein Complexes Struct. Funct.* **2018**, *87*, 229–258.
36. Lau, S.K.P.; Tsang, C.C.; Woo, P.C.Y. *Talaromyces marneffei* genomic, transcriptomic, proteomic and metabolomic studies reveal mechanisms for environmental adaptations and virulence. *Toxins* **2017**, *9*, 192. [CrossRef] [PubMed]
37. Cui, H.; Zhang, C.; Li, C.; Lin, L. Antibacterial mechanism of oregano essential oil. *Ind. Crops Prod.* **2019**, *139*, 111498. [CrossRef]
38. Van Vranken, J.G.; Na, U.; Winge, D.R.; Rutter, J. Protein-mediated assembly of succinate dehydrogenase and its cofactors. *Crit. Rev. Biochem. Mol. Biol.* **2015**, *50*, 168–180. [CrossRef]
39. Mathew, B.P.; Nath, M. Recent approaches to antifungal therapy for invasive mycoses. *ChemMedChem Chem. Enabling Drug Discov.* **2009**, *4*, 310–323. [CrossRef]
40. Zotchev, S.B. Polyene macrolide antibiotics and their applications in human therapy. *Curr. Med. Chem.* **2003**, *10*, 211–223. [CrossRef]
41. Bhatnagar, I.; Kim, S.K. Immense essence of excellence: Marine microbial bioactive compounds. *Mar. Drugs* **2010**, *8*, 2673–2701. [CrossRef] [PubMed]
42. Shi, Y.; Cai, M.J.; Zhou, L.L.; Wang, H.D. The structure and function of cell membranes studied by atomic force microscopy. *Semin. Cell Dev. Biol* **2018**, *73*, 31–44. [CrossRef] [PubMed]
43. Ma, M.M.; Wen, X.F.; Xie, Y.T.; Guo, Z.; Zhao, R.B.; Yu, P.; Gong, D.M.; Deng, S.G.; Zeng, Z.L. Antifungal activity and mechanism of monocaprin against food spoilage fungi. *Food Control* **2018**, *84*, 561–568. [CrossRef]
44. Elsadek, L.A.; Matthews, J.H.; Nishimura, S.; Nakatani, T.; Ito, A.; Gu, T. Genomic and targeted approaches unveil the cell membrane as a major target of the antifungal cytotoxin amantelide A. *ChemBioChem* **2021**, *22*, 1790–1799. [CrossRef] [PubMed]
45. Szomek, M.; Reinholdt, P.; Walther, H.L.; Scheidt, H.A.; Müller, P.; Obermaier, S.; Wüstner, D. Natamycin sequesters ergosterol and interferes with substrate transport by the lysine transporter Lyp1 from yeast. *Biochim. Biophys. Acta (BBA)-Biomembr.* **2022**, *1864*, 184012. [CrossRef] [PubMed]
46. Xiao, L.; Niu, H.J.; Qu, T.L.; Zhang, X.F.; Du, F.Y. Streptomyces sp. FX13 inhibits fungicide-resistant Botrytis cinerea in vitro and in vivo by producing oligomycin A. *Pestic. Biochem. Physiol.* **2021**, *175*, 104834. [CrossRef] [PubMed]
47. Kamble, M.T.; Rudtanatip, T.; Soowannayan, C.; Nambunruang, B.; Medhe, S.V.; Wongprasert, K. Depolymerized Fractions of Sulfated Galactans Extracted from Gracilaria fisheri and Their Antibacterial Activity against *Vibrio parahaemolyticus* and *Vibrio harveyi*. *Mar. Drugs* **2022**, *20*, 469. [CrossRef] [PubMed]
48. Qin, Y.; Wang, J.; Lv, Q.; Han, B. Recent Progress in Research on Mitochondrion-Targeted Antifungal Drugs: A Review. *Antimicrob. Agents Chemother.* **2023**, *67*, e00003-23. [CrossRef]
49. Xin, Z.; OuYang, Q.; Wan, C.; Che, J.; Li, L.; Chen, J.; Tao, N. Isolation of antofine from Cynanchum atratum BUNGE (Asclepiadaceae) and its antifungal activity against *Penicillium digitatum*. *Postharvest Biol. Technol.* **2019**, *157*, 110961. [CrossRef]
50. Zhao, W.B.; Zhao, Z.M.; Ma, Y.; Li, A.P.; Zhang, Z.J.; Hu, Y.M. Antifungal activity and preliminary mechanism of pristimerin against *Sclerotinia sclerotiorum*. *Ind. Crops Prod.* **2022**, *185*, 115124. [CrossRef]
51. Kai-Su, P.; Hong, L.; Dong-Yan, Z.; Yan-Qing, Z.; Andrianopoulos, A.; Latgé, J.P.; Cun-Wei, C. Study on the mechanisms of action of berberine combined with fluconazole against fluconazole-resistant strains of *Talaromyces marneffei*. *Front. Microbiol.* **2022**, *13*, 1033211. [CrossRef] [PubMed]
52. Kang, S.; Kong, F.; Shi, X.; Han, H.; Li, M.; Guan, B. Antibacterial activity and mechanism of lactobionic acid against *Pseudomonas fluorescens* and Methicillin-resistant *Staphylococcus aureus* and its application on whole milk. *Food Control* **2020**, *108*, 106876. [CrossRef]
53. Maliehe, T.S.; Nqotheni, M.I.; Shandu, J.S.; Selepe, T.N.; Masoko, P.; Pooe, O.J. Chemical Profile, Antioxidant and Antibacterial Activities, Mechanisms of Action of the Leaf Extract of *Aloe arborescens* Mill. *Plants* **2023**, *12*, 869. [CrossRef] [PubMed]

Disclaimer/Publisher's Note: The statements, opinions and data contained in all publications are solely those of the individual author(s) and contributor(s) and not of MDPI and/or the editor(s). MDPI and/or the editor(s) disclaim responsibility for any injury to people or property resulting from any ideas, methods, instructions or products referred to in the content.

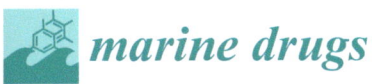 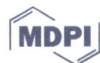

Article

Hepialiamides A–C: Aminated Fusaric Acid Derivatives and Related Metabolites with Anti-Inflammatory Activity from the Deep-Sea-Derived Fungus *Samsoniella hepiali* W7

Zheng-Biao Zou [1,2,†], Tai-Zong Wu [2,†], Long-He Yang [3], Xi-Wen He [3], Wen-Ya Liu [1], Kai Zhang [2], Chun-Lan Xie [2], Ming-Min Xie [2], Yong Zhang [2], Xian-Wen Yang [2,*] and Jun-Song Wang [1,*]

[1] Center for Molecular Metabolism, School of Environmental and Biological Engineering, Nanjing University of Science and Technology, 200 Xiaolingwei Street, Nanjing 210094, China; zhengbiaozou@njust.edu.cn (Z.-B.Z.); wenyaliu2015@163.com (W.-Y.L.)

[2] Key Laboratory of Marine Genetic Resources, Third Institute of Oceanography, Ministry of Natural Resources, 184 Daxue Road, Xiamen 361005, China; wutaizong@tio.org.cn (T.-Z.W.); z18252730063@163.com (K.Z.); xiechunlanxx@163.com (C.-L.X.); xiemingmin@tio.org.cn (M.-M.X.); zhangyong@tio.org.cn (Y.Z.)

[3] Technical Innovation Center for Utilization of Marine Biological Resources, Third Institute of Oceanography, Ministry of Natural Resources, 184 Daxue Road, Xiamen 361005, China; longheyang@tio.org.cn (L.-H.Y.); hexiwen1224@163.com (X.-W.H.)

* Correspondence: yangxianwen@tio.org.cn (X.-W.Y.); wang.junsong@gmail.com (J.-S.W.); Tel.: +86-592-2195319 (X.-W.Y.); +86-25-8431-5512 (J.-S.W.)

† These authors contributed equally to this work.

Abstract: A systematic investigation combined with a Global Natural Products Social (GNPS) molecular networking approach, was conducted on the metabolites of the deep-sea-derived fungus *Samsoniella hepiali* W7, leading to the isolation of three new fusaric acid derivatives, hepialiamides A–C (**1–3**) and one novel hybrid polyketide hepialide (**4**), together with 18 known miscellaneous compounds (**5–22**). The structures of the new compounds were elucidated through detailed spectroscopic analysis. as well as TD-DFT-based ECD calculation. All isolates were tested for anti-inflammatory activity in vitro. Under a concentration of 1 μM, compounds **8**, **11**, **13**, **21**, and **22** showed potent inhibitory activity against nitric oxide production in lipopolysaccharide (LPS)-activated BV-2 microglia cells, with inhibition rates of 34.2%, 30.7%, 32.9%, 38.6%, and 58.2%, respectively. Of particularly note is compound **22**, which exhibited the most remarkable inhibitory activity, with an IC$_{50}$ value of 426.2 nM.

Keywords: deep-sea-derived fungus; fusaric acid derivatives; GNPS molecular networking; inflammation; nitric oxide production

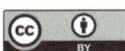

1. Introduction

Secondary metabolites produced by marine-derived fungi have been proven to possess a broad spectrum of bioactivities, such as cytotoxicity, antibacterial, antioxidant, antimalarial, anti-inflammatory, and antiviral properties and have been recognized as significant chemical entities for drug discovery [1–8]. However, continuous investigations on secondary metabolites from marine-derived fungi have led to a high frequency of rediscovery of known compounds, for which, dereplication becomes critical in microbial biodiscovery. Mass spectrometry-based GNPS molecular networking (https://gnps.ucsd.edu, accessed on 1 January 2016) is a strategy that has been proven to be a powerful and promising tool for dereplication. GNPS uses an untargeted metabolomics approach that powerfully processes tandem mass spectrometry (MS/MS) fragmentation data. It is a vector-based workflow that calculates cosine scores (between 0 and 1) to determine the degree of similarity between MS^2 fragments. These fragment ions (nodes) are then organized into relational networks depending on their similarity [9–11]. GNPS has been widely used to identify known compounds and potential new analogs, greatly speeding up the dereplication and structure-based discovery of natural products [12–14].

Fusaric acid (FA), featuring a picolinic acid core, is a well-known mycotoxin commonly found in the metabolites of numerous *Fusarium* species. The biosynthesis of FA and its related analogues has attracted attention since the last century due to the intriguing pyridine moiety, which has been proven to start from an aspartic acid precursor and malonyl-CoA [15–18]. However, naturally occurring amidated derivatives of FA have not been well-described yet in terms of their structural diversity and biological activity, with only two examples reported so far, including atransfusarin from the endophytic fungus *Alternaria atrans* MP-7 [19] and 2-(4-butylpicolinamide) acetic acid from *Fusarium fujikuroi* [20]. Atransfusarin was documented with mild anti-fungi activity while 2-(4-butylpicolinamide) acetic acid was inactive against the tested pathogens.

As part of our ongoing exploration of structurally novel and bioactive secondary metabolites from marine microbes [21–24], we performed a systematic investigation, aided by a GNPS molecular networking approach, on the crude extract of the culture of fungus *Samsoniella epialid* W7, isolated from the sulfide at a depth of 3073 m in the South Atlantic. Prior to isolation, the GNPS network of the extract revealed a big molecular cluster within which none of the nodes were identified by the internal compound library (Figure 1), indicating a certain possibility of new compounds to be found among these metabolites. A further scrutiny of their MS/MS fragmentation pattern (Figure S29), followed by HRMS-based molecular formula analysis, strongly suggested that they were new analogues of fusaric amides [20]. The systematic isolation, along with targeted purification, finally yielded three new fusaric acids, hepialiamides A–C (**1**–**3**), and one novel hybrid polyketide, hepialide (**4**), together with 18 known compounds (**5**–**22**) (Figure 2). The known compounds **8**, **11**, **13**, **21**, and **22** exhibited inhibitory activity against LPS-induced NO production. Herein, we report the fermentation, isolation, structure characterization and bioactivity of these isolates.

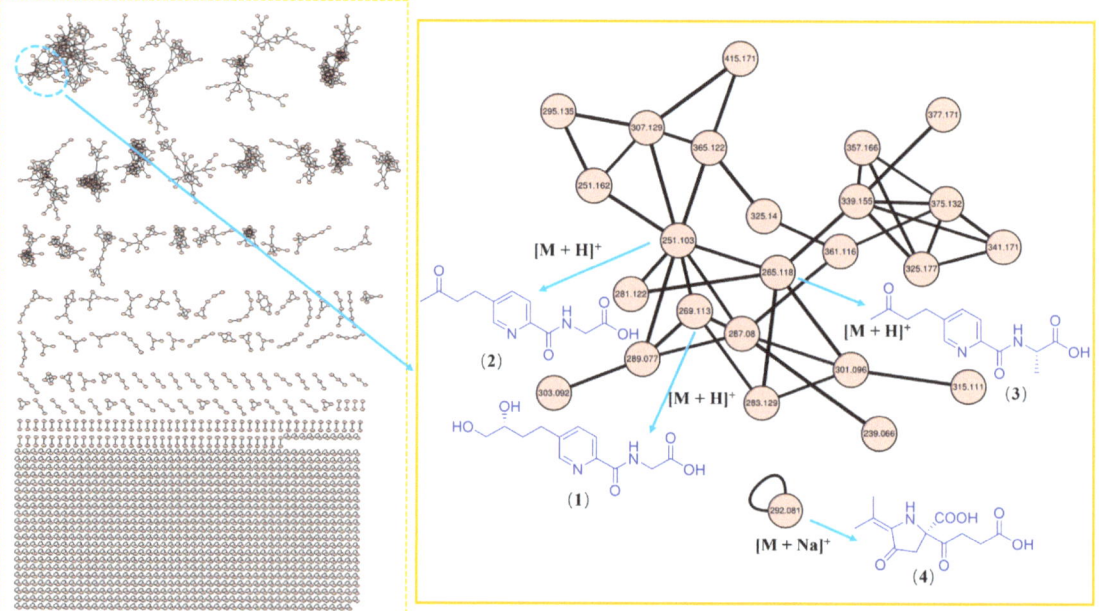

Figure 1. Molecular network of extract of the fungus *Samsoniella hepiali* W7. The cluster of new compounds (**1**–**4**) is expanded, and the nodes are marked with the *m/z* value of the parent ion.

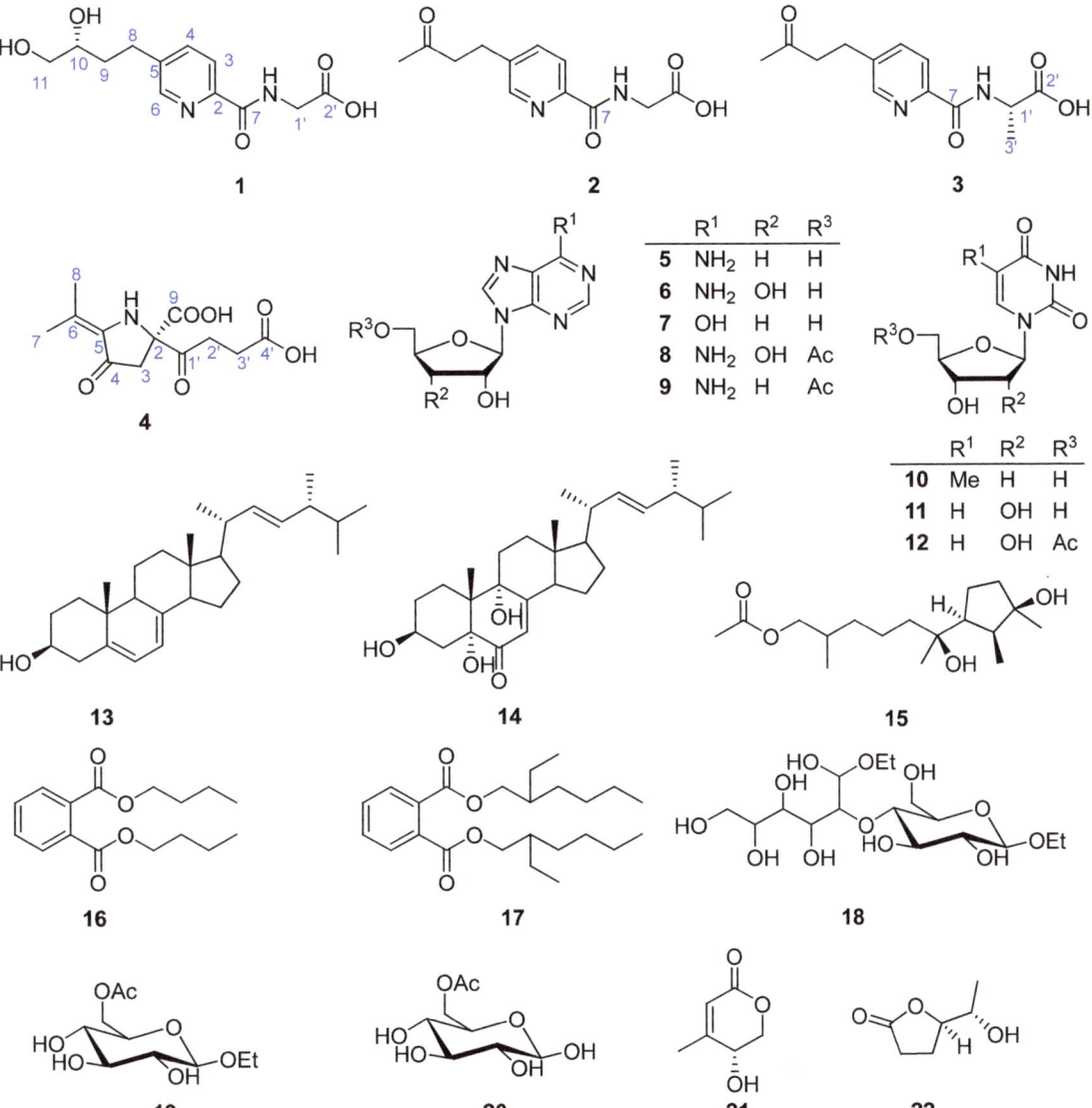

Figure 2. Compounds **1–22** from *Samsoniella hepiali* W7.

2. Results and Discussion

Compound **1** was isolated as a yellow oil. The HRESI(+)MS of **1** exhibited a protonated molecular ion [M + H]$^+$ at m/z 269.1142, indicating a molecular formula of C$_{12}$H$_{17}$N$_2$O$_5$, accounting for seven degrees of unsaturation (DoU). The ^{1}H NMR (Table 1) data of **1** presented the diagnostic signals of three aromatic protons, typically an ABX coupling system at δ_H 8.51 (1H, d, J = 1.5 Hz, H-6), 7.96 (1H, d, J = 8.0 Hz, H-3), and 7.83 (1H, dd, J = 8.0, 2.0 Hz, H-4), indicating the presence of a 2,5-disubstituted pyridine ring in **1**. This was confirmed by the key heteronuclear multiple bond correlation (HMBC) cross-peaks from H-3 to C-5 (δ_C 141.4), from H-4 to C-2 (δ_C 147.3) and C-6 (δ_C 148.5), and from H-6 to C-2 and C-4 (δ_C 137.4), as well as by the correlation spectroscopy (COSY) correlations of H-3/H-4.

Table 1. ^{1}H (400 Hz) and ^{13}C NMR (100 Hz) spectroscopic data of compounds **1–3**.

No.	1 [a] (δ_C, Type)	1 [a] (δ_H, Mult J in Hz)	2 [b] (δ_C, Type)	2 [b] (δ_H, Mult J in Hz)	3 [a] (δ_C, Type)	3 [a] (δ_H, Mult J in Hz)
2	147.3, C		148.4, C		147.4, C	
3	121.7, CH	7.96, d (8.0)	122.8, CH	7.96, d (8.0)	121.6, CH	7.93, d (7.6)
4	137.4, CH	7.83, dd (2.0, 8.0)	138.3, CH	7.77, dd (2.0, 8.0)	137.4, CH	7.82, d (8.0)
5	141.4, C		141.9, C		141.3, C	
6	148.5, CH	8.51, d (1.5)	150.1, CH	8.47, d (1.6)	148.7, CH	8.51, s
7	164.2, C		167.0, C		163.5, C	
8	28.3, CH$_2$	2.71, m; 2.82, m	27.5, CH$_2$	2.90, d (5.2)	26.1, CH$_2$	2.85, m
9	34.7, CH$_2$	1.56, m; 1.77, m	44.6, CH$_2$	2.88, d (5.2)	43.3, CH$_2$	2.84, m
10	70.2, CH	3.39, m	209.8, C		207.3, C	
11	65.8, CH$_2$	3.25, dd (5.7, 10.7) 3.32, dd (5.6, 10.7)	29.9, CH$_3$	2.13, s	29.7, CH$_3$	2.09, s
1′	41.0, CH$_2$	3.97, s	41.9, CH$_2$	4.15, s	47.6, CH	4.46, d (7.1)
2′	171.1, C		172.8, C		173.8, C	
3′					17.5, CH$_3$	1.42, d (7.1)
NH		8.92, t (6.0)		9.04, t (5.4)		8.74, d (7.3)

[a] Measured in DMSO-d_6. [b] Measured in methanol-d_4.

Furthermore, four methylene groups at δ_H 3.97 (2H, s, H-1′), [2.71 (1H, m, H-8), 2.82 (1H, m, H-8)] and [1.56 (1H, m, H-9), 1.77 (1H, m, H-9)], [3.25 (1H, dd, J = 10.7, 5.7 Hz, H-11), 3.32 (1H, dd, J = 10.7, 5.6 Hz, H-11)] and one oxymethine at δ_H 3.39 (1H, m, H-10), were observed (Table 1). The ^{1}H-^{1}H COSY correlations of H-8/H-9/H-10/H-11, together with the HMBC correlations from H-11 to C-10 (δ_C 70.2) and C-9 (δ_C 34.7), from H-10 to C-9 and C-8 (δ_C 28.3), from H-9 to C-8 and C-5, and from H-8 to C-4, C-5, and C-6 indicated a 1,2-butanediol moiety at C-5. Further HMBC correlations of H-1′ to C-7 (δ_C 164.2) and C-2′ (δ_C 171.1) suggested the presence of a glycine moiety (Figure 3). An amido bond between C-2 of the pyridine ring and C-1′ of the glycine unit was confirmed by key HMBC correlations from H-3 and H-1′ to C-7. Thus, compound **1** was identified as a new fusaric acid derivative and given the trivial name hepialiamide A. The comparison of its optical rotation value ($[\alpha]_D^{25}$ + 13) with those of similar known compounds, such as (R)-4-phenyl-1,2-butanediol ($[\alpha]_D^{20}$ + 33) and (S)-4-phenyl-1,2-butanediol ($[\alpha]_D^{20}$ − 34) [25], and comparative analysis of the experimental and theoretically calculated ECD curves established the absolute configuration of hepialiamide A to be 10R (Figure 4).

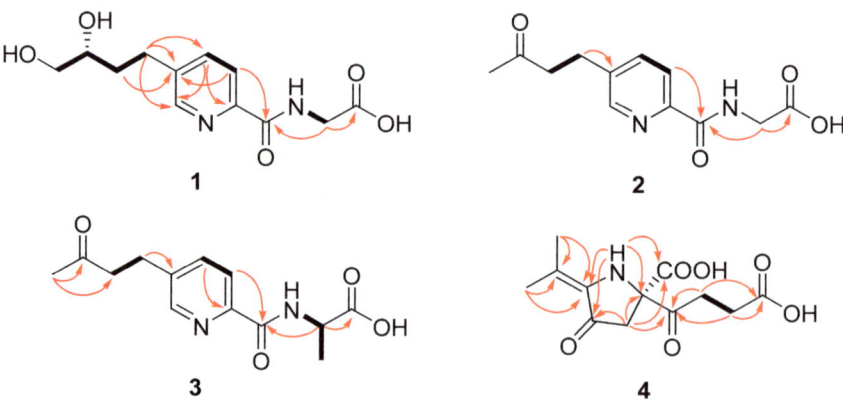

Figure 3. Key HMBC (arrows) and ^{1}H–^{1}H COSY (bold) correlations of compounds **1–4**.

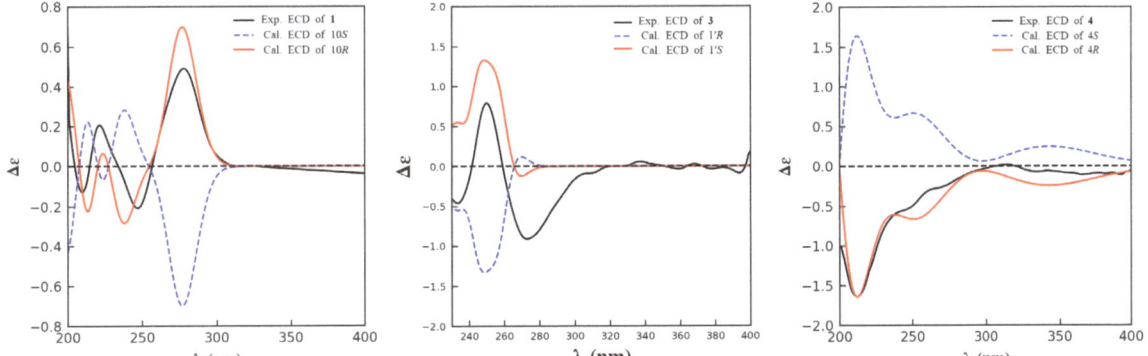

Figure 4. Experimental and calculated ECD spectra of **1**, **3**, and **4**.

Compound **2** was isolated as a yellow oil. The HRESI(+)MS of **2** exhibited a protonated molecular ion [M + H]$^+$ at m/z 251.0950. Analysis of the HRESI(+)MS and ^{13}C NMR data revealed the molecular formula $C_{12}H_{14}N_2O_4$ of **2** indicating seven DoUs. The NMR data (Table 1) of **2** were closely related to those of **1**, except for the presence of a methyl ketone group at (δ_C 209.8, C-10) and (δ_C 29.9, δ_H 2.13, CH$_3$-11) in **2**, which was supported by the HMBC correlations of H$_3$-11 to C-10 and C-9 (δ_C 44.6). The left of the structure was confirmed by 2D NMR correlations, as shown (Figure 3). Therefore, **2** was identified as a new analogue of **1** and named hepialiamide B.

Compound **3** was obtained as a yellow oil with the molecular formula of $C_{13}H_{16}N_2O_4$ implied by its HRESI(+)MS spectrum. The 1D NMR data (Table 1) of **3** were similar to those of **2** except that **3** had an extra methyl group [δ_C 18.2 (C-4′)] at C-2′, which was confirmed by the COSY correlations of NH (δ_H 8.74, d)/H-1′ (δ_H 4.46, d)/H-3′ (δ_H 1.42, d) and the HMBC correlations from H-1′ to C-2′ (δ_C 173.8), C-3′ (δ_C 17.5), and C-7 (δ_C 163.5). The absolute configuration of the chiral center C-1′ in **3** was established to be *S*, as indicated by the agreement between the calculated ECD spectrum of **3** and the experimental data (Figure 4). Hence, compound **3** was identified as another new fusaric acid derivative, and named hepialiamide C.

Compound **4** was obtained as a yellow oil. The HRESI(+)MS of **4** exhibited a sodiated molecular ion [M + Na]$^+$ at m/z 292.0800, suggesting a molecular formula (calculated for $C_{12}H_{15}NO_6Na$, 292.0797) that requires six DoUs. The ^{1}H NMR (Table 2) data of **4** presented the diagnostic signals of three methylene groups at δ_H 2.28 (2H, t, J = 6.3 Hz, H-2′), 2.64 (2H, q, J = 6.9 Hz, H-3′), and 3.10 (2H, q, J = 15.0 Hz, H-3), and two methyl groups at 2.08 (3H, s, H-8) and 1.81 (3H, s, H-9). In the ^{13}C NMR spectrum, 12 carbon signals were observed and classified as two methyl (δ_C 20.8, 18.5), three methylene (δ_C 47.4, 36.3, 27.4), and seven non-protonated carbons (δ_C 207.2, 197.0, 173.5, 171.4, 1129.1, 122.3, 70.3), with the aid of HSQC data. In the ^{1}H-^{1}H COSY spectrum of **4**, homonuclear vicinal coupling correlation (Figure 3) between H-7 and H-8, along with the HMBC correlations from H-7 to C-5/6, from H-8 to C-5/6, indicated an isopropenyl group. The HMBC cross-peaks observed from H-3 to C-2/4/9, H-7/8 to C-4, and the diagnostic signals from an exchangeable proton to C-2/4/5/9 permitted the construction of a five-member ring. Finally, based on the rest of the HMBC correlations from H-3 to C-1′, H-2′ to C-1′/3′/4′, from H-3′ to C-1′/4′, and the COSY signals between H-2′ to H-3′, together with a comparable analysis of the chemical shifts of C-2/5 in **4** and those in literature [26,27], the planar structure of **4** was assigned as shown.

Table 2. ^{1}H (400 Hz) and ^{13}C (100 Hz) NMR spectroscopic data of compound **4** in DMSO-d_6.

No.	δ_C, Type	δ_H, Mult (J in Hz)
2	70.3, C	
3	47.4, CH$_2$	3.15, d (18.0); 3.06, d (18.0)
4	197.0, C	
5	122.3, C	
6	129.1, C	
7	18.5, CH$_3$	2.08, s
8	20.8, CH$_3$	1.81, s
9	171.4, C	
1'	207.2, C	
2'	27.4, CH$_2$	2.28, t (6.3)
3'	36.3, CH$_2$	2.68, m; 2.60, m
4'	173.5, C	
NH		10.27, s

To further assign the absolute configuration of C-2, a theoretical calculation of the ECD spectra of the 4R- and 4S-isomers was conducted. The experimental ECD spectrum of **4** was in good accordance with the calculated result for the 4R-configured **4** (Figure 4). The structure of compound **4** was thus determined and named hepialide.

By comparing the NMR, MS, ECD, and OR data with those reported in the references, 18 previously described components were identified as cordycepin (**5**) [28], adenosine (**6**) [29], 3'-deoxyinosine (**7**) [30], 5'-O-acetyladenosine (**8**) [31], 5'-acetyl-3'-deoxyadenosine (**9**) [32], thymidine (**10**) [33], uridine (**11**) [34], 5'-O-acetyluridine (**12**) [35], ergosterol (**13**) [36], 3β,5α,9α-trihydroxyergosta-7,22-diene-6-one (**14**) [37], 12-acetoxycycloneran-3,7-diol (**15**) [38], dibutyl phthalate (**16**) [39], di-(2-ethylhexyl)phthalate (**17**) [40], oryzasaccharide A (**18**) [41], D-glucopyranoside, ethyl, 6-acetate (**19**) [42], 6-O-acetyl-D-glucose (**20**) [43], walterolactone A (**21**) [44], and (4R,5S)-5-hydroxyhexan-4-olide (**22**) [45]. Among them, **16** and **17** were previously described as plasticizers and common contaminants in natural products [46].

Naturally occurring aminated fusaric acid derivatives are uncommon in fungal metabolites, as mentioned above. Hepialiamides A–C (**1**–**3**) feature an oxidized fusaric acid core structure with a glycine or alanine coupled through an amide bond, representing the third examples of fusaric amides of fungal origin. Hepialide is a novel PKS-NRPS hybrid polyketide with an unusual isopropenylated pyrrolidone moiety that resembles the tetramic acid.

Neuroinflammation, characterized by the activation of microglia cells, is a common denominator in diverse neurological conditions, including neurodegenerative diseases, traumatic brain injury, and neuroinfectious disorders. Microglia cell activation contributes significantly to the progression of these diseases by releasing pro-inflammatory mediators, exacerbating neuronal damage and impairing synaptic plasticity [47]. Hence, inhibiting glial cell activation emerges as a promising therapeutic strategy. The rich diversity and unique chemical structures of marine compounds provide a vast pool of potential drugs. Inflammatory tests were conducted on BV-2 microglia cells. Stimulation of the cells with bacterial products like lipopolysaccharide (LPS) triggers the production of NO and pro-inflammatory cytokines, key mediators in inflammation [48]. Given the significance of high NO levels in inflammation, targeting inducible nitric oxide synthase (iNOS), the enzyme responsible for NO synthesis, has been suggested as an anti-inflammatory therapeutic approach.

In this LPS-induced BV-2 microglia cell model, we evaluated the inhibitory activity of these compounds on NO production at a low concentration (1 μM). The cells were pre-exposed to the compounds for 1 h, followed by LPS stimulation for 24 h, and subsequently, the concentration of nitrite, the primary metabolite derived from NO, was quantified. The results indicated that compounds **8**, **11**, **13**, **21**, and **22** reduced NO production by 34.2 ± 1.6%, 30.7 ± 4.8%, 32.9 ± 1.6%, 38.6 ± 2.1%, and 58.2 ± 2.6%, respectively, with respect to vehicle-treated stimulated cells (Figure 5A). Particularly noteworthy, further analysis revealed that compound **22** exhibited a remarkable dose-dependent inhibitory effect, with an IC$_{50}$ value of 426.2 nM (Figure 5B).

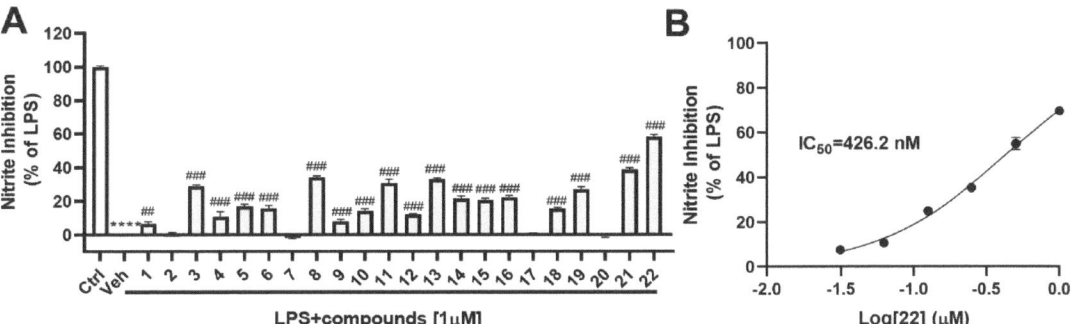

Figure 5. The impact of compounds on NO release in LPS-induced microglia cells: (**A**) Nitrite accumulation in the culture media was quantified using the Griess method, and nitrite production inhibition was calculated compared to the only LPS treated group. Results were normalized to the LPS condition and presented as mean ± SEM (n = 4); **** $p < 0.0001$ vs. Ctrl; ### $p < 0.0001$, ## $p < 0.01$ vs. Veh; (**B**) Inhibitory curve of compound **22** against nitrite production.

These compounds, especially compound **22**, frequently demonstrate anti-inflammatory and immunomodulatory properties, rendering them promising candidates for the development of specific and potent inhibitors that target microglia cell activation pathways. Further research is needed for in-depth evaluation.

3. Materials and Methods

3.1. General Experimental Procedures

Optical rotations were recorded on a Rudolph IV Autopol automatic polarimeter at 25 °C. NMR spectra, including ^{1}H, ^{13}C, DEPT, HSQC, COSY, HMBC, and NOESY were measured on a Bruker Avance 400 MHz spectrometer. Chemical shifts were recorded in δ values using solvent signals (DMSO-d_6: $δ_H$ 2.50/$δ_C$ 39.5; methanol-d_4: $δ_H$ 3.31/$δ_C$ 49.0; CDCl$_3$: $δ_H$ 7.27/$δ_C$ 77.0) as references. HRESIMS data were measured on a Xevo G2 Q-TOF mass spectrometer (Waters Corporation, Milford, MA, USA). Preparative and semipreparative HPLC were performed on an Agilent Technologies 1260 infinity instrument equipped with the DAD detector. UV spectra were recorded on a UV-8000 UV/Vis spectrometer (Shanghai Yuanxi Instrument Co., Ltd., Shanghai, China). Column chromatography (CC) was performed on ODS (50 μm, Daiso, Hiroshima, Japan), silica gel (Qingdao Marine Chemistry Co., Ltd., Qingdao, China), and Sephadex LH-20 (Amersham Pharmacia Biotech AB, Uppsala, Sweden). The TLC plates were visualized under UV light or by spraying with 10% H$_2$SO$_4$. Solvents for isolation were analytical grade. HRMS and MS/MS data were acquired with ultra-high performance liquid chromatography–quadrupole time-of-flight mass spectrometry (UHPLC-Q-TOF MS, AB SCIEX Triple TOF 5600$^+$, Waters Corporation, Milford, MA, USA), with a Phenomenex Kinetex® C18 (100 × 2.1 mm, 2.6 μm).

3.2. Fungal Identification, Fermentation, and Extract

The strain W7 was isolated from a sulfide sample (W 14.52°, S 13.59°) at a depth of 3073 m from the South Atlantic. It was identified as *Samsoniella hepiali* (GenBank accession number OR398925), as the ITS DNA gene sequence alignment demonstrated its similarity to *Samsoniella hepiali* CGMCC 3.17103 (GenBank accession number NR_160318.1). The strain is preserved at the Key Laboratory of Marine Biogenetic Resources, Third Institute of Oceanography, Ministry of Natural Resources (Xiamen, China). The strain *Samsoniella hepiali* was cultured on a PDA plate at 25 °C for 3 days. Fresh mycelia and spores were inoculated into 250 mL Erlenmeyer flasks (×10) containing 30 mL PDB medium and incubated in a 180 rpm rotary shaker at 28 °C for 5 days. Then, the spore cultures were used to inoculate 25 × 1 L Erlenmeyer flasks containing rice medium (80 g rice and 120 mL distilled H_2O for each flask) to perform large-scale fermentation. After 25 days, the fermented culture was extracted with EtOAc three times to provide a crude extract. The extract was redissolved in MeOH and extracted with petroleum ether (PE) three times. The MeOH solution was evaporated under reduced pressure to obtain a defatted extract (25 g).

3.3. UHPLC-Q-TOF and Molecular Networking Analysis

The crude extract was analyzed by LC-MS/MS, equipped with an Atlantis™ Premier BEH C_{18} AX (2.1 × 100 mm, 1.7 μm) column. Samples were dissolved in MeOH with 1 mg/mL. A 10 μL aliquot of each sample was injected and eluted, using a gradient program with water + 0.1% formic acid (A) and CH_3CN + 0.1% formic acid (B). The elution started with a 1% B isocratic phase for 1 min, followed by a gradient from 1% to 99% B in 10 min, maintaining 99% B for 3 min. Then, a gradient from 99% to 1% B in 1 min was applied, and 1% B was maintained for 3 min at a flow rate of 0.4 mL/min, with the temperature maintained at 40 °C. The full mass spectrometry (MS) survey scan was performed in positive electrospray ionization (ESI) mode within the range of 50 to 1000 Da. The MS/MS data were converted to mzXML files using MSConvert software (version 3.01). The converted MS/MS file was submitted to the GNPS platform for molecular networking for dereplication (https://gnps.ucsd.edu, accessed on 1 January 2016). Parameters for molecular network generation were set as follows: both precursor mass and MS/MS fragment ion tolerance were set at 0.02 Da, minimum pairs cosine score 0.6, minimum matched fragment ions 6, minimum cluster size 2, network TopK 10. The spectral networks were imported into Cytoscape 3.9.1 and visualized using the force-directed layout.

3.4. Isolation and Purification

The MeOH extract (25 g) was subjected to CC over silica gel using sequential gradient elution with CH_2Cl_2-MeOH (100:1, 50:1, 30:1, 20:1, 10:1, 5:1, 2:1, and 0:1) to obtain five fractions (Fr.1–Fr.5), based on TLC properties. Fraction Fr.1 (5 g) was chromatographed over ODS using gradient elution of MeOH-H_2O (30 → 80%) to get five subfractions (Fr.1-1–Fr.1-5). Fr.1-1 (625 mg) was subjected to CC on Sephadex LH-20 (MeOH), followed by repeated CC over silica gel, using gradient PE-EtOAc (3:1 → 1:1) to yield **17** (125 mg) and **2** (62 mg). Fr.1-2 (34 mg) was directly separated by Sephadex LH-20 (MeOH) to yield **15** (2 mg). Fr.1-3 (215 mg) was subsequently separated by CC over Sephadex LH-20 (MeOH), silica gel (CH_2Cl_2-MeOH, 100:1 → 50:1), and preparative TLC (PTLC) (CH_2Cl_2-MeOH, 20:1) to obtain **22** (14 mg) and **21** (2 mg). Fr.1-4 (137 mg) was subjected to CC over Sephadex LH-20 (MeOH) and silica gel (CH_2Cl_2-MeOH, 75:1) to yield **3** (40 mg). Fr.1-5 (226 mg) was purified by CC over Sephadex LH-20 (MeOH), silica gel (CH_2Cl_2-MeOH, 100:1), and preparative TLC (PTLC) (CH_2Cl_2-MeOH, 100:1) to afford compound **14** (7 mg).

Fraction Fr.2 (1.3 g) was subjected to CC over ODS with MeOH-H_2O (2% → 30%), followed by purification using CC on Sephadex LH-20 (MeOH), crystallization (MeOH), and silica gel (EtOAc-MeOH, 20:1 → 5:1) to yield **20** (84 mg), **18** (29 mg), **5** (46 mg), **6** (5 mg), **10** (11 mg), **7** (7 mg), **1** (15 mg), and **11** (26 mg).

Fraction Fr.3 (1.5 g) was subjected to CC over ODS with MeOH-H_2O (2% → 50%) and CC on Sephadex LH-20 (MeOH) to yield **19** (4 mg), **4** (11 mg), **12** (11 mg), and **8** (4 mg).

Fraction Fr.4 (9.8 g) was separated by CC over silica gel using sequential gradient elution with PE-EtOAc (100:1, 50:1, 30:1, 20:1, 10:1) and Sephadex LH-20 (CH_2Cl_2-MeOH, 1:1) to yield **13** (320 mg).

Fraction Fr.5 (5.3 g) was subjected to CC over ODS with MeOH-H_2O (10% → 50%), followed by purification using CC on Sephadex LH-20 (MeOH), HPLC (20% → 48%, MeOH-H_2O), crystallization (MeOH), and silica gel (EtOAc-MeOH, 20:1) to yield **9** (2 mg) and **16** (4 mg).

Hepialiamide A (**1**): Yellow oil; $[\alpha]_D^{25}$ + 13 (c 0.10, MeOH), ECD (MeOH) λmax (Δε) 278 (0.07), 245 (−0.09), 217 (0.07); UV (MeOH) λmax (log ε) 229 (2.72), 269 (2.31) nm; HRESIMS m/z 269.1142 [M + H]$^+$ (calcd for $C_{12}H_{17}N_2O_5$, 269.1137).

Hepialiamide B (**2**): Yellow oil; UV (MeOH) λmax (log ε) 230 (2.76), 269 (2.38) nm; ^{1}H and ^{13}C NMR data, Table 1; HRESIMS m/z 251.0950 [M + H]$^+$ (calcd for $C_{12}H_{15}N_2O_4$, 251.1032).

Hepialiamide C (**3**): Yellow oil; $[\alpha]_D^{25}$ + 3 (c 0.10, MeOH); ECD (MeOH) λmax (Δε) 275 (−0.15), 250 (0.13), 213 (−0.17); UV (MeOH) λmax (log ε) 200 (3.06), 269 (2.23) nm; HRESIMS m/z 265.111 [M + H]$^+$ (calcd for $C_{13}H_{17}N_2O_4$, 265.1188).

Hepialide (**4**): Yellow oil; $[\alpha]_D^{25}$ + 5 (c 0.10, MeOH); ECD (MeOH) λmax (Δε) 211 (−0.28); UV (MeOH) λmax (log ε) 228 (2.53), 291 (1.91) nm; HRESIMS m/z 292.0800 [M + Na]$^+$ (calcd for $C_{12}H_{15}NO_6Na$, 292.0797).

3.5. Theoretical ECD Calculation

As reported previously, conformational analysis was first performed via random searching in Sybyl-X 2.0 using the MMFF94S force field with an energy cutoff of 7.0 kcal/mol and an RMSD threshold of 0.2 Å. All conformers were consecutively optimized at PM6 and HF/6-31G(d) levels. Dominant conformers were re-optimized at the B3LYP/6-31G(d) level in the gas phase. The theoretical ECD spectra were calculated using the GIAO method at the MPW1PW91/6-31G (d, p) level in MeOH using Gaussian 09. The ECD spectrum was simulated in SpecDis (version 1.71) by overlapping Gaussian functions for each transition.

3.6. BV-2 Cell Culture and Treatment

BV-2 microglia cells were cultured in DMEM medium containing 10% fetal bovine serum and antibiotics (100 units/mL of penicillin and 100 g/mL of streptomycin) and maintained in a humidified 5% CO_2 incubator at 37 °C. For the experiment, cells were seeded overnight into 24-wells with 2×10^4 cells per well. The next day, cells were incubated with fresh culture medium containing the indicated concentration of compounds for an hour, followed by lipopolysaccharides (LPS) treatment (1 μg/mL). Cells treated with the vehicle (DMSO, 0.1%) served as the control.

3.7. Nitrite Quantification

The concentration of nitrite in the culture medium was determined using the Griess Reagent Kit (Therofisher, Shanghai, China). Briefly, 75 μL of cell culture supernatants was reacted with an equal volume of the Griess Reagent Kit for 30 min at room temperature, and the absorbance of the diazonium compound was obtained at a wavelength of 560 nm. Nitrite production by vehicle stimulation was designated as 100% inhibition (Ctrl) compared to LPS stimulation (Veh) for the experiment.

4. Conclusions

In summary, three new aminated fusaric acid derivatives, hepialiamides A–C (**1**–**3**), and one novel hybrid polyketide, hepialide (**4**), together with 18 known miscellaneous compounds (**5**–**22**), were isolated from the cultures of the deep-sea-derived fungus *Samsoniella hepiali* W7 with the aid of GNPS molecular networking. Hepialiamides A–C feature a glycine/alanine unit embedded in the fusaric acid backbone, representing the third examples of naturally occurring fusaric amides, while hepialide features an uncommon isopropenylated pyrrolidone moiety. Biologically, compound **8**, **11**, **13**, **21**, and **22** showed more than 30% inhibition against NO production induced by LPS at 1 μM, with **22** exhibiting a particularly low nanomole IC_{50}, suggesting potential for developing potent anti-inflammatory drugs.

Supplementary Materials: The following are available online at https://www.mdpi.com/article/10.3390/md21110596/s1. Figures S1–S52: One-dimensional and two-dimensional NMR, UV spectra, ECD calculation details of compounds **1**–**4**, proton NMR spectra of **5**–**22**.

Author Contributions: X.-W.Y. and J.-S.W. designed the project; Z.-B.Z. isolated and purified compounds; Z.-B.Z. and W.-Y.L. performed GNPS analysis; L.-H.Y. and X.-W.H. conducted the biological experiments; K.Z. identified the strains; C.-L.X., M.-M.X. and Y.Z. performed the fermentation; X.-W.Y., Z.-B.Z. and T.-Z.W. analyzed the data and wrote the paper, while critical revisions of the publication were performed by all authors. All authors have read and agreed to the published version of the manuscript.

Funding: This work was financially supported by the Xiamen Southern Oceanographic Center (22GYY007HJ07) and the National Natural Science Foundation of China (22177143).

Institutional Review Board Statement: Not applicable.

Informed Consent Statement: Not applicable.

Data Availability Statement: The data presented in this study are available in Supplementary Materials.

Conflicts of Interest: The authors declare no conflict of interest.

References

1. Newman, D.J.; Cragg, G.M. Natural products as sources of new drugs over the nearly four decades from 01/1981 to 09/2019. *J. Nat. Prod.* **2020**, *83*, 770–803. [CrossRef] [PubMed]
2. Haque, N.; Parveen, S.; Tang, T.; Wei, J.; Huang, Z. Marine natural products in clinical use. *Mar. Drugs* **2022**, *20*, 528. [CrossRef] [PubMed]
3. Teng, Y.F.; Xu, L.; Wei, M.Y.; Wang, C.Y.; Gu, Y.C.; Shao, C.L. Recent progresses in marine microbial-derived antiviral natural products. *Arch. Pharm. Res.* **2020**, *43*, 1215–1229. [CrossRef] [PubMed]
4. Carroll, A.R.; Copp, B.R.; Davis, R.A.; Keyzers, R.A.; Prinsep, M.R. Marine natural products. *Nat. Prod. Rep.* **2021**, *38*, 362–413. [CrossRef]
5. Hai, Y.; Cai, Z.M.; Li, P.J.; Wei, M.Y.; Wang, C.Y.; Gu, Y.C.; Shao, C.L. Trends of antimalarial marine natural products: Progresses, challenges and opportunities. *Nat. Prod. Rep.* **2022**, *39*, 969–990. [CrossRef]
6. Hafez Ghoran, S.; Taktaz, F.; Ayatollahi, S.A.; Kijjoa, A. Anthraquinones and their analogues from marine-derived fungi: Chemistry and biological activities. *Mar. Drugs* **2022**, *20*, 474. [CrossRef] [PubMed]
7. Carroll, A.R.; Copp, B.R.; Davis, R.A.; Keyzers, R.A.; Prinsep, M.R. Marine natural products. *Nat. Prod. Rep.* **2022**, *39*, 1122–1171. [CrossRef]
8. Carroll, A.R.; Copp, B.R.; Davis, R.A.; Keyzers, R.A.; Prinsep, M.R. Marine natural products. *Nat. Prod. Rep.* **2023**, *40*, 275–325. [CrossRef]
9. Yang, J.Y.; Sanchez, L.M.; Rath, C.M.; Liu, X.; Boudreau, P.D.; Bruns, N.; Glukhov, E.; Wodtke, A.; de Felicio, R.; Fenner, A.; et al. Molecular networking as a dereplication strategy. *J. Nat. Prod.* **2013**, *76*, 1686–1699. [CrossRef] [PubMed]
10. Nothias, L.F.; Petras, D.; Schmid, R.; Duhrkop, K.; Rainer, J.; Sarvepalli, A.; Protsyuk, I.; Ernst, M.; Tsugawa, H.; Fleischauer, M.; et al. Feature-based molecular networking in the GNPS analysis environment. *Nat. Methods* **2020**, *17*, 905–908. [CrossRef] [PubMed]
11. Aron, A.T.; Gentry, E.C.; McPhail, K.L.; Nothias, L.F.; Nothias-Esposito, M.; Bouslimani, A.; Petras, D.; Gauglitz, J.M.; Sikora, N.; Vargas, F.; et al. Reproducible molecular networking of untargeted mass spectrometry data using GNPS. *Nat. Protoc.* **2020**, *15*, 1954–1991. [CrossRef]
12. Wei, X.; Su, J.C.; Hu, J.S.; He, X.X.; Lin, S.J.; Zhang, D.M.; Ye, W.C.; Chen, M.F.; Lin, H.W.; Zhang, C.X. Probing indole diketopiperazine-based hybrids as environmental-induced products from *Aspergillus* sp. EGF 15-0-3. *Org. Lett.* **2022**, *24*, 158–163. [CrossRef] [PubMed]
13. Ding, W.J.; Tian, D.M.; Chen, M.; Xia, Z.X.; Tang, X.Y.; Zhang, S.H.; Wei, J.H.; Li, X.N.; Yao, X.S.; Wu, B.; et al. Molecular networking-guided isolation of cyclopentapeptides from the hydrothermal vent sediment derived fungus *Aspergillus pseudoviridinutans* TW58-5 and their anti-inflammatory effects. *J. Nat. Prod.* **2023**, *86*, 1919–1930. [CrossRef] [PubMed]
14. Wang, Y.; Yang, J.; Hu, L.; Bai, R.; Wang, T.; Xing, X.; Chen, L.; Ding, G. LC-MS/MS-guided molecular networking for targeted discovery of undescribed and bioactive ophiobolins from *Bipolaris eleusines*. *J. Agric. Food Chem.* **2023**, *71*, 11982–11992. [CrossRef] [PubMed]
15. Dobson, T.A.; Desaty, D.; Brewer, D.; Vining, L.C. Biosynthesis of fusaric acid in cultures of *Fusarium oxysporum* Schlecht. *Can. J. Biochem.* **1967**, *45*, 809–823. [CrossRef]
16. Stipanovic, R.D.; Wheeler, M.H.; Puckhaber, L.S.; Liu, J.; Bell, A.A.; Williams, H.J. Nuclear magnetic resonance (NMR) studies on the biosynthesis of fusaric acid from *Fusarium oxysporum* f. sp. *vasinfectum*. *J. Agric. Food Chem.* **2011**, *59*, 5351–5356. [CrossRef] [PubMed]
17. Studt, L.; Janevska, S.; Niehaus, E.M.; Burkhardt, I.; Arndt, B.; Sieber, C.M.; Humpf, H.U.; Dickschat, J.S.; Tudzynski, B. Two separate key enzymes and two pathway-specific transcription factors are involved in fusaric acid biosynthesis in *Fusarium fujikuroi*. *Environ. Microbiol.* **2016**, *18*, 936–956. [CrossRef] [PubMed]

18. Hai, Y.; Chen, M.; Huang, A.; Tang, Y. Biosynthesis of mycotoxin fusaric acid and application of a PLP-dependent enzyme for chemoenzymatic synthesis of substituted l-pipecolic acids. *J. Am. Chem. Soc.* **2020**, *142*, 19668–19677. [CrossRef] [PubMed]
19. Yang, Z.; Dan, W.J.; Li, Y.X.; Peng, G.R.; Zhang, A.L.; Gao, J.M. Antifungal metabolites from *Alternaria atrans*: An endophytic fungus in *Psidium guajava*. *Nat. Prod. Commun.* **2019**, *14*, 1934578X19844116. [CrossRef]
20. Hilário, F.; Chapla, V.M.; Araujo, A.R.; Sano, P.T.; Bauab, T.M.; dos Santos, L.C. Antimicrobial screening of endophytic fungi isolated from the aerial parts of *Paepalanthus chiquitensis* (Eriocaulaceae) led to the isolation of secondary metabolites produced by *Fusarium fujikuroi*. *J. Braz. Chem. Soc.* **2016**, *28*, 1389–1395. [CrossRef]
21. Zou, Z.B.; Chen, L.H.; Hu, M.Y.; Xu, L.; Hao, Y.J.; Yan, Q.X.; Wang, C.F.; Xie, C.L.; Yang, X.W. Cladosporioles A and B, two new indole derivatives from the deep-sea-derived fungus *Cladosporium cladosporioides* 170056. *Chem. Biodivers.* **2022**, *19*, e202200538. [CrossRef]
22. Zou, Z.B.; Zhang, G.; Zhou, Y.Q.; Xie, C.L.; Xie, M.M.; Xu, L.; Hao, Y.J.; Luo, L.Z.; Zhang, X.K.; Yang, X.W.; et al. Chemical constituents of the deep-sea-derived *Penicillium citreonigrum* MCCC 3A00169 and their antiproliferative effects. *Mar. Drugs* **2022**, *20*, 736. [CrossRef] [PubMed]
23. He, Z.H.; Xie, C.L.; Wu, T.; Yue, Y.T.; Wang, C.F.; Xu, L.; Xie, M.M.; Zhang, Y.; Hao, Y.J.; Xu, R.; et al. Tetracyclic steroids bearing a bicyclo [4.4.1] ring system as potent antiosteoporosis agents from the deep-sea-derived fungus *Rhizopus* sp. W23. *J. Nat. Prod.* **2023**, *86*, 157–165. [CrossRef]
24. He, Z.H.; Xie, C.L.; Wu, T.; Zhang, Y.; Zou, Z.B.; Xie, M.M.; Xu, L.; Capon, R.J.; Xu, R.; Yang, X.W. Neotricitrinols A-C, unprecedented citrinin trimers with anti-osteoporosis activity from the deep-sea-derived *Penicillium citrinum* W23. *Bioorg. Chem.* **2023**, *139*, 106756. [CrossRef] [PubMed]
25. Wang, F.D.; Yue, J.M. A total synthesis of (+)- and (−)-dihydrokavain with a sonochemical blaise reaction as the key step. *Eur. J. Org. Chem.* **2005**, *2005*, 2575–2579. [CrossRef]
26. Roberts, A.; Beaumont, C.; Manzarpour, A.; Mantle, P. Purpurolic acid: A new natural alkaloid from *Claviceps purpurea* (Fr.) Tul. *Fungal Biol.* **2016**, *120*, 104–110. [CrossRef] [PubMed]
27. Zhang, Z.; He, X.; Wu, G.; Liu, C.; Lu, C.; Gu, Q.; Che, Q.; Zhu, T.; Zhang, G.; Li, D. Aniline-tetramic acids from the deep-sea-derived fungus *Cladosporium sphaerospermum* L3P3 cultured with the HDAC inhibitor SAHA. *J. Nat. Prod.* **2018**, *81*, 1651–1657. [CrossRef] [PubMed]
28. Li, Y.Q.; Park, H.J.; Han, E.S.; Park, D.K. Inhibitory effect on B16/F10 mouse melanoma cell and HT-29 human colon cancer cell proliferation and cordycepin content of the butanol extract of *Paecilomyces militaris*. *J. Med. Plant Res.* **2011**, *5*, 1066–1071.
29. Domondon, D.L.; He, W.; De Kimpe, N.; Hofte, M.; Poppe, J. Beta-adenosine, a bioactive compound in grass chaff stimulating mushroom production. *Phytochemistry* **2004**, *65*, 181–187. [CrossRef]
30. Qiu, W.; Wu, J.; Choi, J.H.; Hirai, H.; Nishida, H.; Kawagishi, H. Cytotoxic compounds against cancer cells from *Bombyx mori* inoculated with *Cordyceps militaris*. *Biosci. Biotechnol. Biochem.* **2017**, *81*, 1224–1226. [CrossRef]
31. Tatani, K.; Hiratochi, M.; Nonaka, Y.; Isaji, M.; Shuto, S. Identification of 8-aminoadenosine derivatives as a new class of human concentrative nucleoside transporter 2 inhibitors. *ACS. Med. Chem. Lett.* **2015**, *6*, 244–248. [CrossRef] [PubMed]
32. Xue, Y.; Wu, L.; Ding, Y.; Cui, X.; Han, Z.; Xu, H. A new nucleoside and two new pyrrole alkaloid derivatives from *Cordyceps militaris*. *Nat. Prod. Res.* **2020**, *34*, 341–350. [CrossRef]
33. Youssef, D.T.A.; Badr, J.M.; Shaala, L.A.; Mohamed, G.A.; Bamanie, F.H. Ehrenasterol and biemnic acid; new bioactive compounds from the Red Sea sponge *Biemna ehrenbergi*. *Phytochem. Lett.* **2015**, *12*, 296–301. [CrossRef]
34. Ma, Y.T.; Qiao, L.R.; Shi, W.Q.; Zhang, A.L.; Gao, J.M. Metabolites produced by an endophyte *Alternaria alternata* isolated from *Maytenus hookeri*. *Chem. Nat. Compd.* **2010**, *46*, 504–506. [CrossRef]
35. Ying, Y.M.; Shan, W.G.; Liu, W.H.; Zhan, Z.J. Alkaloids and nucleoside derivatives from a fungal endophyte of *Huperzia serrata*. *Chem. Nat. Comd.* **2013**, *49*, 184–186. [CrossRef]
36. Kaaniche, F.; Hamed, A.; Abdel-Razek, A.S.; Wibberg, D.; Abdissa, N.; El Euch, I.Z.; Allouche, N.; Mellouli, L.; Shaaban, M.; Sewald, N. Bioactive secondary metabolites from new endophytic fungus *Curvularia*. sp isolated from *Rauwolfia macrophylla*. *PLoS ONE* **2019**, *14*, e0217627. [CrossRef]
37. Sun, Y.; Tian, L.; Huang, J.; Li, W.; Pei, Y.H. Cytotoxic sterols from marine-derived fungus *Pennicilium* sp. *Nat. Prod. Res.* **2006**, *20*, 381–384. [CrossRef] [PubMed]
38. Fang, S.T.; Wang, Y.J.; Ma, X.Y.; Yin, X.L.; Ji, N.Y. Two new sesquiterpenoids from the marine-sediment-derived fungus *Trichoderma harzianum* P1-4. *Nat. Prod. Res.* **2019**, *33*, 3127–3133. [CrossRef]
39. Dearman, R.J.; Cumberbatch, M.; Hilton, J.; Clowes, H.M.; Fielding, I.; Heylings, J.R.; Kimber, I. Influence of dibutyl phthalate on dermal sensitization to fluorescein isothiocyanate. *Fundam. Appl. Toxicol.* **1996**, *33*, 24–30. [CrossRef] [PubMed]
40. Zeiger, E.; Haworth, S.; Mortelmans, K.; Speck, W. Mutagenicity testing of di(2-ethylhexyl)phthalate and related chemicals in Salmonella. *Environ. Mutagen.* **1985**, *7*, 213–232. [CrossRef]
41. Wang, W.; Guo, J.; Zhang, J.; Liu, T.; Xin, Z. New screw lactam and two new carbohydrate derivatives from the methanol extract of rice bran. *J. Agric. Food. Chem.* **2014**, *62*, 10744–10751. [CrossRef]
42. Theil, F.; Schick, H. Enzymes in organic-synthesis. 5. An improved procedure for the regioselective acetylation of monosaccharide derivatives by pancreatin-catalyzed transesterification in organic-solvents. *Synthesis* **1991**, *22*, 533–535. [CrossRef]
43. Park, S.; Kazlauskas, R.J. Improved preparation and use of room-temperature ionic liquids in lipase-catalyzed enantio- and regioselective acylations. *J. Org. Chem.* **2001**, *66*, 8395–8401. [CrossRef] [PubMed]

44. Li, X.B.; Li, Y.L.; Zhou, J.C.; Yuan, H.Q.; Wang, X.N.; Lou, H.X. A new diketopiperazine heterodimer from an endophytic fungus *Aspergillus niger*. *J. Asian Nat. Prod. Res.* **2015**, *17*, 182–187. [CrossRef] [PubMed]
45. Yan, H.J.; Gao, S.S.; Li, C.S.; Li, X.M.; Wang, B.G. Chemical constituents of a marine-derived endophytic fungus *Penicillium commune* G2M. *Molecules* **2010**, *15*, 3270–3275. [CrossRef]
46. Tao, Y.; Feng, C.; Xu, J.; Shen, L.; Qu, J.; Ju, H.; Yan, L.; Chen, W.; Zhang, Y. Di(2-ethylhexyl) phthalate and dibutyl phthalate have a negative competitive effect on the nitrification of black soil. *Chemosphere* **2022**, *293*, 133554. [CrossRef]
47. Silvin, A.; Uderhardt, S.; Piot, C.; Da Mesquita, S.; Yang, K.; Geirsdottir, L.; Mulder, K.; Eyal, D.; Liu, Z.; Bridlance, C.; et al. Dual ontogeny of disease-associated microglia and disease inflammatory macrophages in aging and neurodegeneration. *Immunity* **2022**, *55*, 1448–1465. [CrossRef]
48. Orihuela, R.; McPherson, C.A.; Harry, G.J. Microglial M1/M2 polarization and metabolic states. *Br. J. Pharmacol.* **2016**, *173*, 649–665. [CrossRef]

Disclaimer/Publisher's Note: The statements, opinions and data contained in all publications are solely those of the individual author(s) and contributor(s) and not of MDPI and/or the editor(s). MDPI and/or the editor(s) disclaim responsibility for any injury to people or property resulting from any ideas, methods, instructions or products referred to in the content.

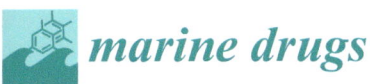

Review

Diversified Chemical Structures and Bioactivities of the Chemical Constituents Found in the Brown Algae Family Sargassaceae

Yan Peng [1], Xianwen Yang [2], Riming Huang [3], Bin Ren [1], Bin Chen [1], Yonghong Liu [4] and Hongjie Zhang [5],*

1. College of Food Science and Engineering, Lingnan Normal University, Zhanjiang 524048, China; py00_2006@126.com (Y.P.); rb2003227@gmail.com (B.R.); 13724755889@139.com (B.C.)
2. Key Laboratory of Marine Biogenetic Resources, Third Institute of Oceanography, Ministry of Natural Resources, 184 Daxue Road, Xiamen 361005, China; yangxianwen@tio.org.cn
3. Guangdong Provincial Key Laboratory of Food Quality and Safety, College of Food Science, South China Agricultural University, Guangzhou 510642, China; huangriming@scau.edu.cn
4. CAS Key Laboratory of Tropical Marine Bio-Resources and Ecology/Guangdong Key Laboratory of Marine Materia Medica, South China Sea Institute of Oceanology, Chinese Academy of Sciences, Guangzhou 510301, China; yonghongliu@scsio.ac.cn
5. School of Chinese Medicine, Hong Kong Baptist University, 7 Baptist University Road, Kowloon Tong, Kowloon, Hong Kong, China
* Correspondence: zhanghj@hkbu.edu.hk

Abstract: Sargassaceae, the most abundant family in Fucales, was recently formed through the merging of the two former families Sargassaceae and Cystoseiraceae. It is widely distributed in the world's oceans, notably in tropical coastal regions, with the exception of the coasts of Antarctica and South America. Numerous bioactivities have been discovered through investigations of the chemical diversity of the Sargassaceae family. The secondary metabolites with unique structures found in this family have been classified as terpenoids, phlorotannins, and steroids, among others. These compounds have exhibited potent pharmacological activities. This review describes the new discovered compounds from Sargassaceae species and their associated bioactivities, citing 136 references covering from March 1975 to August 2023.

Keywords: brown algae; Fucales; Sargassaceae; secondary metabolites; bioactivity

1. Introduction

Seaweeds, a rich renewable resource, are known to produce numerous complex and diverse secondary metabolites with potent bioactivities [1–13]. Based on their thallus pigmentation, seaweeds are typically classified into three groups: brown algae (Phaeophyta), green algae (Chlorophyta), and red algae (Rhodophyta). Sargassaceae, a polyphyletic family of brown seaweed, is comprised of the two former families Sargassaceae and Cystoseiraceae [14,15]. This family encompasses a variety of genera, including *Acrocarpia, Acystis, Anthophycus, Axillariella, Bifurcaria, Carpophyllum, Carpoglossum, Caulocystis, Cladophyllum, Coccophora, Cystoseira, Cystophora, Cystophyllum, Ericaria, Gongolaria, Halidrys, Hormophysa, Landsburgia, Myagropsis, Myriodesma, Nizamuddinia, Oerstedtia, Platythalia, Sargassum, Stolonophrora, Scaberia*, and *Turbinaria*, as listed in the algae database [16]. Among these, the genera with the most species are *Sargassum* (977 species) and *Cystoseira* (288 species), followed by *Turbinaria* (53 species) and *Cystophora* (39 species) [16]. Notably, the former two are the most representative genera of this family and have received significant attention, which has resulted in a wealth of publications [4,17–19].

Since 1973, studies on Sargassaceae species have experienced rapid growth, leading to the discovery of a multitude of novel compounds with potent bioactivities. Valls and Piovetti summarized 134 new diterpenoids isolated from the former Cystoseiraceae family

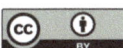

between 1973 and January 1995 [20], and de Sousa et al. [18] and Gouveira et al. [21] compiled the secondary metabolites isolated from various *Cystoseira* species from 1995 to 2016. Chen and Liu [22] and Rushdi et al. [23] reviewed the chemical constituents of *Sargassum* species and their biological activities from 1974 to 2020. Rushdi et al. [24] also provided an overview of secondary metabolites isolated from *Turbinaria* species between 1972 and 2019. Muñoz et al. [4] summarized the linear diterpenes from *Bifurcaria bifurcata*, emphasizing biosynthetic pathways, biological activities, chemotaxonomy, and ecology. This review attempts to summarize the literature data on the new compounds from the Sargassaceae family and their biological activities.

2. Chemistry and Biological Activities of the Compounds from the Sargassaceae Family

Sargassaceae is a family of marine macroalgae comprising over 20 genera and more than 1000 species, and some species are shown in Figure 1. While many genera of this family show a limited distribution, the genera *Bifurcaria*, *Cystophora*, and *Halidrys* display a disjunct distribution [14]. When examining the chemical constituents from Sargassacean species, numerous new structures were obtained, which mainly include terpenoids (encompassing meroterpenoids), phloroglucinol derivatives, steroids, and other types.

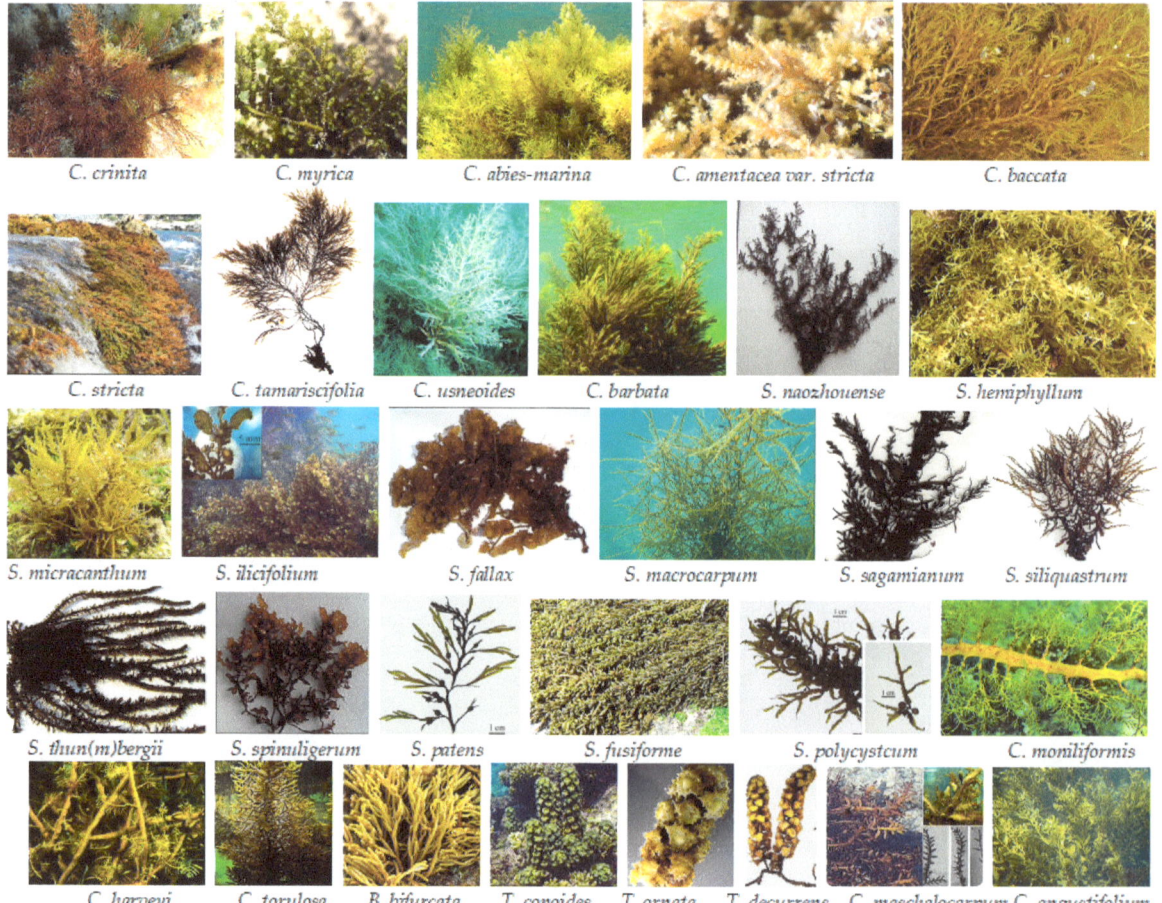

Figure 1. Some Sargassacean species.

2.1. Terpenoids

Terpenoids, a class of predominantly secondary metabolites, have been discovered in the Sargassaceae family [25,26]. Specifically, 223 novel terpenoids have been obtained from five different Sargassacean genera, namely *Cystoseira, Sargassum, Cystophora, Bifurcaria*, and *Turbinaria*. Based on the number of isoprene units and the biosynthesis pathway, these isolated compounds can be categorized into monoterpenoids, sesquiterpenoids, diterpenoids, triterpenes, and meroterpenes.

2.1.1. Monoterpenoids

Two new loliolide-type monoterpenoids, schiffnerilolide (**1**) and sargassumone (**2**) (Figure 2), were isolated from the brown algae *C. schiffneri* and *S. naozhouense*, respectively [27,28]. From the biosynthesis aspect, **1** could be derived from isololiolide through oxidation at carbon-carbon double bond [27,29], while **2** may have been formed from loliolide via various reactions, including selective oxidation, specific reduction, and isomerization [28,30].

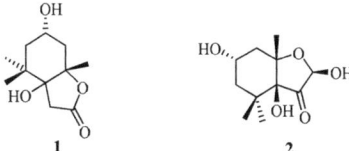

Figure 2. Monoterpenoids isolated from Sargassacean species.

2.1.2. Sesquiterpenoids

A new sesquiterpenoid, oxocrinol (**3**) (Figure 3), was isolated from the Mediterranean alga *C. crinita* [31]. Interestingly, compound **3** was a novel linear terpenoid alcohol, which could potentially originate from farnesol or other possible precursors, such as monoterpenoid and geranylgeraniol [31].

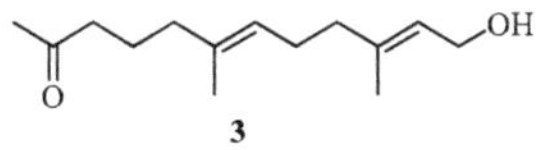

Figure 3. Sesquiterpenoids isolated from Sargassacean species.

2.1.3. Diterpenoids

Sixty-four new diterpenoids, **4–67** (Figures 4–9), were isolated from various Sargassacean species. According to the carbon skeletons, these newly isolated compounds were classified into norditerpenoids, acyclic diterpenes, hydroazulene diterpenes, and xenicane diterpenoids.

Norditerpenoids

Sixteen new norditerpenoid compounds (Figure 4), including three bisnorditerpenes and 13 farnesylacetone derivatives, were obtained from the Sargassaceae family. Among them, 13 were from *Sargassum* sp., while one was from *Cystophora* sp.

Compounds **4–6**, three novel bisnorditerpene isomers featuring an unusual α, β-unsaturated ketone skeleton, were isolated from *S. hemiphyllum*, collected from the Heda coast of the Izu Peninsula, Japan. They appeared to originate from the geranyl geraniol precursor and showed low cytotoxicity against P388 cells [32].

Compounds **7–16**, novel farnesylacetone derivatives categorized as norditerpenes [33], were isolated from the brown alga *S. micracanthum*, harvested at Kominato, Chiba, Japan [33,34]. From a biosynthetic aspect, these compounds could be formed from geranylgeranylquinones and chromenols through selective oxidation.

Compounds **17–19**, also classified as farnesylacetone derivatives belonging to norditerpenoid analogs, were obtained from the brown alga *C. moniliformis*, which was harvested from Port Philip Bay, Australia [35]. Particularly, compounds **18** and **19** were two epimers that were indirectly formed from geranyl acetone [35].

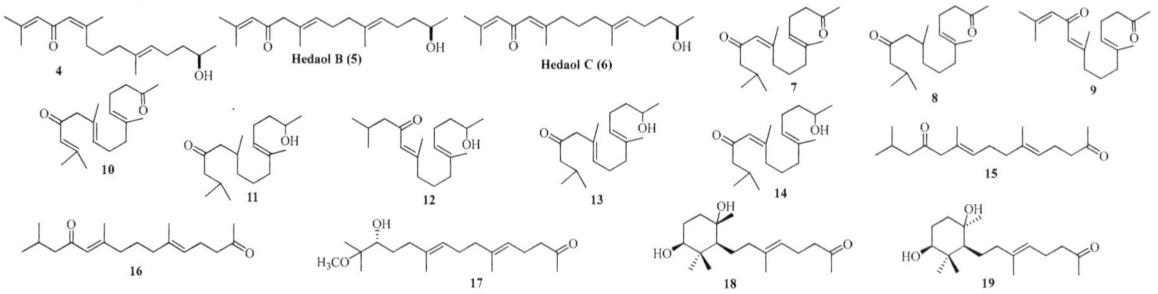

Figure 4. Norditerpenoids isolated from Sargassacean species.

Acyclic Diterpenoids

Though acyclic diterpenoids are seldom found in nature, they are abundantly found in the brown alga B. bifurcata [4]. Notably, 43 new linear diterpenoids (20–62) (Figures 5–7) were obtained from the brown algae B. bifurcata and C. crinita. Based on their biosynthetic origins, these isolates were categorized into three groups: C-12 oxidized congeners, C-13 oxidized congeners, and non-C-12/C-13 oxidized analogs.

- C-12 Oxidized Congeners

Eight new linear diterpenoids, 20–27 (Figure 5), featuring a hydroxyl group at C-12, were isolated from B. bifurcata collected from the Atlantic coasts of Morocco between 1984 and 2002 [36–40]. These compounds exhibited close chemical relationships. Interestingly, compound 20 could undergo epoxidation at the C-6/C-7 double bond, followed by dehydration to produce allylic alcohols 21 and 23, which could be further converted to 22 via a selective reduction at the C-5/C-6 double bond [4,37,38]. In particular, compound 24 was unstable and could slowly transform into its stable isomer 25 at room temperature [39]. Furthermore, 25 could convert into 27, which could undergo methylation to produce 26 [4,39,40]. Compounds 21 and 22 were tested in vitro for cytotoxicity against the NSCLC-N6 cell line and proved to be active [38].

- C-13 Oxidized Congeners

Fourteen new linear diterpenoids, 28–41 (Figure 6), featuring a hydroxyl group at C-13, were isolated from the brown alga B. bifurcata, sourced from various geographical origins [41–45]. These compounds could be formed from 13-hydroxygeranylgeraniol, namely eleganediol [4]. Notably, compound 28, which possesses a furan-3-yl ring formed from eleganediol via terminal cyclization and oxidation, was isolated from the French brown seaweed B. bifurcata, along with compound 29 [41]. Compounds 30–39 were isolated from the brown seaweed B. bifurcata, collected from an intertidal rock pool in County Clare, Ireland [42–44]. Compounds 40 and 41, possibly produced from eleganediol by epoxidation of the C-6/C-7 double bond followed by isomerization to form allylic alcohols, were also obtained from the French brown alga B. bifurcata [45]. Compounds 28, 30, 31, and 35 showed cytotoxic, antiprotozoal, and anticancer activity, respectively [41–44].

Sixteen new acyclic diterpenes, 42–57 (Figure 6), featuring a ketone function at C-13, were isolated from the brown algae C. crinita [46] and B. bifurcata [44,45,47–50]. They could originate from eleganolone. Interestingly, some of these isolates appear to have a close chemical relationship. Specifically, compound 44 could undergo selective reduction of its C-6 ketone group, followed by formation of the corresponding allylic alcohol 42, which could then convert into 46 [46]. Compounds 46 and 47 are two isomers obtained from the France brown alga B. bifurcata, together with compound 48 [45]. Compound 52 could transform into 53 via hydroxylation of C-20 and lactonization, or into 54 following reduction of its C-14/C15 double bond [49]. Compounds 56 and 57 are two eleganolone-type stereoisomers featuring a novel dihydroxy-γ-butyrolactone system [50].

- Non C-12/C-13 Oxidized Analogs

Five new linear diterpenoids, **58–62** (Figure 7), were isolated the brown alga *C. crinita* [31] and *B. bifurcata* [38–40,51]. They are non-C-12/C-13 oxidized congeners, directly or indirectly derived from geranylgeraniol. Among them, compound **58** was isolated from the brown alga *C. crinita*, harvested near Catania, Sicily, Italy [31]. Compound **59**, characterized by a secondary alcohol group at C-10, was isolated from the brown alga *B. bifurcata*, harvested near Oualidia, Morocco [38]. Compound **60**, possessing two conjugated double bonds at C-9 and C-11, was also obtained from the brown alga *B. bifurcata*, collected near Oualidia [39]. Compounds **61** and **62** were isolated from the brown alga *B. bifurcata*, harvested off the Atlantic coast of Morocco [40,51]. Notably, **62** demonstrated potent cytotoxicity to fertilized sea urchin eggs [51].

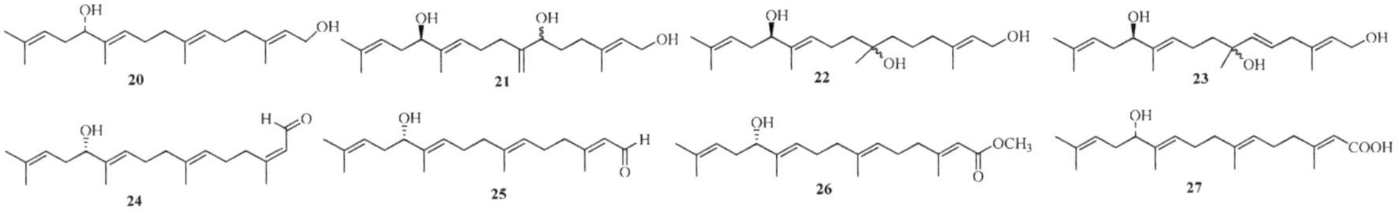

Figure 5. C-12 oxidized linear diterpenoids isolated from Sargassacean species.

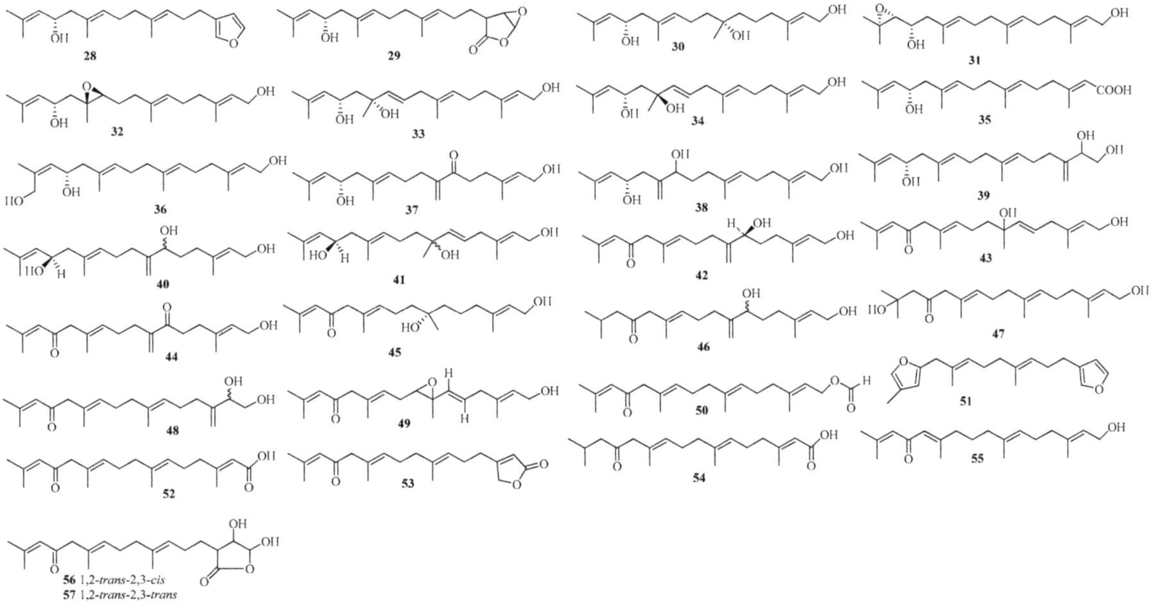

Figure 6. C-13 oxidized linear diterpenoids isolated from Sargassacean species.

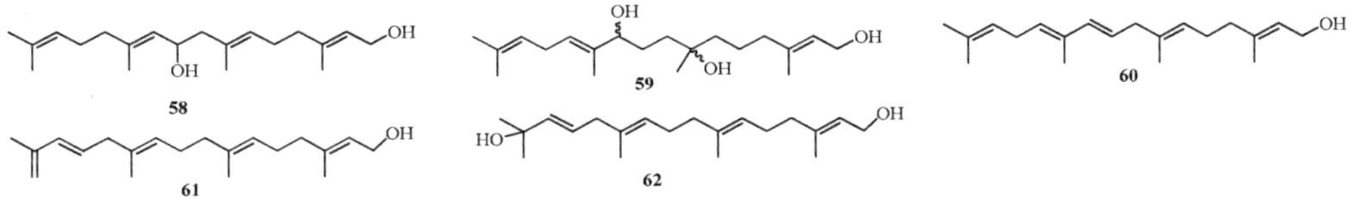

Figure 7. Non C-12/C-13 oxidized linear diterpenoids isolated from Sargassacean species.

Hydroazulene Diterpenoids

Four new diterpenoids, **63–66** (Figure 8), featuring a hydroazulene skeleton, were isolated from the brown alga *C. myrica*, collected at El-Zafrana, Gulf of Suez, Egypt. Their structures were determined by spectroscopic and chemical techniques. The cytotoxicities of these four compounds were tested in vitro against three different mouse cell lines (NIH3T3, SSVNIH3T3, and KA3IT). The results showed moderate cytotoxicity of all isolates against the cancer cell line KA3IT [52].

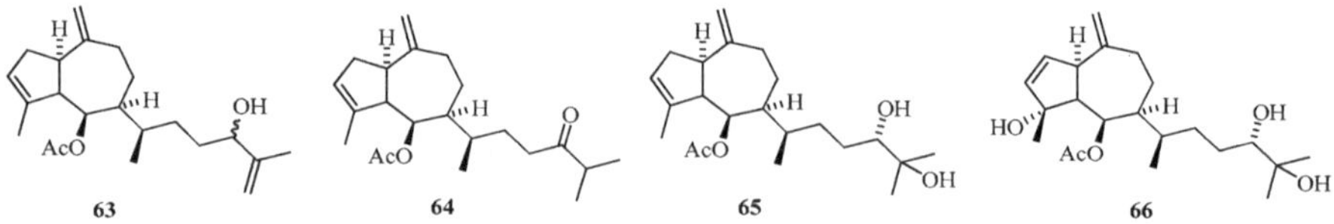

Figure 8. Hydroazulene diterpenes isolated from Sargassacean species.

Xenicane Diterpenoids

A new xenicane-type diterpenoid, **67** (Figure 9), was isolated from the organic extract of the intertidal brown alga *S. ilicifolium*, which was harvested from the Gulf of Manner coast, India. This new metabolite, deduced as sargilicixenicane, showed potential anti-inflammatory and antioxidant activities [53].

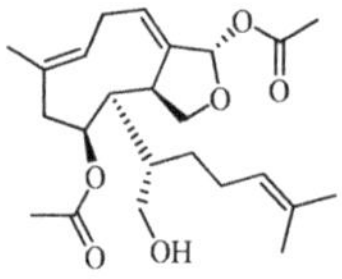

Figure 9. Xenicane diterpenes isolated from Sargassacean species.

2.1.4. Nor-Dammarane Triterpenoids

Two new nor-dammarane triterpenes, decurrencylics A-B (**68** and **69**) (Figure 10), were isolated from the brown alga *T. decurrens*, which was harvested from the Mandapam region in the Gulf of Mannar, Peninsular India, India. Their structures were determined by extensive spectra analysis. The two compounds showed potent anti-inflammatory activities [54].

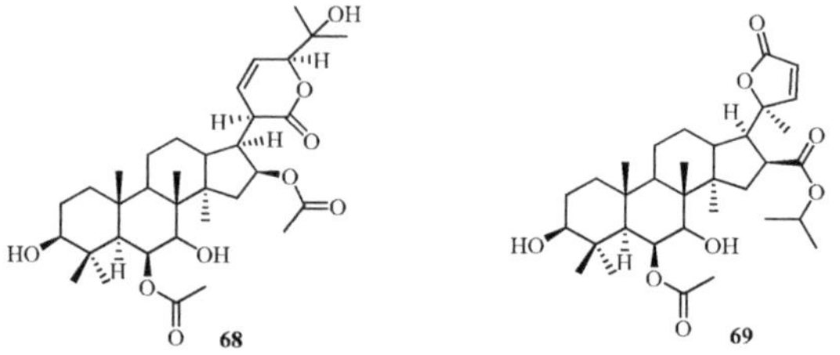

Figure 10. Nor-dammarane triterpenoids isolated from Sargassacean species.

2.1.5. Meroterpenoids

Meroterpenoids represent another major group of terpene metabolites originating from the Sargassaceae family [6,7,18,55–86]. Notably, 154 new meroterpenoids (**70–223**) (Figures 11–13), consisting of an aromatic or substituted aromatic nucleus connected to a terpenoid chain with different degrees of oxidation, were isolated from Sargassaceae species [57–86]. According to the structural characteristics, meroterpenoids can be classified into terpenyl-quinones/hydroquinone analogs, chromenes, and nahocols/isonahocols.

Terpenyl-Quinones/Hydroquinone Analogs

Ninety-six novel terpenyl-quinones/hydroquinones (**70–165**) (Figure 11), which consist of a quinone or hydroquinone nucleus connected to a terpenyl moiety, were isolated from three Sargassacean genera, namely *Cystoseira*, *Sargassum*, and *Cystophora*.

Three novel tetraprenyl-toluquinone derivatives (**70–72**), seven new tetraprenyltoluquinols congeners (**73–79**), two new triprenyltoluquinol derivatives (**80** and **81**), and one new O-methyltoluquinol diterpenoid (**82**) were isolated from two distinct samples of *C. crinita*, one collected from the south coast of Sardinia [57] and another from the French Riviera coasts [58]. Compounds **70/71, 73/74, 75/76, 77/78,** and **80/81** belong to five pairs of Δ^6 stereoisomers and showed antioxidant activities [57]. Particularly, **77** could be formed from **75** via dihydroxylation at C-13′ [57]. Compound **82** could be further converted into **72** and **79** [58].

Four new meronorsesquiterpenoids (**83–86**) and two new meroditerpenoids (**87** and **88**) were isolated from the brown alga *C. abies-marina* [59,60]. Of them, **83/84** and **85/86** represent two pairs of Δ^6 diastereomers characterized by a C14 terpenoid side chain, which were possibly formed from the diterpenoid side chain through oxidative degradation [61]. Compounds **87** and **88** contain two methoxyl groups in the aromatic nucleus, which were formed from geranylgeranyltoluquinol via various reaction cascades, such as methylation and/or oxidation [59]. Compounds **83, 84, 87,** and **88** were evaluated for their cytotoxic and antioxidant activities in vitro. The results revealed that **83, 84,** and **87** showed inhibitory activities against Hela cells, while **88** exhibited moderate antioxidant activity against DPPH radicals [59].

A new meroditerpene, 4′-methoxy-2(E)-bifurcarenone (**89**), was isolated from the brown alga *C. amentacea* var. *stricta*, harvested at Le Brusc, France. This new isolate showed cytotoxic effects against the development of the fertilized eggs of sea urchin *Paracentrotus lividus* [62].

Two novel meroditerpenoids (**90** and **91**) were obtained from the brown alga *C. baccata* collected on the Moroccan Atlantic coast. They share the same *trans*-fusion bicyclic [4.3.0] nonane ring system, making the first instance of such a system reported from marine Sargassaceae algae [63].

Two new meroditerpenoids, preamentol triacetate (**92**) and 14-epi-amentol triacetate (**93**), were isolated from the acetone extract of an unidentified *Cystoseira* specimen harvested at the Spanish Canary Islands [64]. The two compounds could be formed from geranylgeranyltoluquinol via oxidation and cyclization [65].

A novel tetraprenylhydroquinol, balearone (**94**), was isolated from the chloroform extract of the brown alga *C. balearica*, collected at Portopalo, Sicily, Italy. Its chemical structure was deduced by single-crystal X-ray diffraction analysis [66].

Fifteen new tetraprenyl-toluquinol derivatives (**95–109**) were isolated from the Mediterranean seaweed *C. stricta*, harvested from three different locations on the Sicilian coasts [67–72]. They exhibit structural similarities. Especially, selective methylation of phenolic hydroxyl in **95** could produce the methyl ether **96** [67]. Compounds **99** and **100** are the Z-2-isomers of **103** and **94**, respectively [68,70]. The oxidation of **101** with silver oxide could lead to *p*-benzoquinone **102**, which could also undergo reduction to produce **101** [69]. Compound **104**, derived from **107** via the removal of its acidic proton at C-11 and subsequent formation of the C-11 to C-7 bond, could be converted into **105** by selective methylation, or into **106** via isomerization [71]. Compounds **108** and **109** present two new irregular tetraprenyltoluquinol epimers [72].

Four unique phloroglucinol-meroterpenoid hybrids, named cystophloroketals A–D (**110–113**), were isolated from the Mediterranean alga *C. tamariscifolia*, harvested in the Mediterranean Sea near Tipaza, Algeria. They represent the first example of meroterpenoids with a 2,7-dioxabicyclo [3.2.1] octane unit fused to a phloroglucinol. Their antifouling activities were assessed against several marine species involved in the biofouling process, and the results showed that they were active [73].

Twenty-two new meroterpenoids, namely cystodiones A–M (**114–125**), cystones A–F (**126–131**), usneoidones E and Z (**132** and **133**), and usneoidoles Z and E (**134** and **135**), were isolated from the brown alga *C. usneoides* collected from the Moroccan, Spanish, and Portuguese coasts [74–77]. Of which, **114**, **115**, and **118–135** consist of a toluquinol core and a diterpenoid chain with various oxygenated functionalities and unsaturation, while **116** and **117** consist of a C_{14}-side chain attached to an *O*-methyltoluquinol ring [74–77]. Interestingly, compounds **114/115**, **116/117**, **118/119**, **123/124**, **128/129**, **130/131**, **132/133**, and **134/135** form eight pairs of Δ^6 stereoisomers. Compounds **114–117** displayed antioxidant activities in the ABTS radical-scavenging assay, along with **120–131** [74–77]. Compounds **120**, **125**, and **128** also showed significant inhibitory activities on production of the proinflammatory cytokine TNF-α in LPS-stimulated THP-1 human macrophages [75]. Furthermore, compounds **132–135** exhibited antitumor and antiviral activities [76,77].

A pair of novel tetraprenyltoluquinol isomers, **136** and **137**, were isolated from the brown alga *C. sauvageuana*, collected at Aci Castello, Sicily, Italy. It was determined that **136** could be converted into **137** after photoisomerization [78].

A novel, linearly fused 6,6,5-tricyclic geranyltoluquinone, pycnanthuquinone C (**138**), was isolated from the acetone extract of the Western Australian marine brown alga *Cystophora harveyi*. This marks the second report of prenylated quinone with a linear 6,6,5-cyclic skeleton from marine organisms [79].

Two new meroditerpenoids, fallahydroquinone (**139**) and fallaquinone (**140**), were isolated from the brown alga *S. fallax*, collected from Port Philip Bay, Victoria, Australia [80]. Compound **140** is likely to be an artifact compound, as it could be produced from **139** by oxidation upon exposure to air. The absolute stereochemistry for **139** and **140** could not be established, owing to their instability and rapid decomposition. The two isolates displayed weak antitumor activities in a P388 assay [80].

Three new meroterpenoids, macrocarquinoids A–C (**141–143**), were isolated from the EtOH extract of the brown alga *S. macrocarpum*, harvested on the coast of Tsukumo Bay, Japan. Compound **142** possesses a γ-lactone ring at C-9′ to C-11′ and C-18′ of the terpenyl chain, while **143** has a δ-lactone ring at C-11′ to C-14′ and C-18′ [81]. All of these compounds showed inhibitory activity against AGE that were either comparable to, or more potent than, activity of aminoguanidine, which was used as a positive control [81].

Four new plastoquinones **144–147** were isolated from the brown alga *S. micracanthum*, collected from the Toyama Bay coast of Japan. Their structures were determined by spectroscopic analysis and chemical conversions. Compounds **144–146** showed both antioxidant and cytotoxic activities [82].

Four new meroditerpenoids—sargahydroquinal (**148**), paradoxhydroquinone (**149**), paradoxquinol (**150**), and paradoxquinone (**151**)—were isolated from the brown alga *S. paradoxum*, collected from Governor Reef near Indented Head, Port Philip Bay, Australia. They consisted of a diterpenoid chain attached to hydroquinone or *p*-benzoquinone rings. Their structures were determined by spectroscopic techniques. Particularly, **148** was identified by HPLC-NMR and HPLC-MS, coupled with comparison with the known compound due to its instability. Compounds **149–151** showed weak antibacterial activities against *Streptococcus pyogenes* [83].

Three new sargaquinoic acid derivatives, 15′-hydroxysargaquinolide (**152**), (2′E,5′E)-2-methyl-6-(7′-oxo-3′-methylocta-2′,5′-dienyl)-1,4-benzoquinone (**153**), and 15′-methylenesargaquinolide (**154**), and two new plastoquinone analogs, sargahydroquinoic acid (**155**) and yezoquinolide (**156**), were isolated from the brown algae *S. sagamianum* [84] and *S. sagamianum* var. *yezoense* [85]. Noticeably, **153** and **154** are a selectively oxidized analog and a dehydration derivative of **152**, respectively [83]. Compound **155** is a hydroquinone derivative of sargaquinoic acid [53], while **156** features an α, β-unsaturated γ-lactone moiety, marking the first example of a plastoquinone with a butenolide unit [85]. Compounds **152** and **153** showed antibacterial activities and cytotoxicities against Hela S3 cells [84].

Two new meroditerpenoids (**157** and **158**) were isolated from the brown alga *S. siliquastrum*, collected from Jeju Island, Korea [86]. Compound **157**, a derivative of sargahydroquinoic acid, exhibited significant radical-scavenging activity as well as slight inhibitory activity against isocitrate lyase from *Candida albicans*. The stereochemistry at C-13′ of **157** remained uncertain due to the limited quantity. Compound **158**, representing the first reported meroditerpenoid with a modified dihydroquinone unit from marine brown algae, exhibited weak activity against transpeptidase sortase A from *Staphylococcus aureus* [86]. Interestingly, **158** was presumed to be a biosynthetic precursor of nahocols and isonahocols, based on a 1,3-migration of its methyl acetate group.

Seven new geranylgeranylbenzoquinone derivatives (**159–165**) were separated from the Japanese marine alga *S. tortile* harvested at Awa-Kominato, Chiba, Japan. These isolates consist of a hydroquinone or benzoquinone core linked to a diterpenoid moiety. Among them, compounds **159/160** and **162/163** constitute two pair of isomers. Compound **161** could be converted into quinone **164** by selective oxidation [87].

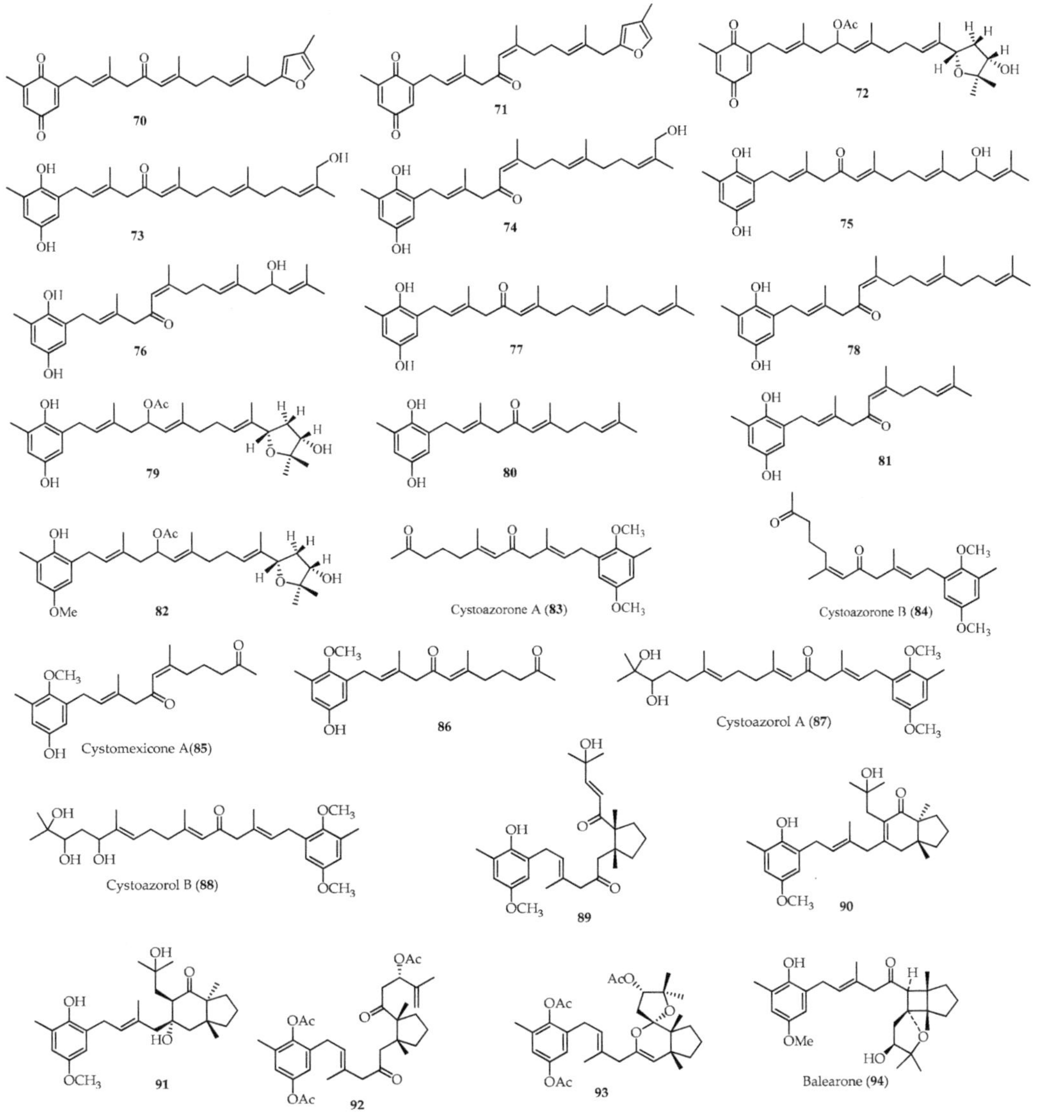

Figure 11. *Cont.*

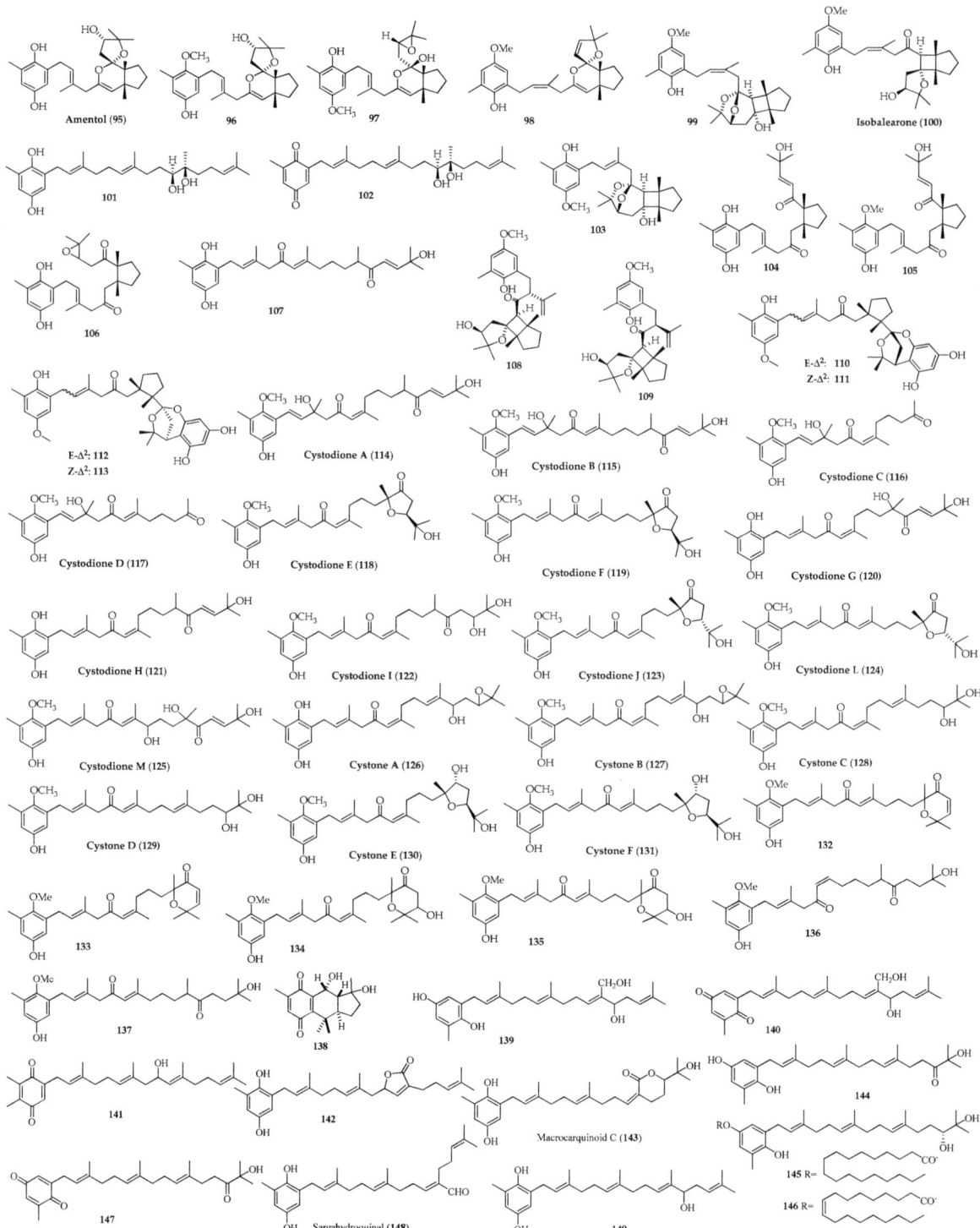

Figure 11. *Cont.*

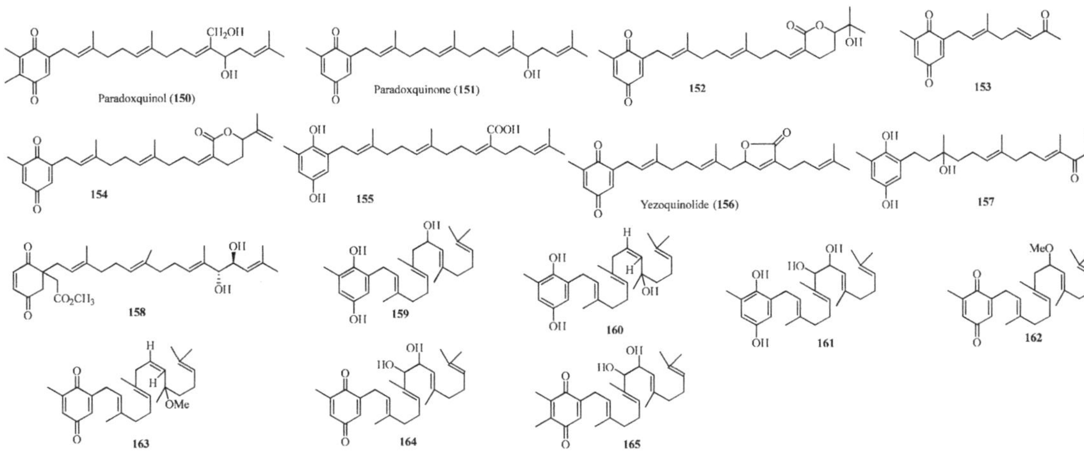

Figure 11. Terpenyl-quinones/hydroquinones isolated from Sargassacean species.

Chromenes

Forty-nine new chromene meroterpenods (Figure 12) were isolated from certain species of Sargassaceae. Their structures are similar to that of vitamin E.

A new chromene meroditerpene (**166**) was isolated from the brown alga *C. amentacea* var. *stricta* mentioned above. It is a derivative of 4′-methoxy-2(E)-bifurcarenone originated from the same species [62].

Two novel chromene meroditerpenoid isomers (**167** and **168**) and their derivatives (**169–171**), together with two new chromane meroditerpenoid epimers (**172** and **173**), were isolated from the brown alga *C. baccata* and *S. muticum* [63,87–89]. Among them, compounds **167–171** share the same *trans*-fused carbon skeleton, marking the first report of such a structure in the Sargassaceae family [63]. Compounds **172** and **173** also possess the same *trans*-fused bicyclic system and were found to exhibit photodamage attenuation effects [89,90]. Compounds **168**, **169**, and **171** showed antifouling activities against the settlement of certain macroalgae, the growth of microalgae, and the activities of mussels [63].

Three new chromane meroditerpenes (**174–176**) were isolated from the previously mentioned unidentified *Cystoseira* specimen. Due to their inherent instability, **175** and **176** were only obtained in the acetate form. In particular, **175** represented the first example of meroditerpene containing a newly rearranged structure, featuring a novel ether linkage in the diterpene chain. The structure is likely formed from **176** via an oxidation process of the enol-ether system, followed by rearrangement [64].

A new phloroglucinol-meroditerpenoid hybrid (**177**), consisting of a chromane meroditerpenoid linked to a phloroglucinol through a 2,7-dioxabicylo [3.2.1] octane unit, was isolated from the brown alga *C. tamariscifolia* mentioned above. This isolate showed moderate to weak antifouling activities against several marine colonizing species such as bacteria, fungi, micro- and macroalgae [73].

A new chromene meroditerpenoid, fallachromenoic acid (**178**), featuring a carboxylic group and a chlorine atom, was isolated from the brown alga *S. fallax* described above. Its absolute configuration could not be assigned due to its instability [80]. Compound **178** showed weak antitumor activity against P388 murine leukemia cells [80].

Two new chromane meroterpenoids (**179** and **180**) were obtained from the brown alga *S. micracanthum*, harvested on the Toyama Bay coast, Japan. Their structures were determined by extensive spectroscopic analysis and chemical conversion [91].

Two new chromene meroditerpenoids (**181** and **182**), characterized by a lactone ring, were isolated from the Japanese alga *S. sagamianum* mentioned above [84]. Their structures were determined by extensive spectrometric analysis and comparison with published data. Particularly, **181** exhibited antibacterial and weak cytotoxic activities [84].

Twenty-four chromene meroterpenoids (**183–206**) were isolated from two distinct samples of *S. siliquastrum*, one collected from the seashore of Pusan [92], and another from Jeju Island (Korea) [93–96]. Among them, **186–188** and **206** contain a linear triprenyl moiety, while the rest possess a tetraprenyl moiety [93,94]. Notably, **198–201** contained a rearranged tetraprenyl carbon skeleton, while **202** had a cyclized tetraprenyl chain, reported for the first time [94]. Compounds **183–202, 205**, and **206** showed antioxidant activities [92–94,96], while **193** and **201** were found to display inhibitory activities toward butylcholine esterase [94]. Additionally, **203** and **204** exhibited cytotoxic activities against AGS, HT-29, and HT-1080 cell lines [95].

A novel furanyl-substituted isochromanyl derivative, turbinochromanone (**207**), was isolated from the ethyl acetate-methanolic extract of the brown seaweed *Turbinaria conoides*, collected from the coasts of Peninsular India. Compound **207** exhibited potential attenuation properties against 5-lipoxygenase and cyclooxygenase-2-enzyme. Furthermore, its antioxidant properties supported its potential use as an anti-inflammatory agent [97].

Two new tetraprenyltoluquinol isomers, thunbergol A (**208**) and B (**209**), were obtained from the brown alga *S. thunbergii* collected along the Busan coast of Korea. The two compounds showed antioxidant effects against DPPH radical and authentic/induced $ONOO^-$ [98].

Four new chromene compounds (**210–213**), along with a new isoprenoid chromenol (**214**), were isolated from two distinct samples of *S. tortile*, one collected from the coast of Tanabe Bay, Japan [99], and the other from Wakasa Bay, Fukui Prefecture, Japan [100,101]. Compounds **210–213** showed cytotoxic activities toward cultured P-388 lymphocytic leukemia cells [99].

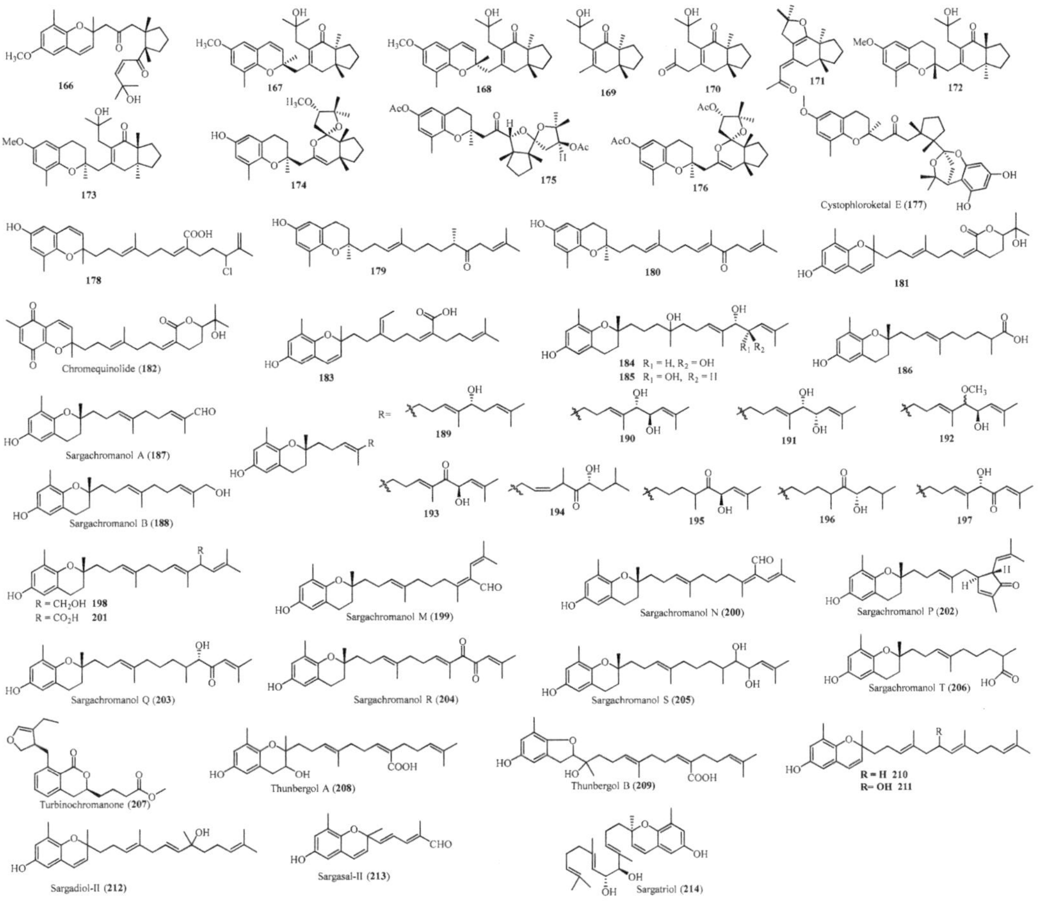

Figure 12. Chromene meroterpenoids isolated from Sargassacean species.

Nahocols/Isonahocols

Five new nahocols (**215–219**) and four novel isonahocols (**220–223**) were isolated from the brown alga *S. siliquastrum* mentioned above [86,102]. Their structures are shown in Figure 13. They share structural similarities to **158** [86]. Especially, **219** contains a cyclopentenone moiety, the characteristic cyclization pattern of which has only been reported for the second time in marine algae. All of them exhibited radical-scavenging activity against DPPH free radicals. Furthermore, isonahocols **220–223** showed a 100-fold increase in radical-scavenging activities compared with nahocols **215–219**, indicating the crucial role of the phenolic group in DPPH radical scavenging activity. In addition, **215–219** showed still-weak activities against isocitrate lyase from *Candida albicans*, while **220–223** exhibited inhibitory effects on transpeptidase sortase A derived from *Staphylococcus aureus*.

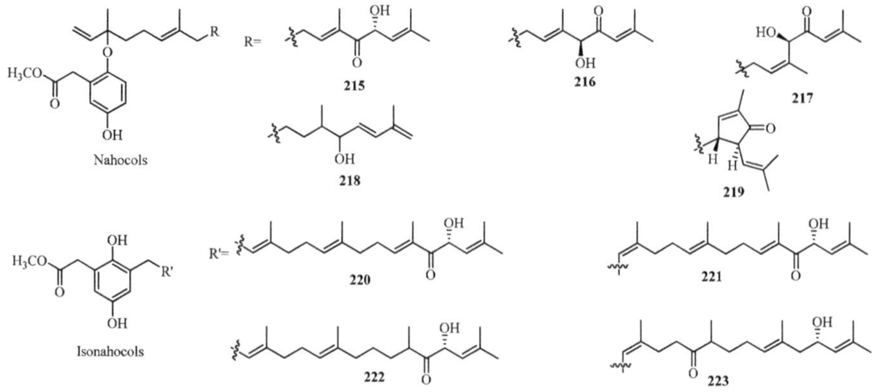

Figure 13. Nahocol/isonahocol meroterpenoids isolated from Sargassacean species.

2.2. Phloroglucinols

To date, numerous phloroglucinol derivatives have been identified in brown seaweed species [103,104]. Notably, some new phloroglucinols were obtained from Sargassaceae species [105–116]. Based on the number of phloroglucinol units, phloroglucinols may be conveniently classified into monomeric phloroglucinols and phlorotannins.

2.2.1. Monomeric Phloroglucinols

Five new monomeric phloroglucinols, **224–228** (Figure 14), were isolated from the brown algae *S. nigrifoloides*, *S. micracanthum*, and *S. spinuligerum* [105–107]. Among them, compounds **224–226** are classified as acyphloroglycinols, and they were isolated from the brown alga *S. nigrifoloides* collected at Nanji Island of Zhejiang, China [105]. These three compounds exhibited inhibitory activities against CDK5 and GSK3β [105].

Compound **227**, consisting of a hydroxyphloroglucinol unit and a sargassumketone moiety, was obtained from the brown alga *S. micracanthum*, collected at Wando County, Korea. It showed radical-scavenging activity against ABTS$^+$ radicals [106].

Compound **228**, containing a phloroglucinol unit and an ascorbic acid moiety, was isolated from the ethanolic extract of the brown alga *S. spinuligerum* as a novel phloroglucinol derivate. Its stereochemistry was determined through NOE experiments and molecular modeling [107].

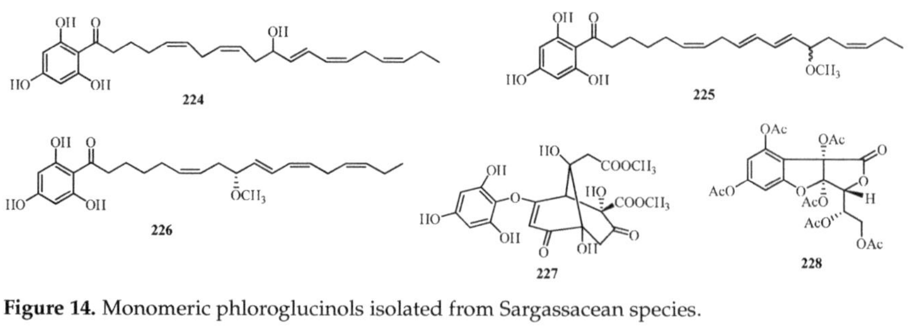

Figure 14. Monomeric phloroglucinols isolated from Sargassacean species.

2.2.2. Phlorotannins

Phlorotannins, a major class in the unique phloroglucinol-based polyphenols, were predominantly found in the Sargassaceae family [103,104]. These compounds were mainly isolated as their acetates due to their instability. Over recent decades, a great number of phlorotannins have been isolated from various Sargassacean species [108–116]. According to the types of linkages between the phloroglucinol units, phlorotannins have been systematically categorized into groups such as fucophlorethols, hydroxyphlorethols, carmalols, phlorethofuhalols, and fuhalols, among others.

Fucophlorethols

Twenty-three new phloroglucinol derivatives (**229–251**) (Figure 15), belonging to the class of fucophlorethols with three to fourteen rings, were isolated from three distinct Sargassaceae species, namely *Carpophyllum maschalocarpum*, *S. spinuligerum*, and *Cystophora torulosa*. Among these, **229–234** were obtained from the brown alga *C. maschalocarpum* collected at Torbay, north of Auckland, New Zealand [108]. Interestingly, **234** is the largest fucophlorethol, characterized by 14 phloroglucinol units. Due to the presence of extra hydroxyl groups, **229**, **231**, and **233** were also categorized as hydroxyfucophlorethols.

Compounds **235–239** were isolated from the brown alga *S. spinuligerum*, collected from Wangaparoa Island, district Auckland, New Zealand [109]. Notably, **238** and **239** were once again obtained from the brown alga *C. torulosa*, collected at Whangaparoa, New Zealand [109]. Interestingly, **239** was found as a chlorine-containing fucophlorethol.

Compounds **240–251** were obtained from the brown algae *C. torulosa* and *S. spinuligerum* harvested at Whangaparoa, New Zealand [109,110]. Among them, **240–242** and **245–251** contain additional hydroxy groups, leading to their classification as hydroxyfucophlorethols as well [110,111]. Compounds **243** and **244**, however, are bis-fucophlorethols that lack a 1,2,3-triphenoxy-5-acetoxybenzene unit [110].

Hydroxyphlorethols

Five new phloroglucinol derivatives belonging to the class of hydroxyphlorethols, **252–256** (Figure 16), were isolated from two *Carpophyllum* species, namely *C. maschalocarpum* and *C. angustifolium* [112,113]. Specifically, **252** and **253**, which contain an additional hydroxyl group, were isolated from the brown alga *C. maschalocarpum* collected at Torbay, north of Auckland [112].

Compounds **254–256** feature three additional hydroxyl groups as well as two 1,2-diphoxylated 3,4,5-triacetoxybenzene rings linked by an ether bond, leading to their designation as trihydroxyphlorethols. All of them were isolated from the brown alga *C. angustifolium* harvested at Panetiki Island, Cape Rodney [113].

Carmalols

Two new phloroglucinol derivatives belonging to the class of carmalols (**257** and **258**) (Figure 17) were isolated from the brown alga *C. maschalocarpum* mentioned above [112,114]. Compound **257** contains two phloroglucinol units and an additional hydroxyl group, and it was named diphlorethohydroxycarmalol nonaacetate. Meanwhile, **258**, which possesses three phloroglucinol units and one additional hydroxyl group, was designated as triphlorethohydroxycarmalol undecaacetate [114].

Phlorethofuhalols

Three new phloroglucinol derivatives (**259–261**) (Figure 18), which are part of the phlorethofuhalol class containing an increased number of 1,4-diphenoxylated 3,5-diacetoxybenzene rings compared with their corresponding fuhalol counterparts, were isolated from the brown alga *C. maschalocarpum*. Among them, **259** and **260** were two isomers composed of six phloroglucinol units linked by ether bonds, whereas **261** consisted of seven phloroglucinol elements linked by ether bonds and contained one additional 1,4-diphenoxylated 3,5-diacetoxybenzene moiety [114].

Fuhalols and Others

A new phloroglucinol derivative belonging to the class of fuhalols, **262** (Figure 19), together with two new phlorotannins with a chlorine atom (**263** and **264**), were isolated from the brown alga *C. angustifolium*, collected at Panetike Island/Cape Rodney/New Zealand [115]. Among them, **262** consists of eight phloroglucinol units linked by ether bonds and contains additional hydroxyl groups. Compound **263** is a chlorinated bifuhalol derivative, whereas **264** is a chlorinated difucol derivative.

In addition, a new phloroglucinol derivative, DDBT (**265**) (Figure 19), was isolated from the brown alga *S. patens*, harvested from the coast of the Noto Peninsula, Japan. This compound showed inhibitory effects against α-amylase and α-glucosidase [116].

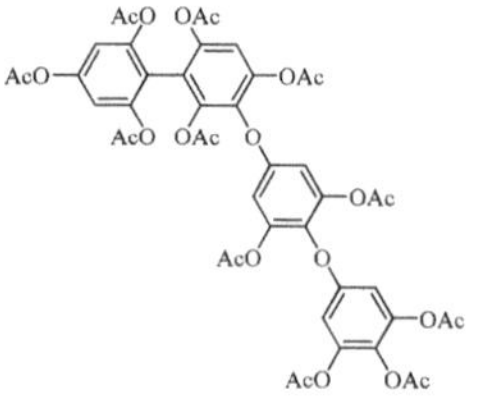

229

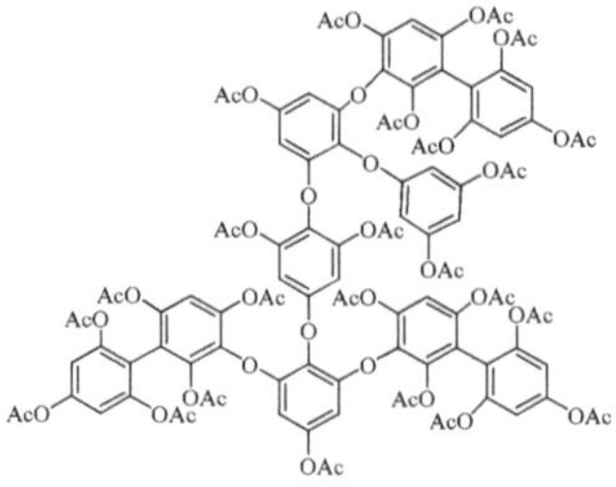

230

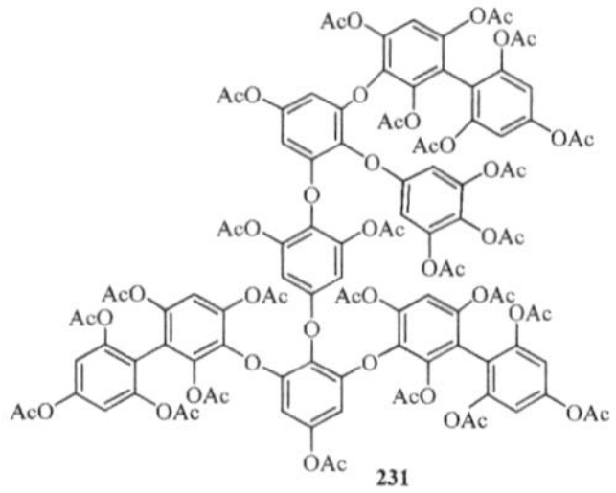

231

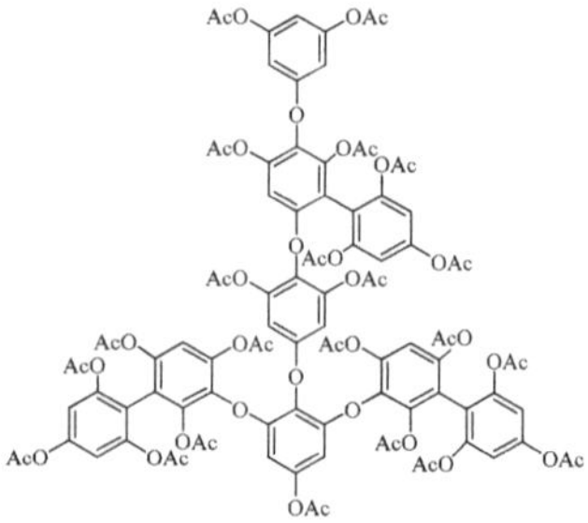

232

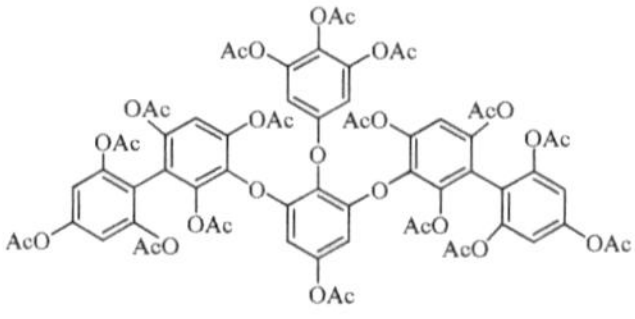

233

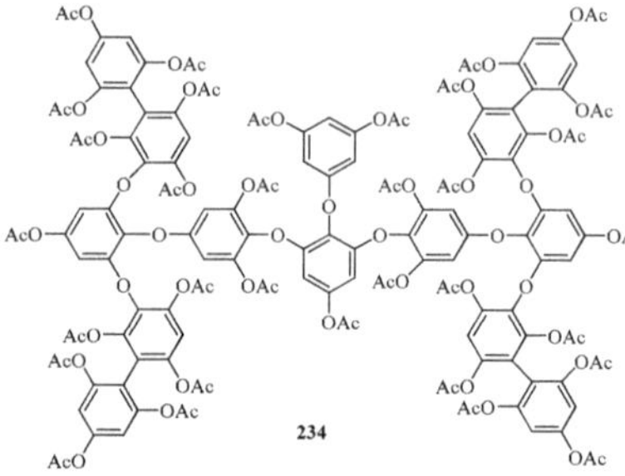

234

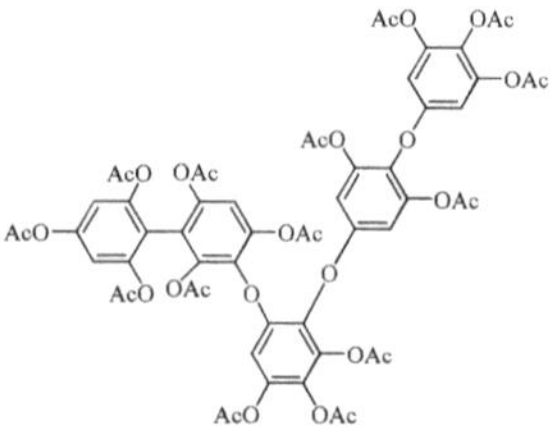

235

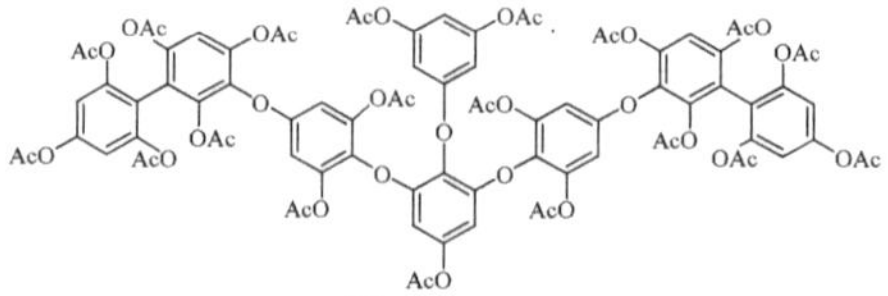

236

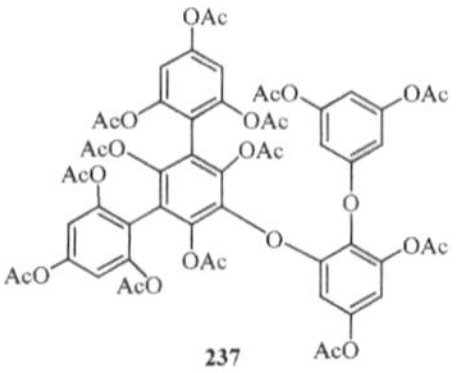

237

Figure 15. *Cont.*

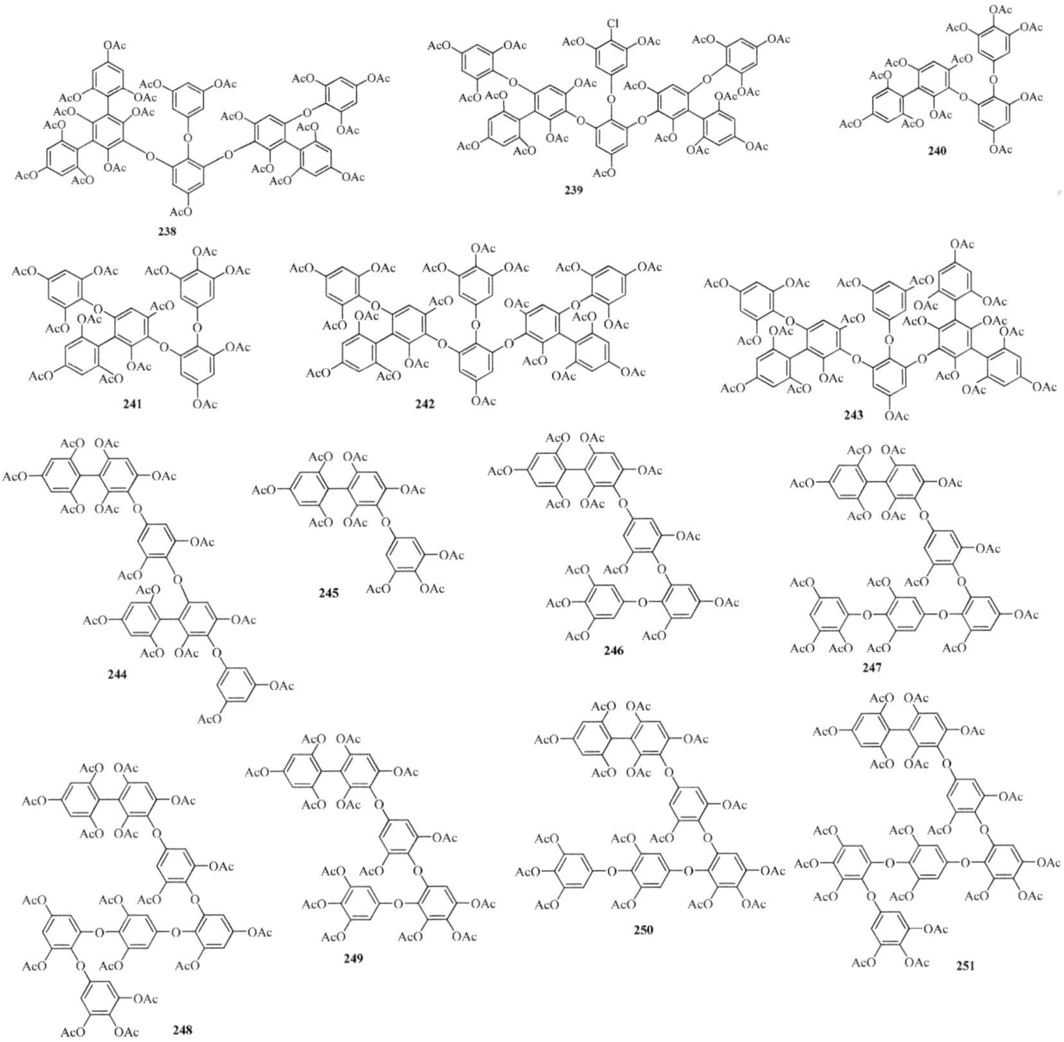

Figure 15. Phloroglucinol derivatives belonging to the class of fucophlorethols.

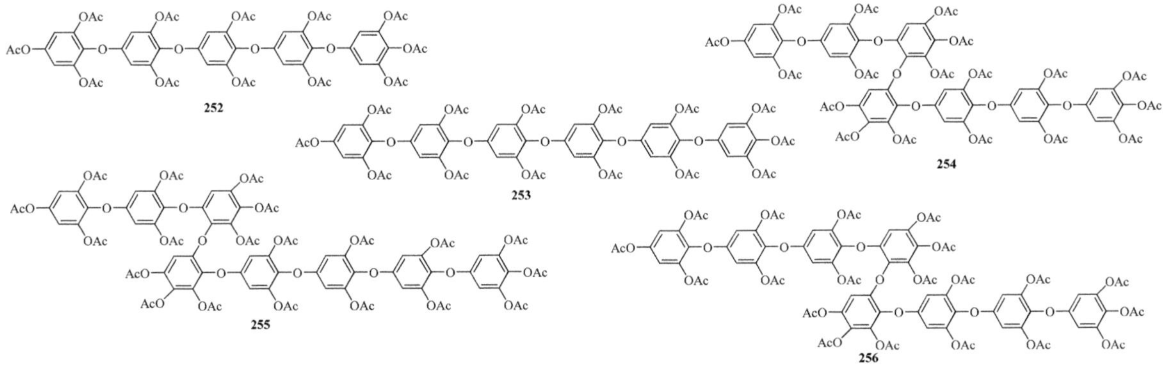

Figure 16. Phloroglucinol derivatives belonging to the class of hydroxyphlorethols.

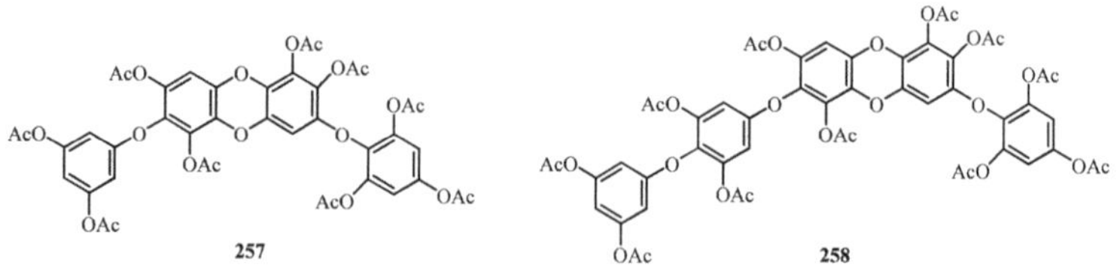

Figure 17. Phloroglucinol derivatives belonging to the class of carmalols.

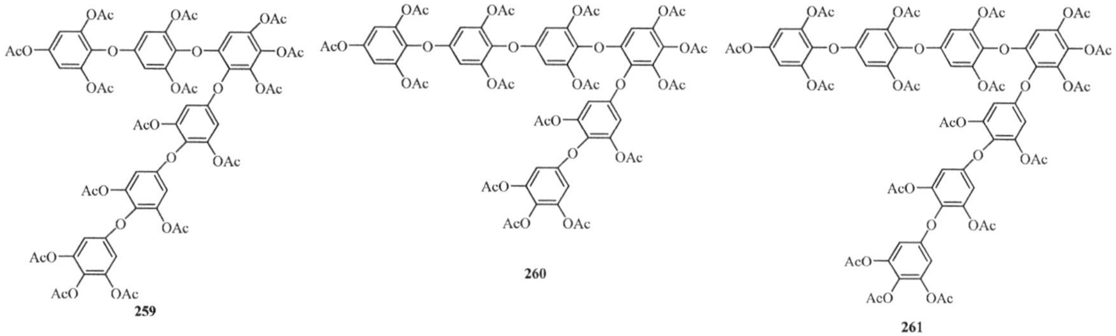

Figure 18. Phloroglucinol derivatives belonging to the class of phlorethofuhalols.

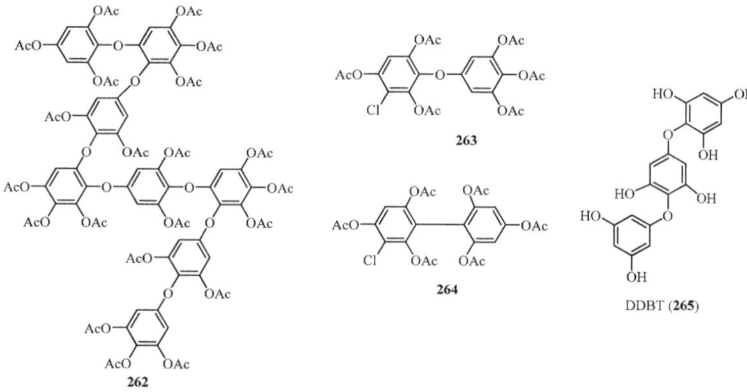

Figure 19. Phloroglucinol derivatives belonging to the class of fuhalols and others.

2.3. Steroids

Steroids are another class of unique metabolites discovered in the Sargassaceae family. Seventeen new sterols (**266–282**) (Figure 20) were isolated from various species of Sargassaceae [117–125]. Interestingly, they are C_{23}-, C_{27}-, and C_{29}- steroids, characterized by keto and hydroxy groups. Among these steroids, one was obtained from *Cystoseira* sp., eight from *Sargassum* sp., and eight from *Turbinaria* sp.

Compound **266**, a C_{27}-brassinosteroid with two keto groups and a hydroxy group, was isolated from the brown alga *C. myrica*, harvested from the region of Fayed, Egypt. It represented the first report of brassinosteroid analogs derived from seaweed. Compound **266** showed cytotoxic effects against HEPG-2 and HCT116 cell lines [117].

Compound **267**, a C_{29}-steroid with an α, β-unsaturated carbonyl group and a tertiary hydroxyl group, was isolated from the brown alga *S. asperifolium*, collected at Hurghada, Egypt. From a biosynthetic perspective, **267** could potentially be derived from saringosterol via an oxidation process involving 3β-OH, followed by the formation of an α, β-unsaturated ketone [118].

Compounds **268** and **269**, two polyoxygenated steroids, were isolated from the brown alga *S. carpophyllum*, harvested from the coasts of the South China Sea in Beihai, China. Specifically, **268** is a C_{29}-polyoxygenated steroid, while **269** is a C_{27}-dinorsteroid, representing only the second example of ring A-dinorsteroid analogs found in natural organisms. Both compounds could induce morphological abnormalities of *Pyricularia oryzae* mycelia. In addition, **268** exhibited cytotoxic activity against HL-60 cell lines [119].

Compounds **270** and **271** are two cholestane-type sterols, each featuring an α, β-unsaturated ketone moiety. Among them, **270** is a C_{27}-steroid, while **271** is a C_{29}-steroid. Both were isolated from the brown alga *S. fusiforme*, harvested from Anhui Bozhou Xiancheng Pharmaceutical Limited Company of China. Their absolute configurations were determined by comparing the calculated and experimental ECD spectra [120].

Compound **272**, a stigmastane-type sterol characterized by three double bonds and one hydroxyl group, was isolated from the brown alga *S. polycystcum*, collected from the North China Sea, China [121].

Compound **273**, a tri-unsaturated C_{29}-sterol with a 3β-hydroxy-Δ^5-steroid skeleton and a vinyloxy group, was isolated from the brown alga *S. thumbergii*, harvested at Muroran, Japan. Its structure was determined by combining NMR spectroscopy and chemical conversion [122].

Compound **274**, a C_{29}-sterol with a 3-hydroxy-2,5-dien-4-carbonyl fragment, was isolated from the brown alga *S. thunbergii*, harvested along the coasts of Nanji Island in the East China Sea of China. It was the first sterol example discovered to contain a 3-hydroxy-2,5-dien-4-carbonyl moiety. Compound **274** showed significant inhibitory activity against PTP1B with an IC_{50} of 2.24 μg/mL [123].

Compounds **275–282**, which are oxygenated steroids, were isolated from two separate samples of *Turbinaria conoides*, one collected at Salin Munthal (India) [124] and another at the coast of Kenting (Taiwan). Notably, **276** is identified as a cardenolide-type C_{23} steroid with an aromatic ring, while the remaining compounds are either stigmasterol or fucosterol derivatives, comprised of 29 carbons. Compounds **275** and **276** showed antimicrobial activities [124], whereas **279–282** exhibited cytotoxic effects against cancer cell lines P-388, KB, A-549, and HT-29 [125].

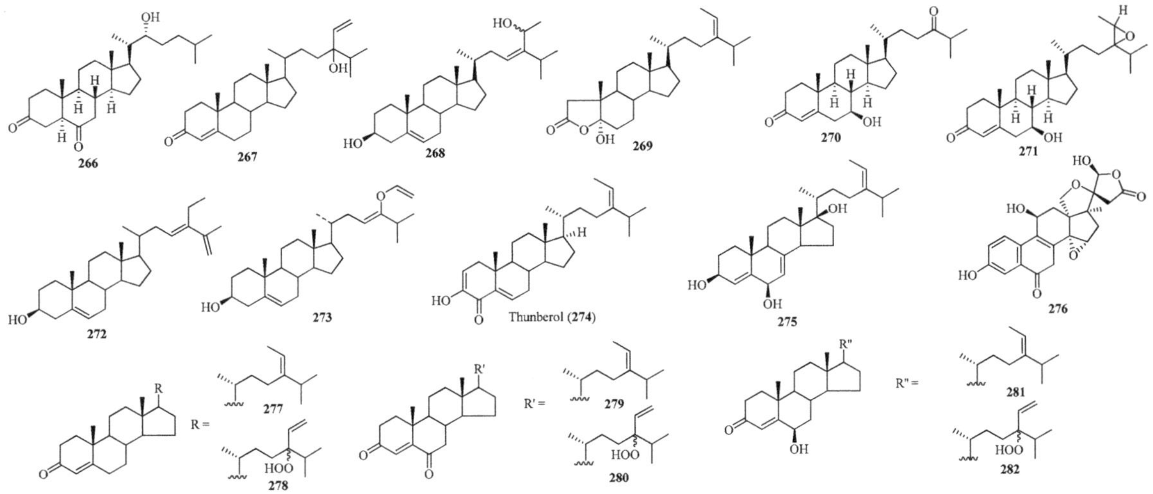

Figure 20. Steroids isolated from the family Sargassaceae.

2.4. Others

Apart from producing an abundance of unique terpenoids, phloroglucinols, and steroids, Sargassaceae species also generate a variety of other metabolites, including macrocyclic lactones, pyran derivatives, furanones, spiroketals, glycerol derivatives, phenol derivatives, amide derivatives, and lipids (Figure 21).

Three new macrolide compounds, conoidecyclics A–C (**283–285**), along with three novel 2H-pyranoids (**286–288**), were isolated from the brown alga *T. conoides*, harvested from the Gulf of Mannar, India [126,127]. These isolates showed anti-inflammatory and radical scavenging activities. Specifically, compounds **283–285** also exhibited antihypertensive and antidiabetic activities [126].

Three new terpenic cyclooctafuranones, turbinafuranones A–C (**289–291**), together with three novel 6,6-spiroketals, spirornatas A–C (**292–294**), were isolated from the marine alga *T. orata*, collected from the Gulf of Manner of India [128,129]. The six compounds showed scavenging activities against DPPH and ABTS radicals. Notably, **289–291** also exhibited in vitro antidiabetic properties [128], while **292–294** showed antihypertensive activities [129].

Five new glycerol derivatives, identified as **295–299**, were isolated from three different *Sargassum* species [130–132]. Among them, **295** and **296** were identified from *S. parvivesiculosum* in Sanya, China, **297** was obtained from *S. sagamianum* on Jeju Island, Korea [131], and **298** and **299** were derived from *S. thunbergii* in the West Sea, Korea [132]. Particularly, **296** and **297** were determined to be monoglycerides, whereas **298** and **299** were glycolipids. Compound **297** exhibited inhibitory activities against COX-2 and sPLA2-IIA [131].

Two novel resorcinols, 1-(5-acetyl-2,4-dihydroxyphenyl)-3-methylbutan-1-one (**300**) and 1-(5-acetyl-2-hydroxy-4-methoxyphenyl)-3-methylbutan-1-one (**301**), were isolated from the brown alga *S. thunbergii*, supplied by the Guanghua Algae Company in Weihai, Shandong, China. Their structures were determined by extensive spectrometric analysis [133].

Two new aryl cresol isomers (**302** and **303**) were isolated from the brown alga *S. cinereum*, harvested along the coasts of the Red Sea in Hurghada, Egypt. Interestingly, the two isolates showed antiproliferative activities against certain cancer cell lines and inhibitory effects against 5-LOX and 15-LOX, the enzymes that have a vital effect on the viability of tumor cells [134].

A novel ketone hybrid of mix biogenesis (**304**), consisting of a four-carbon chain attached to a hydroquinol ring, was isolated from the aforementioned brown alga *C. abies* [60]. Its structure was determined by spectroscopic analysis, including NMR, MS, and UV.

A new amide derivative, sargassulfamide A (**305**), was obtained from the brown alga *S. naozhouense*, harvested from the Leizhou Peninsula, China. Its structure was established by spectrometric analysis and single-crystal X-ray diffraction [135].

Two new unsaturated lipids, (10Z,13Z)-hexadeca-10,13-dienal (**306**) and Ethyl-(10Z,13Z)-hexadeca-10,13-dienoate (**307**), were isolated from the brown alga *C. barbata*, harvested from Salses, France. Compound **306** showed anticancer effects against P388 cells in mice at 40 mg/kg [136].

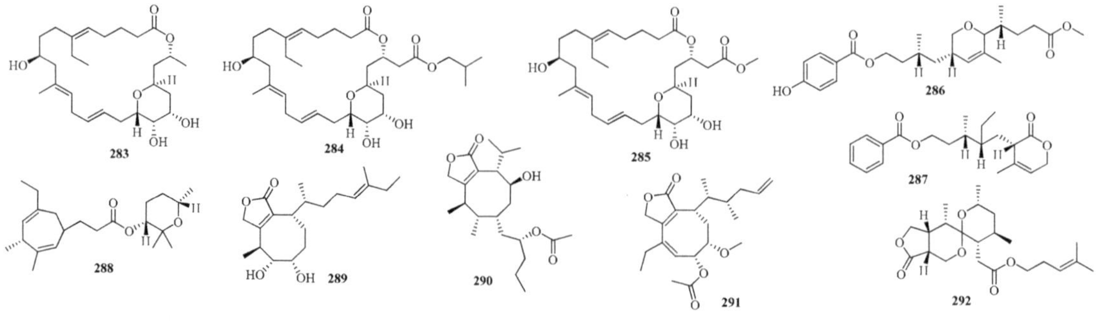

Figure 21. *Cont.*

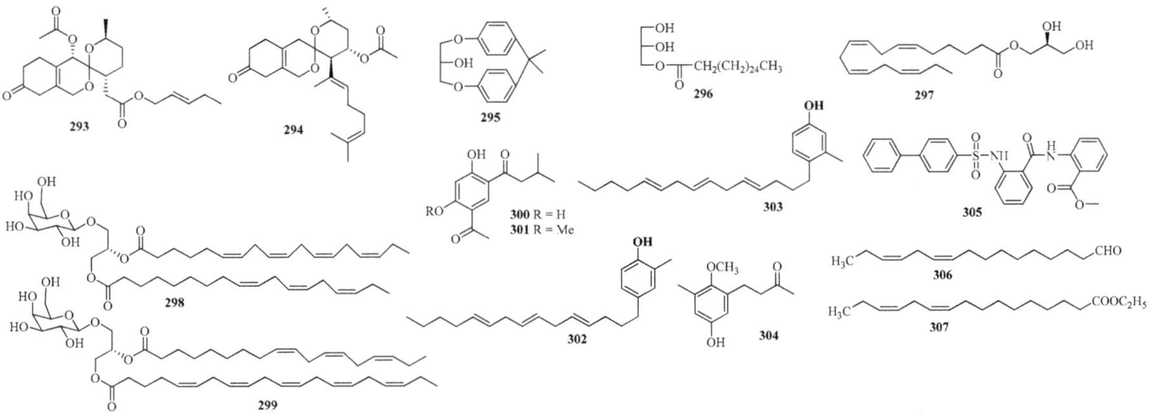

Figure 21. Other types of compounds isolated from Sargassacean species.

3. Conclusions

The merging of the former Cystoseiraceae and Sargassaceae families has resulted in Sargassaceae becoming the largest family in Fucale. To date, more than 60 species of Sargassaceae have been chemically studied, leading to the identification of more than 400 metabolites. Based the available literature, this review summarizes a total of 307 new compounds obtained from 44 Sargassaceae species spanning six genera, and newly discovered compounds derived from the 44 species collected from diverse locations along the Tunisian, Chinese, Italian, Japanese, Australian, Moroccan, Irish Atlantic, Spanish, French, Indian, Egyptian, Portuguese, Algerian, Korean, and New Zealand coasts (Table 1). These include 223 terpenoids, 42 phloroglucinols, 17 steroids, and 25 other types of compounds.

Table 1. Chemical compounds studied in the Sargassaceae species in this review.

Species	Sampling Locations	Compounds and Types	Ref.
Cystoseira schiffneri	Chebba, Tunisia	1 (monoterpenoid)	[27]
C. crinita	Catania, Sicily, Italy	3, 42–44, 58 (sesquiterpenoid and diterpenoids)	[31,46]
	South coast of Sardinia, Italy	70, 71, 73–78, 80, 81 (meroterpenoids)	[57]
	Toulon, France	72, 79, 82 (meroterpenoids)	[58]
C. myrica	El-Zaafarana, Egypt	63–66 (diterpenoids)	[52]
	Fayed, Egypt	266 (steroids)	[117]
C. abies-marina	Mosteiros, Portugal	83, 84, 87, 88 (meroterpenoids)	[59]
	Punta del Hidalgo, Spain	85, 86, 304 (meroterpenoids, ketone)	[60]
C. amentacea var. stricta	Le Brusc, Toulon, France	89, 166 (meroterpenoids)	[62]
C. baccata	El Jadida, Morocco	90, 91, 167–173 (meroterpenoids)	[63,88]
Cystoseira sp.	Montaña Clara Island, Spain	92, 93, 174–176 (meroterpenoids)	[64]
C. balearica	Portopalo, Sicily, Italy	94 (meroterpenoid)	[66]
C. stricta var. amentacea	Castelluccio, Syracuse, Sicily, Italy	95, 96, 104–107 (meroterpenoids)	[67,71]
C. stricta	Acicastello, Catania, Sicily, Italy	97–100, 108, 109 (meroterpenoids)	[67,68,72]
	Portopalo, Sicily, Italy	103 (meroterpenoid)	[70]
C. stricta var. spicata	near Cava d'Aliga, Italy	101, 102 (meroterpenoids)	[69]
C. tamariscifolia	Mediterranean Sea, Algeria	110–113, 177 (meroterpenoids)	[73]
C. usneoides	Mediterranean coast, Morocco	114–119 (meroterpenoids)	[74]
	Tarifa, Spain	120–131 (meroterpenoids)	[75]
	Sesimbra and Cabo Espichel, Portugal	132–135 (meroterpenoids)	[76,77]
C. sauvageuana	Aci Castello, Sicily, Italy	136, 137 (meroterpenoids)	[78]
C. barbata	Salses, France	306, 307 (lipids)	[136]
Sargassum naozhouense	Leizhou Peninsula, China	2, 305 (monoterpenoid and amide)	[28,135]
S. hemiphyllum	Heda Coast, Izu Peninsula, Japan	4–6 (norditerpenoids)	[32]

Table 1. *Cont.*

Species	Sampling Locations	Compounds and Types	Ref.
S. micracanthum	Kominato, Chiba, Japan	7–14 (norditerpenoids)	[33]
	Coast of Gosa, Japan	15, 16 (norditerpenoids)	[34]
	Coast of Toyama Bay, Japan	144–147, 179, 180 (meroterpenoids)	[82,91]
	Wando County, Korea	227 (phloroglucinol)	[106]
S. ilicifolium	Gulf of Manner, India	67 (diterpenoid)	[53]
S. fallax	Governor Reef near Indented Head, Port Phillip Bay, Australia	139, 140, 178 (meroterpenoids)	[80]
S. macrocarpum	Coast of Tsukumowan, Japan	141–143 (meroterpenoids)	[81]
S. paradoxum	Governor Reef near Indented Head, Australia	148–151 (meroterpenoids)	[83]
S. sagamianum	Manazuru, Japan	152–154, 181, 182 (meroterpenoids)	[84]
	Jeju Island, South Korea	297 (glyceride)	[131]
S. sagamianum var. yezoense	Oshoro Bay, Japan	155, 156 (meroterpenoids)	[85]
S. siliquastrum	Jeju Island, Korea	157, 158, 215–223, 184–206 (meroterpenoids)	[86,93–96]
	Seashore of Pusan, Korea	183 (meroterpenoids)	[92]
S. tortile	Awa-Kominato, Chiba, Japan	159–165 (meroterpenoids)	[87]
	Tanabe Bay, Japan	210–213 (meroterpenoids)	[99]
	Wakasa Bay, Japan	214 (meroterpenoid)	[100,101]
	Coast of Busan, Korea	208, 209 (meroterpenoids)	[98]
S. thun(m)bergii	Muroran, Japan	273 (steroid)	[122]
	Nanji Island, East China Sea, China	274 (steroid)	[123]
	West Sea, Korea	298, 299 (glycolipids)	[132]
	Weihai, Shandong, China	300, 301 (resorcinols)	[133]
S. nigrifoloides	Nanji Island, Zhejiang, China	224–226 (phloroglucinols)	[105]
S. spinuligerum	Wangaparoa Island, New Zealand	228, 235–239 (phloroglucinols)	[107,109]
	Auckland Harbour, New Zealand	245, 249 (phlorotannins)	[111]
S. patens	Coast of Noto Peninsula, Japan	265 (phlorotannins)	[116]
S. asperifolium	Hurghada, Egypt	267 (steroid)	[118]
S. carpophyllum	South China Sea, Beihai, China	268, 269 (steroids)	[119]
S. fusiforme	Anhui Bozhou Xiancheng Pharmaceutical Limited Company, China	270, 271 (steroids)	[120]
S. polycystcum	Weizhou Island, Beihai, China	272 (steroid)	[121]
S. parvivesiculosum	Sanya, Hainan, China	295, 296 (glycerols)	[130]
S. cinereum	Red Sea, Hurghada, Egypt	302, 303 (aryl cresols)	[134]
Cystophora moniliformis	Port Phillip Bay, Victoria, Australia	17–19 (norditerpenoids)	[35]
C. harveyi	East of Cape Leeuwin Lighthouse, Australia	138 (meroterpenoid)	[79]
C. torulosa	Whangaparoa, New Zealand	238–251 (phlorotannins)	[109–111]
Bifurcaria bifurcata	Atlantic coasts of Morocco	20–22, 24–26, 60, 62 (linear diterpenoids)	[36,37,39,51]
	Oualidia, Morocco	23, 27, 59, 61 (linear diterpenoids)	[38,40]
	Roscoff, Brittany, France	28, 29, 50–57 (linear diterpenoids)	[41–50]
	Kilkee, County Clare of Ireland	30–39, 45 (linear diterpenoids)	[42–44]
	Quiberon, Brittany, France	40, 41, 46–48 (linear diterpenoids)	[45]
	Near Piriac, France	49 (linear diterpenoid)	[47]
Turbinaria conoides	Gulf of Manner, India	207, 283–288 (meroterpenoid, macrolides, and pyranoids)	[97,126,127]
	Salin Munthal, Gulf of Mannar, India	275, 276 (steroids)	[124]
	Kenting, Taiwan, China	277–282 (steroids)	[125]
T. ornata	Indian peninsular, India	289–291 (furanones)	[128]
	Gulf of Manner, India	292–294 (spiroketals)	[129]
T. decurrens	Mandapam region, India	68, 69 (triterpenes)	[54]
Carpophyllum maschalocarpum	Torbay, north of Auckland, New Zealand	229–234, 252, 253, 257–261 (phlorotannins)	[108,112,114]
C. angustifolium	Panetiki Island, Cape Rodney, New Zealand	254–256, 262–264 (phlorotannins)	[113,115]

The majority of the secondary metabolites are meroterpenoids, diterpenoids, and phloroglucinols (Figure 22). *Sargassum* and *Cystoseira* are the most studied genera, reported by 42 and 27 articles, respectively, and are rich in meroterpenoids (Figure 23). *Bifurcaria*, investigated in 15 articles, is rich in linear diterpenoids, followed by *Turbinaria*, *Cystophora*, and *Carpophyllum*, which were discussed by eight, five, and five articles, respectively. Notably, the most productive species were *B. bifurcata* and *S. siliquastrum*, which have yielded 39 and 35 new compounds, respectively. They were followed by *C. usneoides*, *C. crinita* and *S. micracanthum*, which produced 22, 18, and 17 new compounds, respectively (Table 1).

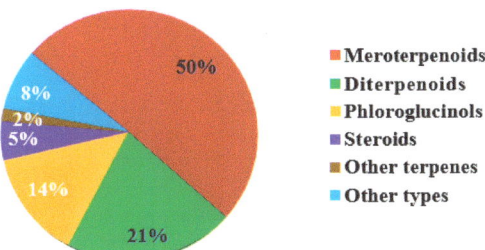

Figure 22. Distribution of compounds from Sargassacean species.

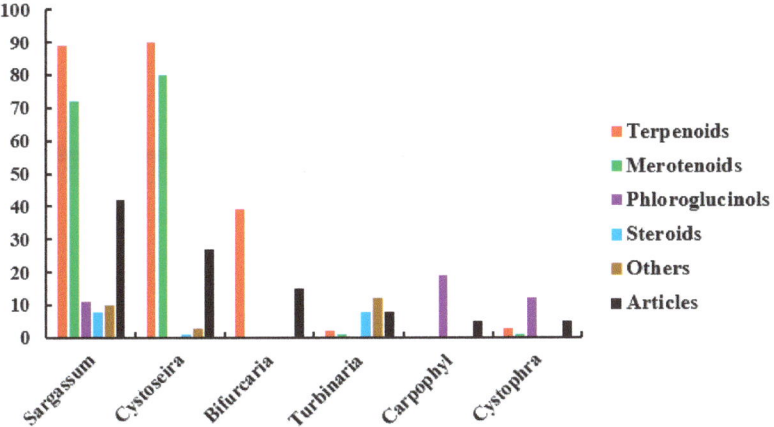

Figure 23. Numbers of compounds and publications from Sargassacean genus.

Notably, from a chemical viewpoint, *B. bifurcata* is clearly distinguishable from other Sargassaceae species due to its extensive production of linear diterpenes. In contrast, the remaining species, with the exception of *C. crinita*, do not produce acyclic diterpenoids. Interestingly, the linear diterpenes yielded by *B. bifurcata* belong to mono-, dio-, and trioxygenated geranylgeraniol derivatives with the oxygenated function located at C-12, C-13, or C-10, depending on the specific sampling locations.

Remarkably, a total of 134 compounds (Table 2), including 85 meroterpenoids, 16 diterpenoids, 2 triterpenoids, 5 phloroglucinols, 10 steroids, 3 macrolides, 3 pyran derivatives, 3 furanones, 3 spiroketals, 3 phenols, and one glycerol derivative, showed various biological activities, such as cytotoxic, antiprotozoal, antioxidant, antifouling, antiviral, antiglycation, antimicrobial, anti-Alzheimer's disease, antidiabetic, antihypertensive, and antiphotoaging effects. Among them, 34 showed cytotoxicities against multiple cancer cell lines, including P388, A-549, L-1210, KB, HT-29, NSCLC-N6, MDA-MB-231, KA3IT, Colon26-L5, AGS, HT-1080, HEPG-2, HCT116, MCF-7, Caco-2, and HL-60. Structure-activity relationships indicated that the configuration of the double bond and positions/quantities/oxidation of hydroxyl groups played key roles in their cytotoxic activities. Additionally, 74 of them demonstrated potent radical-scavenging effects in the DPPH and ABTS assay, while 22 of them showed superior attenuation potential against cyclooxygenase-1/2 and 5-lipoxygenase, and TNF-α.

Table 2. Bioactive compounds reported from Sargassaceae species in this review.

Activity Class	Compounds	Biological Activities	Ref.
Cytotoxicity	4–6	against P388, IC_{50}: 5.1, 2.2, and 50 μg/mL	[32]
	132, 133	against P388, IC_{50}: 0.8 and 1.5 μg/mL	[76]
		against A-549, IC_{50}: 1.25 and 1.4 μg/mL	[76]
	134, 135	against P-388, IC_{50}: 3.2 and 6.8 μg/mL	[77]
		against L-1210, inhibition rate: 50–100%, 10–20 μg/mL	[77]
		against A-549, inhibition rate: 50–70%, 20 μg/mL	[77]
	139, 140, 178	against P388, IC_{50} > 27–29 μM	[80]
	210–213	against P388, ED_{50}: 20.8, 14.0, 16.8 and 5.7 μg/mL	[99]
	279–282	against P-388, ED_{50}: 0.6, 0.8, 0.9 and 0.4 μg/mL	[125]
		against KB, ED_{50}: 5.9, 4.0, 4.6 and 1.8 μg/mL	[125]
		against A-549, ED_{50}: 3.1, 2.5, 2.3 and 1.8 μg/mL	[125]
		against HT-29, ED_{50}: 0.4, 1.4, 1.2 and 1.7 μg/mL	[125]
	307	against P388 in mice in vivo at 40 mg/kg	[136]
	21, 22	against NSCLC-N6, IC_{50}: 12.3 and 9.5 μg/mL	[37]
	31	against MDA-MB-231, inhibition rate: 78.8%, 100 μg/mL	[43]
	35	against MDA-MB-231, IC_{50}: 30.7 μg/mL	[44]
	63–66	against KA3IT, IC_{50}: 10, 5, 5 and 5 μg/mL	[52]
	83, 84, 87	against Hela in Log and Lag phases, IC_{50}: 17.3–25.0, 20.1–32.0 and 2.8–10.2 μg/mL	[59]
	152, 153, 181	against Hela S3, IC_{50}: 10, 4.0 and 10 μg/mL	[84]
	144–146	against Colon 26-L5, IC_{50}: 1.51, 17.5 and 1.69 μg/mL	[82]
	204	against AGS, HT-29 and HT-1080, IC_{50}: 6.5, 3.4 and 13.9 μg/mL	[95]
	266	against HEPG-2 and HCT116, IC_{50}: 2.96 and 12.38 μM	[117]
	302	against HepG2, MCF-7 and Caco-2, IC_{50}: 14.5, 17.6 and 18.2Mm	[134]
	303	against HepG2, MCF-7, and Caco-2, IC_{50}: 13.1, 12.7 and 11.2 μM	[134]
	268	against HL-60, IC_{50}: 2.96 μg/mL	[119]
		causing morphological abnormality of *Pyricularia oryzae* mycelia, MMDC: 63 μg/mL	[119]
	269	causing morphological abnormality of *P. oryzae* mycelia, MMDC: 250 μg/mL	[119]
	28, 62, 89	against *Paracentrotus lividus*, ED_{50}: 12, 4 and 12 μg/mL	[41,51,62]
Anti-inflammatory	67	inhibit COX-1/2 and 5-LOX, IC_{50}: 3.52, 2.47 and 4.70 mM	[53]
	68, 69	inhibit COX-1, IC_{50}: 21.62 and 22.02 μM	[54]
		inhibit COX-2, IC_{50}: 15.51 and 13.98 μM	[54]
		inhibit 5-LOX, IC_{50}: 3.92 and 3.02 μM	[54]
	207	inhibit COX-2 and 5-LOX, IC_{50}: 1.47 and 3.70 μM	[97]
	283–288	inhibit COX-1, IC_{50}: 3.13, 3.19, 3.35, 4.06, 5.11 and 5.23 mM	[126,127]
		inhibit COX-2, IC_{50}: 1.75, 1.93, 1.99, 2.15, 2.93 and 3.27 mM	[126,127]
		inhibit 5-LOX, IC_{50}: 4.24, 4.88, 5.07, 2.41, 2.99 and 3.22 mM	[126,127]
	297	inhibit COX-2 and sPLA2-IIA, inhibition rate: 35.6%, 50 μM; 26.1%, 10 μM	[131]
	114, 115, 117	TNF-α inhibition, inhibition rate: 11–33%, 6–10 μM	[74]
	120	TNF-α inhibition, inhibition rate: 81%, 10 μM	[75]
	121, 123, 127, 129, 130	TNF-α inhibition, inhibition rate: 21–35%, 8–10 μM	[75]
	125	TNF-α inhibition, inhibition rate: 79%, 8 μM	[75]
	128	59% inhibition against TNF-α at 5 μM	[75]

Table 2. *Cont.*

Activity Class	Compounds	Biological Activities	Ref.
Antioxidant	67	scavenge DPPH and ABTS$^+$ radicals, IC$_{50}$: 1.26 and 1.38 mM	[53]
	70, 71, 73–78, 80, 81	scavenge DPPH radicals, scavenging rate: 29.0–96.7%, 164–230 µM	[57]
	87, 88	scavenge DPPH radicals, scavenging rate: 29–30%, 500 µg/mL	[59]
	114–117	scavenge ABTS$^{\cdot+}$ radicals, EC$_{50}$: 22.5–55.9 µM	[72]
	120–125, 127–130	scavenge ABTS$^{\cdot+}$ radicals, EC$_{50}$: 14.81–32.41 µM	[75]
	144–146	inhibition lipid peroxidation, IC$_{50}$: 0.95–44.3 µg/mL	[82]
		scavenge DPPH radicals, IC$_{50}$: 3.00–52.6 µg/mL	[82]
	157	scavenge DPPH radicals, RC$_{50}$: 0.24 µg/mL	[86]
	183	scavenge DPPH radicals, scavenging rate: 96.07%, 0.5 mg/mL	[92]
	187–202	scavenge DPPH radicals, scavenging rate: 87–91%, 100 µg/mL	[94]
	205, 206	scavenge DPPH radicals, EC$_{50}$: 31.1–57.1 mM	[96]
		scavenge ABTS$^+$ radicals, EC$_{50}$: 15.8–28.1 µM	[96]
	207	scavenge DPPH and ABTS$^+$ radicals, IC$_{50}$: 24.25 and 24.32 µM	[97]
	208, 209	scavenge DPPH radicals, EC$_{50}$: 30 and 31 µg/mL	[98]
		scavenge authentic/induced ONOO-, scavenging rate: 60/98.6%, 57.1/90.6%	[98]
	215–219	scavenge DPPH radicals, RC$_{50}$: 11.72–23.23 µg/mL	[86]
	220–223	scavenge DPPH radicals, RC$_{50}$: 0.10–0.33 µg/mL	[86]
	227	scavenge ABTS+ radicals, IC$_{50}$: 47 µM	[106]
	283–285	scavenge DPPH radicals, IC$_{50}$: 1.20, 1.35 and 1.54 mM	[126]
		scavenge ABTS$^+$ radicals, IC$_{50}$: 1.48, 1.54, and 1.81mM	[126]
	286–288	scavenge DPPH radicals, IC$_{50}$: 0.54, 0.54 and 0.68 mg/mL	[127]
		scavenge ABTS$^+$ radicals, IC$_{50}$: 0.58, 0.58 and 0.76 mg/mL	[127]
	289–291	scavenge DPPH radicals, IC$_{50}$: 1.16, 1.05 and 1.21 mM	[128]
		scavenge ABTS$^+$ radicals, IC$_{50}$: 1.38, 1.24 and 1.41 mM	[128]
	292–294	scavenge DPPH radicals, IC$_{50}$: 1.14, 1.25 and 1.42 mM	[129]
		scavenge ABTS$^+$ radicals, IC$_{50}$: 1.28, 1.34 and 1.71 mM	[129]
	184–186	reduce ROS formation in HT 1080 cells by over 67.2% at 5 µg/mL	[93]
		inhibit lipid peroxidation induced by H$_2$O$_2$	[93]
		increase GSH levels in HT1080 cells at 5 µg/mL	[93]
Antifouling	110–113, 177	against *Pseudoalteromonas elyakovii*, *Vibrio aesturianus*, *Polaribacter irgensii*, *Halosphaeriopsis mediosetigera*, *Asteromyces cruciatus*, and *Lulworthia uniseptate*, MIC: 0.1–10 µg/mL	[73]
		against *Exanthemachrysis gayraliae*, *Cylindrotheca closterium*, *Pleurochrysis roscoffensis*, *Ulva intestinalis*, and *Undaria pinnatifida*, MIC: 0.1–10 µg/mL	[73]
	168	against *Sargassum muticum* and phenoloxidase, IC$_{50}$: 2.5 and 1 µg/mL	[63]
	169	against *S. muticum*, *U. intestinalis*, phenoloxidase, and *E. gayraliae*, IC$_{50}$: 1 µg/mL	[63]
	171	against *U. intestinalis* and phenoloxidase, IC$_{50}$: 2.5 and 2.5 µg/mL	[63]
Antimicrobial	149–151	against *Streptococcus pyogenes* (345/1), zones of inhibition: 1–3 mm, 1 mg/mL	[83]
	152, 153, 181	against *Bacillus subtilis* and *Staphylococcus aureus*, inhibition rate: ca. 30 and 80%	[84]
	157	slight inhibition against isocitrate lyase from *S. aureus*	[86]
	158, 215–223	weak inhibition AGAINST sortase A from *Candida albicans*	[86]
	275	against *Staphylococcus aureus*, *S. epidermidis*, *Escherichia coli* and *Pseudomonas aeruginosa*, MIC: 32–128 µg/mL	[124]
		against *Candida albicans* and *Aspergillus niger*, MIC: 16 µg/mL	[124]
	276	against *S. aureus*, *S. epidermidis*, *E. coli* and *P. aeruginosa*, MIC: 32–128 µg/mL	[124]
		against *C. albicans* and *A. niger*, MIC: 4 and 2 µg/mL	[124]

Table 2. Cont.

Activity Class	Compounds	Biological Activities	Ref.
Anti-Alzheimer's disease	193, 201	butylcholine esterase inhibition, inhibition rates: 82.7 or 80%	[94]
	224–226	against CDK5, IC_{50}: 12, 18 and 17 µM	[105]
		against GSK3β, IC_{50}: 1.6, 1.1 and 1.8 µM	[105]
Antidiabetic	265	against α-amylase and α-glucosidase with IC_{50} values of 3.2 and 25.4–114 µg/mL, respectively	[116]
	274	PTP1B inhibition, IC_{50}: 2.24 mM	[123]
	283–285	PTP-1B inhibition, IC_{50}: 1.39, 2.33 and 3.13 mM	[126]
	289–291	PTP-1B inhibition, IC_{50}: 2.58, 2.42 and 2.77 mM	[128]
		α-amylase inhibition, IC_{50}: 0.39, 0.31 and 0.48 mM	[128]
		α-glucosidase inhibition, IC_{50}: 0.34, 0.27 and 0.44 mM	[128]
Antihypertensive	283–285	ACE-I inhibition, IC_{50}: 1.23, 1.89 and 2.23 mM	[126]
	292–294	ACE-I inhibition, IC_{50}: 4.55, 4.72 and 4.86 mM	[129]
Antiprotozoal	30	against *Plasmodium falciparum*, IC_{50}: 0.65 µg/mL	[42]
Antiviral	132–135	against CV-1, IC_{50}: 4.0, 1.0, 3.6 and 4.0 µg/mL	[76,77]
		against BHK, IC_{50}: 6.2, 1.1, 3.7 and 6.2 µg/mL	[76,77]
Antiglycation	141–143	AGEs inhibition, IC_{50}: 2.1, 2.6 and 1.0 mM	[81]
Antiphotoaging	172, 173	photodamage attenuation effect, cell viability value: 82.6–95.1%, 5–20 µg/mL	[90]

Therefore, Sargassacean algae are an important source of bioactive secondary metabolites. Given the great number of species of this family that remain chemically and pharmacologically underexplored, it is thus worthy to further investigate novel lead compounds from Sargassacean algae.

Author Contributions: Y.P. collected the references and wrote the review. X.Y. and R.H. completed the word processing and graphics. B.R., B.C. and Y.L. analyzed data from the references. H.Z. conceived of and greatly revised the manuscript. All authors have read and agreed to the published version of the manuscript.

Funding: This project was financially supported by grants from the Overseas Scholarship Program for Elite Young and Middle-aged Teachers of Lingnan Normal University (No. 20151170129), Zhanjiang City-Science and Technology Program (No. 2016A03025), and Natural Science Foundation of Lingnan Normal University (No. KYB2114).

Institutional Review Board Statement: Not applicable.

Data Availability Statement: The data presented in this study are available.

Acknowledgments: We thank the people who helped with this work and Enyi Xie of Fisheries College, Guangdong Ocean University.

Conflicts of Interest: The authors declare no conflicts of interest.

References

1. Kumari, P.; Kumar, M.; Gupta, V.; Reddy, C.R.K.; Jha, B. Tropical marine macroalgae as potential sources of nutritionally important PUFAs. *Food Chem.* **2010**, *120*, 749–757. [CrossRef]
2. Anis, M.; Ahmed, S.; Hasan, M.M. Algae as nutrition, medicine and cosmetic: The forgotten history, present status and future trends. *World J. Pharm. Sci.* **2017**, *6*, 1934–1959.
3. Yende, S.R.; Harle, U.N.; Chaugule, B.B. Therapeutic potential and health benefits of *Sargassum* species. *Phcog. Rev.* **2014**, *8*, 1–7. [CrossRef] [PubMed]
4. Muñoz, J.; Culioli, G.; Köck, M. Linear Diterpenes from the Marine Brown Alga *Bifurcaria bifurcata*: A chemical perspective. *Phytochem. Rev.* **2013**, *12*, 407–424. [CrossRef]
5. Remya, R.R.; Samrot, A.V.; Kumar, S.S.; Mohanavel, V.; Karthick, A.; Chinnaiyan, V.K.; Umapathy, D.; Muhibbullah, M. Bioactive potential of brown algae. *Adsorpt. Sci. Technol.* **2022**, *2022*, 1–13. [CrossRef]

6. Arrieche, D.; Carrasco, H.; Olea, A.F.; Espinoza, L.; San-Martín, A. Secondary metabolites isolated from Chilean Marine Algae: A Review. *Mar. Drugs* **2022**, *20*, 337. [CrossRef] [PubMed]
7. Máximo, P.; Ferreira, L.M.; Branco, P.; Lima, P.; Lourenço, A. Secondary metabolites and biological activity of invasive macroalgae of Southern Europe. *Mar. Drugs* **2018**, *16*, 265. [CrossRef] [PubMed]
8. Peng, Y.; Hu, J.; Yang, B.; Lin, X.P.; Zhou, X.F.; Yang, X.W.; Liu, Y.H. Chemical Composition of Seaweed. In *Seaweed Sustainability: Food and Non-Food Applications*, 1st ed.; Tiwari, B.K., Troy, D.J., Eds.; Academic Press: Amsterdam, The Netherlands, 2015; pp. 79–124.
9. Balboa, E.M.; Conde, E.; Moure, A.; Falqué, E.; Domínguez, H. *In vitro* antioxidant properties of crude extracts and compounds from brown algae. *Food Chem.* **2013**, *138*, 1764–1785. [CrossRef]
10. Generalić Mekinić, I.; Skroza, D.; Šimat, V.; Hamed, I.; Čagalj, M.; Popović Perković, Z. Phenolic content of brown algae (*Pheophyceae*) species: Extraction, identification, and quantification. *Biomolecules* **2019**, *9*, 244. [CrossRef]
11. Huang, B.; Ding, L.; Luan, R.; Sun, Z. New classification system of marine brown algae of China. *Guangxi Sci.* **2015**, *22*, 189–200.
12. Carroll, A.R.; Copp, B.R.; Davis, R.A.; Keyzers, R.A.; Prinsep, M.R. Marine natural products. *Nat. Prod. Rep.* **2022**, *39*, 1122–1171. [CrossRef] [PubMed]
13. Blunt, J.W.; Carroll, A.R.; Copp, B.R.; Davis, R.A.; Keyzers, R.A.; Prinsep, M.R. Marine natural products. *Nat. Prod. Rep.* **2017**, *34*, 235–294. [CrossRef] [PubMed]
14. Draisma, S.G.A.; Ballesteros, E.; Rousseau, F.; Thibaut, T. DNA sequence data demonstrate the polyphyly of the genus *Cystoseira* and other *Sargassaceae genera* (Phaeophyceae). *J. Phycol.* **2010**, *46*, 1329–1345. [CrossRef]
15. Rousseau, F.; de Reviers, B. Phylogenetic relationships within the Fucales (Phaeophyceae) based on combined partial SSU + LSU rDNA sequence data. *Eur. J. Phycol.* **1999**, *34*, 53–64.
16. Guiry, M.D.; Guiry, G.M. AlgaeBase. World-Wide Electronic Publication, National University of Ireland, Galway. Available online: http://www.algaebase.org (accessed on 7 August 2023).
17. Liu, L.; Heinrich, M.; Myers, S.; Dworjanyn, S.A. Towards a better understanding of medicinal uses of the brown seaweed *Sargassum* in Traditional Chinese Medicine: A phytochemical and pharmacological review. *J. Ethnopharmacol.* **2012**, *142*, 591–619. [CrossRef] [PubMed]
18. de Sousa, C.B.; Gangadhar, K.N.; Macridachis, J.; Pavão, M.; Morais, T.R.; Campino, L.; Varela, J.; Lago, J.H.G. *Cystoseira* algae (Fucaceae): Update on their chemical entities and biological activities. *Tetrahedron: Asymmetry* **2017**, *28*, 1486–1505. [CrossRef]
19. Catarino, M.D.; Pires, S.M.G.; Silva, S.; Costa, F.; Braga, S.S.; Pinto, D.C.G.A.; Silva, A.M.S.; Cardoso, S.M. Overview of phlorotannins' constituents in *Fucales*. *Mar. Drugs* **2022**, *20*, 754. [CrossRef]
20. Valls, R.; Piovetti, L. The chemistry of the *Cystoseiraceae* (Fucales: Pheophyceae): Chemotaxonomic relationships. *Biochem. Syst. Ecol.* **1995**, *23*, 723–745. [CrossRef]
21. Gouveia, V.; Seca, A.M.L.; Barreto, M.C.; Pinto, D.C.G.A. Di- and sesquiterpenoids from *Cystoseira* genus: Structure, intramolecular transformations and biological activity. *Mini-Rev. Med. Chem.* **2013**, *13*, 1150–1159. [CrossRef]
22. Chen, Z.; Liu, H.B. Recent Advance on the Chemistry and Bioactivity of Genus *Sargassum*. *Chin. J. Mar. Drugs* **2012**, *31*, 41–51.
23. Rushdi, M.I.; Abdel-Rahman, I.A.M.; Saber, H.; Attia, E.Z.; Abdelraheem, W.M.; Madkour, H.A.; Hassan, H.M.; Elmaidomy, A.H. Pharmacological and natural products diversity of the brown algae genus *Sargassum*. *RSC Adv.* **2020**, *10*, 24951–24972. [CrossRef] [PubMed]
24. Rushdi, M.I.; Abdel-Rahman, I.A.M.; Saber, H.; Attia, E.Z.; Abdelraheem, W.M.; Madkour, H.A.; Abdelmohsen, U.R. The genus *Turbinaria*: Chemical and pharmacological diversity. *Nat. Prod. Res.* **2021**, *35*, 4560–4578. [CrossRef] [PubMed]
25. Xu, R.S.; Ye, Y.; Zhao, W.M. *Natural Products Chemistry*, 2nd ed.; Beijing Press: Beijing, China, 2004; pp. 166–374.
26. Roberts, S.C. Production and engineering of terpenoids in plant cell culture. *Nat. Chem. Biol.* **2007**, *3*, 387–395. [CrossRef] [PubMed]
27. Salem, A.B.; Di Giuseppe, G.; Anesi, A.; Hammami, S.; Mighri, Z.; Guella, G. Natural products among brown algae: The case of *Cystoseira schiffneri* Hamel (Sargassaceae, Phaeophyceae). *Chem. Biodivers.* **2017**, *14*, e1600333. [CrossRef] [PubMed]
28. Peng, Y.; Huang, R.M.; Lin, X.P.; Liu, Y.H. Norisoprenoids from the brown alga *Sargassum naozhouense* Tseng et Lu. *Molecules* **2018**, *23*, 348. [CrossRef]
29. Smith, A.B.; Branca, S.J.; Pilla, N.N.; Guaciaro, M.A. Stereocontrolled total synthesis of (±)-pentenomycins. I-III, their epimers, and dehydropentenomycin I. *J. Org. Chem.* **1982**, *47*, 1855–1869. [CrossRef]
30. Kimura, J.; Maki, N. New loliolide derivatives from the brown alga *Undaria pinnatifa*. *J. Nat. Prod.* **2002**, *65*, 57–58. [CrossRef] [PubMed]
31. Fattorusso, E.; Magno, S.; Mayol, L.; Santacroce, C.; Sica, D.; Amico, V.; Oriente, G.; Piattelli, M.; Tringal, C. Oxocrinol and Crinitol, novel linear terpenoids from the brown alga *Cystoseira crinita*. *Tetrahedron Lett.* **1976**, *17*, 937–940. [CrossRef]
32. Takada, N.; Watanabe, R.; Suenaga, K.; Yamada, K.; Uemura, D. Isolation and structures of hedaols A, B, and C, new bisnorditerpenes from a Japanese brown alga. *J. Nat. Prod.* **2001**, *64*, 653–655. [CrossRef]
33. Kusumi, T.; Ishitsuka, M.; Nomura, Y.; Konno, T.; Kakisawa, H. New farnesylacetone derivatives from *Sargassum micracanthum*. *Chem. Lett.* **1979**, *8*, 1181–1184. [CrossRef]
34. Shizuri, Y.; Matsukawa, S.; Ojika, M.; Yamada, K. Two new farnesylacetone derivatives from the brown alga *Sargassum micracanthum*. *Phytochemistry* **1982**, *21*, 1808–1809. [CrossRef]

35. Reddy, P.; Urban, S. Linear and cyclic C18 terpenoids from the Southern Australian marine brown alga *Cystophora moniliformis*. *J. Nat. Prod.* **2008**, *71*, 1441–1446. [CrossRef] [PubMed]
36. Valls, R.; Banaigs, B.; Francisco, C.; Codomier, L.; Cave, A. An acyclic diterpene from the brown alga *Bifurcaria bifurcata*. *Phytochemistry* **1986**, *25*, 751–752. [CrossRef]
37. Culioli, G.; Ortalo-Magné, A.; Daoudi, M.; Thomas-Guyon, H.; Valls, R.; Piovetti, L. Trihydroxylated linear diterpenes from the brown alga *Bifurcaria bifurcata*. *Phytochemistry* **2004**, *65*, 2063–2069. [CrossRef]
38. El Hattab, M.; Ben Mesaoud, M.; Daoudi, M.; Ortalo-Magné, A.; Culioli, G.; Valls, R.; Piovetti, L. Trihydroxylated linear diterpenes from the brown alga *Bifurcaria bifurcata* (Fucales, Phaeophyta). *Biochem. Syst. Ecol.* **2008**, *36*, 484–489. [CrossRef]
39. Culioli, G.; Daoudi, M.; Ortalo-Magné, A.; Valls, R.; Piovetti, L. (S)-12-hydroxygeranylgeraniol-derived diterpenes from the brown alga *Bifurcaria bifurcata*. *Phytochemistry* **2001**, *57*, 529–535. [CrossRef] [PubMed]
40. Semmak, L.; Zerzouf, A.; Valls, R.; Banaigs, B.; Jeanty, G.; Francisco, C. Acyclic diterpenes from *Bifurcaria bifurcata*. *Phytochemistry* **1988**, *27*, 2347–2349. [CrossRef]
41. Valls, R.; Piovetti, L.; Banaigs, B.; Archavlis, A.; Pellegrini, M. (S)-13-hydroxygeranylgeraniol-derived furanoditerpenes from *Bifurcaria bifurcata*. *Phytochemistry* **1995**, *39*, 145–149. [CrossRef]
42. Smyrniotopoulos, V.; Merten, C.; Kaiser, M.; Tasdemir, D. Bifurcatriol, a new antiprotozoal acyclic diterpene from the brown alga *Bifurcaria bifurcata*. *Mar. Drugs* **2017**, *15*, 245. [CrossRef]
43. Smyrniotopoulos, V.; Firsova, D.; Fearnhead, H.; Grauso, L. Density functional theory (DFT)-aided structure elucidation of linear diterpenes from the Irish brown seaweed *Bifurcaria bifurcata*. *Mar. Drugs* **2021**, *19*, 42. [CrossRef]
44. Smyrniotopoulos, V.; Merten, C.; Firsova, D.; Fearnhead, H.; Tasdemir, D. Oxygenated acyclic diterpenes with anticancer activity from the Irish brown seaweed *Bifurcaria bifurcata*. *Mar. Drugs* **2020**, *18*, 581. [CrossRef] [PubMed]
45. Ortalo-Magné, A.; Culioli, G.; Valls, R.; Pucci, B.; Piovetti, L. Polar acyclic diterpenoids from *Bifurcaria bifurcata*. *Phytochemistry* **2005**, *66*, 2316–2323. [CrossRef] [PubMed]
46. Amico, V.; Oriente, G.; Piattelli, M.; Ruberto, G.; Tringali, C. Novel acyclic diterpenes from the brown alga *Cystoseira crinita*. *Phytochemistry* **1981**, *20*, 1085–1088. [CrossRef]
47. Combaut, G.; Piovetti, L. A novel acyclic diterpene from the brown alga *Bifurcaria bifurcata*. *Phytochemistry* **1983**, *22*, 1787–1789. [CrossRef]
48. Göthel, Q.; Muñoz, J.; Köck, M. Formyleleganolone and bibifuran, two metabolites from the brown alga *Bifurcaria bifurcata*. *Phytochem. Lett.* **2012**, *5*, 693–695. [CrossRef]
49. Göthel, Q.; Lichte, E.; Köck, M. Further eleganolone-derived diterpenes from the brown alga *Bifurcaria bifurcata*. *Tetrahedron Lett.* **2012**, *53*, 1873–1877. [CrossRef]
50. Hougaard, L.; Anthoni, U.; Christophersen, C. Two new diterpenoid dihydroxy-γ-butyrolactones from *Bifurcaria bifurcata* (Cystoseiraceae). *Tetrahedron Lett.* **1991**, *32*, 3577–3578. [CrossRef]
51. Valls, R.; Banaigs, B.; Piovetti, L.; Archavlis, A.; Artaud, J. Linear diterpene with antimitotic activity from the brown alga *Bifurcaria bifurcata*. *Phytochemistry* **1993**, *34*, 1585–1588. [CrossRef]
52. Ayyad, S.E.N.; Abdel-Halim, O.B.; Shier, W.T.; Hoye, T.R. Cytotoxic hydroazulene diterpenes from the brown alga *Cystoseira myrica*. *Z. Naturforsch. C* **2003**, *58*, 33–38. [CrossRef]
53. Dhara, S.; Chakraborty, K. Anti-inflammatory xenicane-type diterpenoid from the intertidal brown seaweed *Sargassum ilicifolium*. *Nat. Prod. Res.* **2021**, *35*, 5699–5709. [CrossRef]
54. Thambi, A.; Chakraborty, K. Anti-inflammatory decurrencyclics A-B, two undescribed nor-dammarane triterpenes from triangular sea bell *Turbinaria decurrens*. *Nat. Prod. Res.* **2023**, *37*, 713–724. [CrossRef] [PubMed]
55. Joung, E.-J.; Gwon, W.-G.; Shin, T.; Jung, B.-M.; Choi, J.; Kim, H.-R. Anti-inflammatory action of the ethanolic extract from *Sargassum serratifolium* on lipopolysaccharide-stimulated mouse peritoneal macrophages and identification of active components. *J. Appl. Phycol.* **2017**, *29*, 563–573. [CrossRef]
56. Azam, M.S.; Choi, J.; Lee, M.-S.; Kim, H.-R. Hypopigmenting effects of brown algae-derived phytochemicals: A review on molecular mechanisms. *Mar. Drugs* **2017**, *15*, 297. [CrossRef] [PubMed]
57. Fisch, K.M.; Böhm, V.; Wright, A.D.; König, G.M. Antioxidative meroterpenoids from the brown alga *Cystoseira crinita*. *J. Nat. Prod.* **2003**, *66*, 968–975. [CrossRef] [PubMed]
58. Praud, A.; Valls, R.; Piovetti, L.; Banaigs, B.; Benaïm, J.-Y. Meroditerpenes from the brown alga *Cystoseira crinita* off the French Mediterranean coast. *Phytochemistry* **1995**, *40*, 495–500. [CrossRef]
59. Gouveia, V.L.M.; Seca, A.M.L.; Barreto, M.C.; Neto, A.I.; Kijjoa, A.; Silva, A.M.S. Cytotoxic meroterpenoids from the macroalga *Cystoseira abies-marina*. *Phytochem. Lett.* **2013**, *6*, 593–597. [CrossRef]
60. Fernández, J.J.; Navarro, G.; Norte, M. Novel metabolites from the brown alga *Cystoseira abies-marina*. *Nat. Prod. Lett.* **1998**, *12*, 285–291. [CrossRef]
61. García, P.A.; Hernández, Á.P.; San Feliciano, A.; Castro, M.Á. Bioactive prenyl- and terpenyl-quinones/hydroquinones of marine origin. *Mar. Drugs* **2018**, *16*, 292. [CrossRef]
62. Mesguiche, V.; Valls, R.; Piovetti, L.; Banaigs, B. Meroditerpenes from *Cystoseira amentacea* var. *stricta* collected off the Mediterranean coasts. *Phytochemistry* **1997**, *45*, 1489–1494.

63. Mokrini, R.; Mesaoud, M.B.; Daoudi, M.; Hellio, C.; Maréchal, J.-P.; El Hattab, M.; Ortalo-Magné, A.; Piovetti, L.; Culioli, G. Meroditerpenoids and derivatives from the brown alga *Cystoseira baccata* and their antifouling properties. *J. Nat. Prod.* **2008**, *71*, 1806–1811. [CrossRef]
64. Navarro, G.; Fernández, J.J.; Norte, M. Novel meroditerpenes from the brown alga *Cystoseira* sp. *J. Nat. Prod.* **2004**, *67*, 495–499. [CrossRef] [PubMed]
65. Amico, V. Marine brown algae of family Cystoseiraceae: Chemistry and chemotaxonomy. *Phytochemistry* **1995**, *39*, 1257–1279. [CrossRef]
66. Amico, V.; Cunsolo, F.; Piattelli, M.; Ruberto, G.; Fronczek, F.R. Balearone, a metabolite of the brown alga *Cystoseira balearica*. *Tetrahedron* **1984**, *40*, 1721–1725. [CrossRef]
67. Amico, V.; Piattelli, M.; Neri, P.; Ruberto, G.; Mayol, L. Novel metabolites from the marine genus *cystoseira*-application of two-dimensional ^{1}H-^{13}C correlation to the structure elucidation. *Tetrahedron* **1986**, *42*, 6015–6020. [CrossRef]
68. Amico, V.; Cunsolo, F.; Piattelli, M.; Ruberto, G. Prenylated O-methyltoluquinols from *Cystoseira stricta*. *Phytochemistry* **1987**, *26*, 1719–1722. [CrossRef]
69. Amico, V.; Oriente, G.; Piattelli, M.; Ruberto, G.; Tringali, C. A quinone-hydroquinone couple from the brown alga *Cystoseira stricta*. *Phytochemistry* **1982**, *21*, 421–424. [CrossRef]
70. Amico, V.; Cunsolo, F.; Piattelli, M.; Ruberto, G.; Mayol, L. Strictaketal, a new tetraprenyltoluquinol with a heterotetracyclic diterpene moiety from the brown alga *Cystoseira stricta*. *J. Nat. Prod.* **1987**, *50*, 449–454. [CrossRef]
71. Amico, V.; Oriente, G.; Neri, P.; Piattelli, M.; Ruberto, G. Tetraprenyltoluquinols from the brown alga *Cystoseira stricta*. *Phytochemistry* **1987**, *26*, 1715–1718. [CrossRef]
72. Amico, V.; Piattelli, M.; Cunsolo, F.; Neri, P.; Ruberto, G. Two epimeric, irregular diterpenoid toluquinols from the brown alga *Cystoseira stricta*. *J. Nat. Prod.* **1989**, *52*, 962–969. [CrossRef]
73. El Hattab, M.; Genta-Jouve, G.; Bouzidi, N.; Ortalo-Magné, A.; Hellio, C.; Maréchal, J.-P.; Piovetti, L.; Thomas, O.P.; Culioli, G. Cystophloroketals A-E, unusual phloroglucinol-meroterpenoid hybrids from the brown alga *Cystoseira tamariscifolia*. *J. Nat. Prod.* **2015**, *78*, 1663–1670. [CrossRef]
74. de los Reyes, C.; Zbakh, H.; Motilva, V.; Zubía, E. Antioxidant and anti-inflammatory meroterpenoids from the brown alga *Cystoseira usneoides*. *J. Nat. Prod.* **2013**, *76*, 621–629. [CrossRef] [PubMed]
75. de los Reyes, C.; Ortega, M.J.; Zbakh, H.; Motilva, V.; Zubía, E. *Cystoseira usneoides*: A brown alga rich in antioxidant and anti-inflammatory meroditerpenoids. *J. Nat. Prod.* **2016**, *79*, 395–405. [CrossRef]
76. Urones, J.G.; Basabe, P.; Marcos, I.S.; Pineda, J.; Lithgow, A.M.; Moro, R.F.; Palma, F.M.S.B.; Araújo, M.E.M.; Gravalos, M.D.G. Meroterpenes from *Cystoseira usneoides*. *Phytochemistry* **1992**, *31*, 179–182. [CrossRef]
77. Urones, J.G.; Araujo, M.E.M.; Palma, F.M.S.B.; Basabe, P.; Marcos, I.S.; Moro, R.F.; Lithgow, A.M.; Pineda, J. Meroterpenes from *Cystoseira usneoides* II. *Phytochemistry* **1992**, *31*, 2105–2109. [CrossRef]
78. Amico, V.; Cunsolo, F.; Piattelli, M.; Ruberto, G. Acyclic tetraprenyltoluquinols from *Cystoseira sauvageuana* and their possible role as biogenetic precursors of the cyclic *Cystoseira* metabolites. *Phytochemistry* **1985**, *24*, 2663–2668. [CrossRef]
79. Laird, D.W.; Poole, R.; Wikström, M.; van Altena, I.A. Pycnanthuquinone C, an unusual 6,6,5-tricyclic geranyltoluquinone from the Western Australian brown alga *Cystophora harveyi*. *J. Nat. Prod.* **2007**, *70*, 671–674. [CrossRef] [PubMed]
80. Reddy, P.; Urban, S. Meroditerpenoids from the southern Australian marine brown alga *Sargassum fallax*. *Phytochemistry* **2009**, *70*, 250–255. [CrossRef]
81. Niwa, H.; Kurimoto, S.; Kubota, T.; Sekiguchi, M. Macrocarquinoids A–C, new meroterpenoids from *Sargassum macrocarpum*. *J. Nat. Med.* **2021**, *75*, 194–200. [CrossRef]
82. Mori, J.; Iwashima, M.; Wakasugi, H.; Saito, H.; Matsunaga, T.; Ogasawara, M.; Takahashi, S.; Suzuki, H.; Hayashi, T. New plastoquinones isolated from the brown alga, *Sargassum micracanthum*. *Chem. Pharm. Bull.* **2005**, *53*, 1159–1163. [CrossRef]
83. Brkljača, R.; Urban, S. Chemical profiling (HPLC-NMR & HPLC-MS), isolation, and identification of bioactive meroditerpenoids from the southern Australian marine brown alga *Sargassum paradoxum*. *Mar. Drugs* **2015**, *13*, 102–127.
84. Horie, S.; Tsutsumi, S.; Takada, Y.; Kimura, J. Antibacterial quinone metabolites from the brown alga, *Sargassum sagamianum*. *Bull. Chem. Soc. Jpn.* **2008**, *81*, 1125–1130. [CrossRef]
85. Segawa, M.; Shirahama, H. New plastoquinones from the brown alga *Sargassum sagamianum* var. *yezoense*. *Chem. Lett.* **1987**, *16*, 1365–1366. [CrossRef]
86. Jung, M.; Jang, K.H.; Kim, B.; Lee, B.H.; Choi, B.W.; Oh, K.-B.; Shin, H. Meroditerpenoids from the brown alga *Sargassum siliquastrum*. *J. Nat. Prod.* **2008**, *71*, 1714–1719. [CrossRef] [PubMed]
87. Ishitsuka, M.; Kusumi, T.; Nomura, Y.; Konno, T.; Kakisawa, H. New geranylgeranylbenzoquinone derivatives from *Sargassum tortile*. *Chem. Lett.* **1979**, *8*, 1269–1272. [CrossRef]
88. Valls, R.; Piovetti, L.; Banaigs, B.; Praud, A. Secondary metabolites from Morocco brown algae of the genus *Cystoseira*. *Phytochemistry* **1993**, *32*, 961–966. [CrossRef]
89. Fuentes-Monteverde, J.C.C.; Nath, N.; Forero, A.M.; Balboa, E.M.; Navarro-Vázquez, A.; Griesinger, C.; Jiménez, C.; Rodríguez, J. Connection of isolated stereoclusters by combining ^{13}C-RCSA, RDC, and J-based configurational analyses and structural revision of a tetraprenyltoluquinol chromane meroterpenoid from *Sargassum muticum*. *Mar. Drugs* **2022**, *20*, 462. [CrossRef]

90. Balboa, E.M.; Li, Y.-X.; Ahn, B.-N.; Eom, S.-H.; Domínguez, H.; Jiménez, C.; Rodríguez, J. Photodamage attenuation effect by a tetraprenyltoluquinol chromane meroterpenoid isolated from *Sargassum muticum*. *J. Photochem. Photobiol. B.* **2015**, *148*, 51–58. [CrossRef]
91. Iwashima, M.; Tako, N.; Hayakawa, T.; Matsunaga, T.; Mori, J.; Saito, H. New chromane derivatives isolated from the brown alga, *Sargassum micracanthum*. *Chem. Pharm. Bull.* **2008**, *56*, 124–128. [CrossRef]
92. Cho, S.H.; Cho, J.Y.; Kang, S.E.; Hong, Y.K.; Ahn, D.H. Antioxidant activity of mojabanchromanol, a novel chromene, isolated from brown alga *Sargassum siliquastrum*. *J. Environ. Biol.* **2008**, *29*, 479–484.
93. Lee, J.I.; Seo, Y. Chromanols from *Sargassum siliquastrum* and their antioxidant activity in HT1080 cells. *Chem. Pharm. Bull.* **2011**, *59*, 757–761. [CrossRef]
94. Jang, K.H.; Lee, B.H.; Choi, B.W.; Lee, H.S.; Shin, J. Chromenes from the brown alga *Sargassum siliquastrum*. *J. Nat. Prod.* **2005**, *68*, 716–723. [CrossRef] [PubMed]
95. Lee, J.-I.; Park, B.J.; Kim, H.; Seo, Y. Isolation of two new meroterpenoids from *Sargassum siliquastrum*. *Bull. Korean. Chem. Soc.* **2014**, *35*, 2867–2869. [CrossRef]
96. Kang, H.-S.; Kim, J.-P. New chromene derivatives with radical scavenging activities from the brown alga *Sargassum siliquastrum*. *J. Chem. Res.* **2017**, *41*, 116–119. [CrossRef]
97. Dhara, S.; Chakraborty, K. Novel furanyl-substituted isochromanyl class of anti-inflammatory turbinochromanone from brown seaweed *Turbinaria conoides*. *Chem. Biodivers.* **2022**, *19*, e202100723. [CrossRef] [PubMed]
98. Seo, Y.; Park, K.E.; Kim, Y.A.; Lee, H.-J.; Yoo, J.-S.; Ahn, J.-W.; Lee, B.-J. Isolation of tetraprenyltoluquinols from the brown alga *Sargassum thunbergii*. *Chem. Pharm. Bull.* **2006**, *54*, 1730–1733. [CrossRef] [PubMed]
99. Numata, A.; Kanbara, S.; Takahashi, C.; Fujiki, R.; Yoneda, M.; Usami, Y.; Fujita, E. A cytotoxic principle of the brown alga *Sargassum tortile* and structures of chromenes. *Phytochemistry* **1992**, *31*, 1209–1213. [CrossRef]
100. Kikuchi, T.; Mori, Y.; Yokoi, T.; Nakazawa, S.; Kuroda, H.; Masada, Y.; Kitamura, K.; Umezaki, I. Structure of sargatriol, a new isoprenoid chromenol from a marine alga: *Sargassum tortile*. *Chem. Pharm. Bull.* **1975**, *23*, 690–692. [CrossRef]
101. Kikuchi, T.; Mori, Y.; Yokoi, T.; Nakazawa, S.; Kuroda, H.; Masada, Y.; Kitamura, K.; Kuriyama, K. Structure and absolute configuration of sargatriol, a new isoprenoid chromenol from a brown alga, *Sargassum tortile* C. Agardh. *Chem. Pharm. Bull.* **1983**, *31*, 106–113. [CrossRef]
102. Jung, M.; Jang, K.H.; Kim, B.; Lee, B.H.; Choi, B.W.; Oh, K.-B.; Shin, H. Meroditerpenoids from the brown alga *Sargassum siliquastrum*. *J. Nat. Prod.* **2009**, *72*, 1723. [CrossRef]
103. Gunathilake, T.; Akanbi, T.O.; Suleria, H.A.R.; Nalder, T.D.; Francis, D.S.; Barrow, C.J. Seaweed phenolics as natural antioxidants, aquafeed additives, veterinary treatments and cross-linkers for microencapsulation. *Mar. Drugs* **2022**, *20*, 445. [CrossRef]
104. Singh, I.P.; Bharate, S.B. Phloroglucinol compounds of natural origin. *Nat. Prod. Rep.* **2006**, *23*, 558–591. [CrossRef] [PubMed]
105. Jiang, C.-S.; Wang, Y.-Y.; Song, J.-T.; Yu, J.-H. Acylphloroglucinols as kinase inhibitors from *Sargassum nigrifoloides*. *J. Asian Nat. Prod. Res.* **2018**, *21*, 619–626. [CrossRef] [PubMed]
106. Kim, C.; Lee, I.-K.; Cho, G.Y.; Oh, K.-H.; Lim, Y.W.; Yun, B.-S. Sargassumol, a novel antioxidant from the brown alga *Sargassum micracanthum*. *J. Antibiot.* **2012**, *65*, 87–89. [CrossRef] [PubMed]
107. Keusgen, M.; Falk, M.; Walter, J.A.; Glombitza, K.-W. A phloroglucinol derivative from brown alga *Sargassum spinuligerum*. *Phytochemistry* **1997**, *46*, 1–8. [CrossRef]
108. Glombitza, K.-W.; Li, S.-M. Fucophlorethols from the brown alga *Carpophyllum maschalocarpum*. *Phytochemistry* **1991**, *30*, 3423–3427. [CrossRef]
109. Glombitza, K.-M.; Keusgen, M.; Hauperich, S. Fucophlorethols from the brown algae *Sargassum spinuligerum* and *Cystophora torulosa*. *Phytochemistry* **1997**, *46*, 1417–1422. [CrossRef]
110. Glombitza, K.-W.; Hauperich, S. Phlorotannins from the brown alga *Cystophora torulosa*. *Phytochemistry* **1997**, *46*, 735–740. [CrossRef]
111. Glombitza, K.-M.; Hauperich, S.; Keusgen, M. Phlorotannins from the brown algae *Cystophora torulosa* and *Sargassum spinuligerum*. *Nat. Toxins* **1997**, *5*, 58–63. [CrossRef]
112. Glombitza, K.-W.; Li, S.-M. Hydroxyphlorethols from the brown alga *Carpophyllum maschalocarpum*. *Phytochemistry* **1991**, *30*, 2741–2745. [CrossRef]
113. Glombitza, K.-M.; Schmidt, A. Trihydroxyphlorethols from the brown alga *Carpophyllum angustifolium*. *Phytochemistry* **1999**, *51*, 1095–1100. [CrossRef]
114. Li, S.-M.; Glombitza, K.-W. Carmalols and phlorethofuhalols from the brown alga *Carpophyllum maschalocarpum*. *Phytochemistry* **1991**, *30*, 3417–3421. [CrossRef]
115. Glombitza, K.-W.; Schmidt, A. Nonhalogenated and halogenated phlorotannins from the brown alga *Carpophyllum angustifolium*. *J. Nat. Prod.* **1999**, *62*, 1238–1240. [CrossRef] [PubMed]
116. Kawamura-Konishi, Y.; Watanabe, N.; Saito, M.; Nakajima, N.; Sakaki, T.; Katayama, T.; Enomoto, T. Isolation of a new phlorotannin, a potent inhibitor of carbohydrate-hydrolyzing enzymes, from the brown alga *Sargassum patens*. *J. Agric. Food Chem.* **2012**, *60*, 5565–5570. [CrossRef] [PubMed]
117. Hamdy, A.-H.A.; Aboutabl, E.A.; Sameer, S.; Hussein, A.A.; Díaz-Marrero, A.R.; Darias, J.; Cueto, M. 3-Keto-22-epi-28-norcathasterone, a brassinosteroid-related metabolite from *Cystoseira myrica*. *Steroids* **2009**, *74*, 927–930. [CrossRef]

118. Ayyad, S.-E.N.; Sowellim, S.Z.A.; El-Hosini, M.S.; Abo-Atia, A. The structural determination of a new steroidal metabolite from the brown alga *Sargassum asperifolium*. *Z. Naturforsch. C.* **2003**, *58*, 5–6. [CrossRef]
119. Tang, H.-F.; Yi, Y.-H.; Yao, X.-S.; Xu, Q.-Z.; Zhang, S.-Y.; Lin, H.-W. Bioactive steroids from the brown alga *Sargassum carpophyllum*. *J. Asian Nat. Prod. Res.* **2002**, *4*, 95–101. [CrossRef]
120. Wang, S.-Y.; Xiang, J.; Huang, X.-J.; Wei, X.; Zhang, Q.; Du, X.-H.; Hu, J.-S.; Wang, Y.-M.; Zhang, C.-X. Chemical constituents from *Sargassum fusiforme* (Harv.) Setch. *Chem. Biodivers.* **2020**, *17*, e2000182. [CrossRef]
121. Xu, S.-H.; Ding, L.-S.; Wang, M.-K.; Peng, S.-L.; Liao, X. Studies on the chemical constituents of the algae *Sargassum polycystcum*. *Chin. J. Org. Chem.* **2002**, *22*, 138–140.
122. Kobayashi, M.; Hasegawa, A.; Mitsuhashi, H. Marine sterols. XV. Isolation of 24-vinyloxycholesta-5,23-dien-3β-ol from the brown alga *Sargassum thumbergii*. *Chem. Pharm. Bull.* **1985**, *33*, 4012–4013. [CrossRef]
123. He, W.-F.; Yao, L.-G.; Liu, H.-L.; Guo, Y.-W. Thunberol, a new sterol from the Chinese brown alga *Sargassum thunbergii*. *J. Asian Nat. Prod. Res.* **2014**, *16*, 685–689. [CrossRef]
124. Kumar, S.S.; Kumar, Y.K.; Khan, M.S.Y.; Gupta, V. New antifungal steroids from *Turbinaria conoides* (J.Agardh) Kutzing. *Nat. Prod. Res.* **2010**, *24*, 1481–1487. [CrossRef] [PubMed]
125. Sheu, J.-H.; Wang, G.-H.; Sung, P.-J.; Duh, C.-Y. New cytotoxic oxygenated fucosterols from the brown alga *Turbinaria conoides*. *J. Nat. Prod.* **1999**, *62*, 224–227. [CrossRef] [PubMed]
126. Chakraborty, K.; Dhara, S. Conoidecyclics A–C from marine macroagla *Turbinaria conoides*: Newly described natural macrolides with prospective bioactive properties. *Phytochemistry* **2021**, *191*, 112909. [CrossRef] [PubMed]
127. Chakraborty, K.; Dhara, S. First report of substituted 2H-pyranoids from brown seaweed *Turbinaria conoides* with antioxidant and anti-inflammatory activities. *Nat. Prod. Res.* **2020**, *34*, 3451–3461. [CrossRef] [PubMed]
128. Dhara, S.; Chakraborty, K. Turbinafuranone A–C, new 2-furanone analogures from marine macroalga *Turbinaria ornata* as prospective anti-hyperglycemic agents attenuate tyrosine phosphatase-1B. *Med. Chem. Res.* **2021**, *30*, 1635–1648. [CrossRef]
129. Chakraborty, K.; Dhara, S. Spirornatas A–C from brown alga *Turbinaria ornata*: Anti-hypertensive spiroketals attenuate angiotensin-I converting enzyme. *Phytochemistry* **2022**, *195*, 113024. [CrossRef]
130. Qi, S.-H.; Zhang, S.; Huang, J.-S.; Xiao, Z.-H.; Wu, J.; Long, L.-J. Glycerol derivatives and sterols from *Sargassum parvivesiculosum*. *Chem. Pharm. Bull.* **2004**, *52*, 986–988. [CrossRef]
131. Chang, H.W.; Jang, K.H.; Lee, D.; Kang, H.R.; Kim, T.-Y.; Lee, B.H.; Choi, B.W.; Kim, S.; Shin, J. Monoglycerides from the brown alga *Sargassum sagamianum*: Isolation, synthesis, and biological activity. *Bioorg. Med. Chem. Lett.* **2008**, *18*, 3589–3592. [CrossRef]
132. Kim, Y.H.; Kim, E.-H.; Lee, C.; Kim, M.-H.; Rho, J.-R. Two new monogalactosyl diacylglycerols from brown alga *Sargassum thunbergii*. *Lipids* **2007**, *42*, 395–399. [CrossRef]
133. Cai, Y.-P.; Xie, C.-B.; Wang, B.-C.; Li, P.-L.; Li, B.-F. Two new resorcinols from *Sargassum thunbergii*. *J. Asian Nat. Prod. Res.* **2010**, *12*, 1001–1104. [CrossRef]
134. Alzarea, S.I.; Elmaidomy, A.H.; Saber, H.; Musa, A.; Al-Sanea, M.M.; Mostafa, E.M.; Hendawy, O.M.; Youssif, K.A.; Alanazi, A.S.; Alharbi, M.; et al. Potential anticancer lipoxygenase inhibitors from the Red Sea-derived brown algae *Sargassum cinereum*: An in-silico-supported in-vitro study. *Antibiotics* **2021**, *10*, 416. [CrossRef] [PubMed]
135. Peng, Y.; Cao, L.; Liu, Y.; Huang, R. Sargassulfamide A, an unprecedented amide derivative from the seaweed *Sargassum naozhouense*. *Chem. Nat. Compd.* **2020**, *56*, 98–100. [CrossRef]
136. Banaigs, B.; Francisco, C.; Gonzalez, E.; Codomier, L. Lipids from the brown alga *Cystoseira barbata*. *Phytochemistry* **1984**, *23*, 2951–2952. [CrossRef]

Disclaimer/Publisher's Note: The statements, opinions and data contained in all publications are solely those of the individual author(s) and contributor(s) and not of MDPI and/or the editor(s). MDPI and/or the editor(s) disclaim responsibility for any injury to people or property resulting from any ideas, methods, instructions or products referred to in the content.

MDPI AG
Grosspeteranlage 5
4052 Basel
Switzerland
Tel.: +41 61 683 77 34

Marine Drugs Editorial Office
E-mail: marinedrugs@mdpi.com
www.mdpi.com/journal/marinedrugs

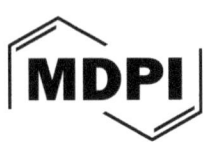

Disclaimer/Publisher's Note: The statements, opinions and data contained in all publications are solely those of the individual author(s) and contributor(s) and not of MDPI and/or the editor(s). MDPI and/or the editor(s) disclaim responsibility for any injury to people or property resulting from any ideas, methods, instructions or products referred to in the content.